WHO Technical Repo
996

CW01240413

WHO Expert Committee on Specifications for Pharmaceutical Preparations

Fiftieth report

This report contains the views of an international group of experts, and does not necessarily represent the decisions or the stated policy of the World Health Organization

World Health Organization

WHO Library Cataloguing-in-Publication Data

Fiftieth report of the WHO Expert Committee on specifications for pharmaceutical preparations.

(WHO technical report series ; no. 996)

1.Pharmaceutical Preparations - standards. 2.Technology, Pharmaceutical - standards.
3.Drug Industry - legislation. 4.Quality Control.
I.World Health Organization. II.Series.

ISBN 978 92 4 120996 0 (NLM classification: QV 771)
ISBN 978 92 4 069548 1 (PDF)
ISSN 0512-3054

© World Health Organization 2016

All rights reserved. Publications of the World Health Organization are available on the WHO website (www.who.int) or can be purchased from WHO Press, World Health Organization, 20 Avenue Appia, 1211 Geneva 27, Switzerland (tel.: +41 22 791 3264; fax: +41 22 791 4857; email: bookorders@who.int).

Requests for permission to reproduce or translate WHO publications – whether for sale or for non-commercial distribution– should be addressed to WHO Press through the WHO website (www.who.int/about/licensing/copyright_form/en/index.html).

The designations employed and the presentation of the material in this publication do not imply the expression of any opinion whatsoever on the part of the World Health Organization concerning the legal status of any country, territory, city or area or of its authorities, or concerning the delimitation of its frontiers or boundaries. Dotted and dashed lines on maps represent approximate border lines for which there may not yet be full agreement.

The mention of specific companies or of certain manufacturers' products does not imply that they are endorsed or recommended by the World Health Organization in preference to others of a similar nature that are not mentioned. Errors and omissions excepted, the names of proprietary products are distinguished by initial capital letters.

All reasonable precautions have been taken by the World Health Organization to verify the information contained in this publication. However, the published material is being distributed without warranty of any kind, either expressed or implied. The responsibility for the interpretation and use of the material lies with the reader. In no event shall the World Health Organization be liable for damages arising from its use.

This publication contains the collective views of an international group of experts and does not necessarily represent the decisions or the policies of the World Health Organization.

Printed in Italy

Contents

WHO Expert Committee on Specifications for Pharmaceutical Preparations

Geneva, 12–16 October 2015

Members[1]

Professor Saleh A. Bawazir, Consultant, College of Pharmacy, King Saud Unit, Riyadh, Saudi Arabia (*Rapporteur*)

Professor Theo G. Dekker, Professor Emeritus, Research Institute for Industrial Pharmacy, North-West University, Potchefstroom, South Africa

Professor Jos Hoogmartens, Leuven, Belgium (*Co-chairperson*)

Professor Jin Shaohong, Chief Expert for Pharmaceutical Products, National Institutes for Food and Drug Control, Beijing, People's Republic of China

Professor Henning G. Kristensen, Vedbaek, Denmark

Ms Gugu N. Mahlangu, Director-General, Medicines Control Authority of Zimbabwe, Harare, Zimbabwe (*Chairperson*)

Dr Justina A. Molzon, Bethesda, MD, USA

Mrs Lynda Paleshnuik, Arnprior, Ontario, Canada

Dr Jitka Sabartova, Prague, Czech Republic (*Rapporteur*)

Temporary advisers[2]

Professor Erwin Adams, Laboratorium voor Farmaceutische Analyse, Leuven, Belgium

Dr Marius Brits, Director, WHO Collaborating Centre for the Quality Assurance of Medicines, North-West University, Potchefstroom, South Africa

Dr Mônica da Luz Carvalho Soares, Expert Health Regulation, Brazilian Health Surveillance Agency (ANVISA), Brasilia, Brazil

Mr David Churchward, Expert Good Manufacturing and Distribution Practice Inspector, Inspection, Enforcement and Standards, Medicines & Healthcare products Regulatory Agency (MHRA), London, England

---

[1] Unable to attend: Ms Nilka M. Guerrero Rivas, Technical Director, Radiopharmacy, Radiofarmacia de Centroamérica, SA, Ciudad del Saber, Panama; Dr Toru Kawanishi, Director General, National Institute of Health Sciences, Tokyo, Japan; Dr Adriaan J. van Zyl, Cape Town, South Africa.

[2] Unable to attend: Dr Jean-Louis Robert, Luxembourg; Dr Jan Welink, Medicines Evaluation Board, Utrecht, Netherlands.

Dr Alfredo García Arieta, Head of Service on Pharmacokinetics and Generic Medicines, Division of Pharmacology and Clinical Evaluation, Department of Human Use Medicines, Agencia Española de Medicamentos y Productos Sanitarios (AEMPS), Madrid, Spain

Dr John Gordon, Wolfville, Nova Scotia, Canada

Dr Olivier Le Blaye, Inspector, Trials and Vigilance Inspection Department, Agence nationale de sécurité du médicament (ANSM) et des produits de santé, Saint-Denis, France

Dr John Miller, Ayr, Scotland

Professor Alain Nicolas, Radiopharmacist, Pharmacie, Hôpital Brabois Adultes, Vandoeuvre, France

Mr Salim Akbaralli Veljee, Director, Food and Drugs Administration, Directorate of Food and Drugs Administration, Goa, India

Mr John Wilkinson, Director of Devices, Medicines & Healthcare products Regulatory Agency (MHRA), London, England

Ms Caroline Munyimba-Yeta, Director, Operations (Plant), NRB Pharma Zambia Limited, Lusaka, Zambia

Representation from United Nations offices[3]

United Nations Children's Fund (UNICEF)

Dr Peter Svarrer Jakobsen, Quality Assurance Specialist, UNICEF Supply Division, Copenhagen, Denmark

Representation from specialized agencies and related organizations[4]

World Trade Organization (WTO)

Ms Daria Novozhilkina, Research Associate, Intellectual Property Division, Geneva, Switzerland

Representation from intergovernmental organizations[5]

Council of Europe

Dr Stefan Almeling, Deputy Head, Laboratory Department, European Directorate for the Quality of Medicines & HealthCare (EDQM), Strasbourg, France

---

[3] Unable to attend: United Nations Development Programme (UNDP), New York, NY, USA.

[4] Unable to attend: United Nations Industrial Development Organization (UNIDO), Vienna, Austria; World Intellectual Property Organization (WIPO), Geneva, Switzerland; World Bank, Washington, DC, USA; International Atomic Energy Agency (IAEA), Vienna, Austria.

[5] Unable to attend: World Customs Organization (WCO), Brussels, Belgium; European Commission (EC), Directorate-General for Health and Consumer Protection, Brussels, Belgium.

European Medicines Agency (EMA)
Mr Andrei Spinei, London, England

Representation from nongovernmental organizations[6]

Active Pharmaceutical Ingredients Committee (APIC)
Dr Landry Le Chevanton, Team Leader, Global Regulatory Affairs and Quality Management, DSM Nutritional Products Ltd, Switzerland

The Stop TB Partnership
Dr Nigorsulton Muzafarova, Product Quality Officer, Global Drug Facility (GDF), Geneva, Switzerland

Dr Kaspars Lunte, Team Leader, Sourcing and Special Project, GDF, Geneva

International Federation of Pharmaceutical Manufacturers and Associations (IFPMA)
Dr Betsy Fritschel, Director, Quality & Compliance, Johnson & Johnson, New Brunswick, NJ, USA

Ms Valérie Faillat-Proux, Regulatory Affairs Senior Director, Access to Medicines & Malaria Programme, Sanofi, Gentilly, France

International Generic Pharmaceutical Alliance (IGPA)
Dr Koen Nauwelaerts, Quality and Regulatory Affairs Manager, EGA-European Generic and Biosimilar Medicines Association, Brussels, Belgium

International Pharmaceutical Excipients Council (IPEC)
Dr Eckart Krämer , SE Tylose GmbH & Co., Cologne, Germany

International Pharmaceutical Federation (FIP)
Ms Zuzana Kusynová, Policy Analyst and Project Coordinator, The Hague, Netherlands

Observers[7]

Dr C. Michelle Limoli, Senior International Health Advisor, Center for Biologics Evaluation and Research, US Food and Drug Administration, Silver Spring, MD, USA

Ms Wei Ningyi, Associate Researcher, Division of Chemical Drugs, National Institutes for Food and Drug Control, Beijing, People's Republic of China

Dr Gabriela Zenhäusern, Senior Case Manager, Sector Authorisation, Swissmedic, Berne, Switzerland

6 Unable to attend: Commonwealth Pharmacists Association (CPA), London, England; Global Fund to Fight AIDS, Tuberculosis and Malaria, Geneva, Switzerland; International Society for Pharmaceutical Engineering (ISPE), Tampa, FL, USA; World Self-Medication Industry (WSMI), Ferney-Voltaire, France.

7 Unable to attend: Pharmaceutical Inspection Co-operation Scheme (PIC/S), Geneva, Switzerland.

Professor Zhang Mei, Deputy Director and Vice Chairman, Institutes for Food and Drug Control, Jiangsu, People's Republic of China/Antibiotic Subcommittee, Chinese Pharmacopoeia Commission, People's Republic of China

Pharmacopoeias[8]

Farmacopéia Brasileira

Mr Varley Dias Sousa, Coordinator, Coordination of Brazilian Pharmacopoeia, Brazilian Health Surveillance Agency (ANVISA), Brasilia, Brazil

British Pharmacopoeia

Ms Helen Corns, British Pharmacopoeia and Laboratory Services, Medicines & Healthcare products Regulatory Agency (MHRA), London, England

Pharmacopoeia of the People's Republic of China

Dr Wang Fei, Beijing, People's Republic of China

European Pharmacopoeia[9]

Council of Europe, Strasbourg, France

Japanese Pharmacopoeia

Dr Yoshihiro Matsuda, Deputy Director, Pharmaceutical and Medical Devices Agency, Division of Pharmacopoeia and Standards for Drugs, Office of Standards and Guidelines Development, Pharmaceuticals and Medical Devices Agency, Tokyo, Japan

Pharmacopoeia of the Republic of Korea

Dr Kwangmoon Lee, Deputy Director, Drug Research Division, Pharmaceutical Standardization Research and Drug Research Division, National Institute of Food and Drug Safety Evaluation, Ministry of Food and Drug Safety, Chungcheongbuk-do, Republic of Korea

State Pharmacopoeia of the Russian Federation

Dr Elena Sakanyan, Director, Centre of Pharmacopoeia and International Collaboration, Scientific Centre for Expert Evaluation of Medicinal Products of the Ministry of Health of the Russian Federation, Moscow, Russian Federation

Ms Olga Gubareva, Head, International Cooperation Department, Moscow, Russian Federation

United States Pharmacopeia

Dr Kevin Moore, Manager, Pharmacopeial Harmonization, Rockville, MD, USA

Dr Kelly S. Willis, Senior Vice President, Global Public Health, Rockville, MD, USA

---

[8] Unable to attend: Farmacopea Argentina; Indian Pharmacopoeia Commission; Indonesian Pharmacopoeia Commission; Pharmacopoeia of Ukraine.

[9] See under *Council of Europe*.

Representation from WHO Regional Offices[10]

Regional Office for the Western Pacific
Ms Uhjin Kim, Essential Medicines and Health Technology, Division of Health Systems, WHO Regional Office for the Western Pacific, Manila, Philippines

WHO Secretariat[11]

Health Systems and Innovation (HIS)
Dr M.-P. Kieny, Assistant Director-General

Essential Medicines and Health Products (HIS/EMP)
Mr C. de Joncheere, Director, Essential Medicines and Health Products (*EMP*)

Regulation of Medicines and other Health Technologies (EMP/RHT)
Dr L. Rägo, Head

Technologies, Standards and Norms (EMP/RHT/TSN)
Dr D.J. Wood, Coordinator

Medicines Quality Assurance (EMP/RHT/TSN)
Dr S. Kopp, Group Lead, Medicines Quality Assurance (*Secretary*)

Dr H. Schmidt, TSN

Dr H. Chen, TSN (*volunteer*)

International Nonproprietary Name (INN/RHT/TSN)
Dr R.G. Balocco, Group Lead

Policy, Access and Use (EMP/PAU)
Ms Bernadette Cappello

Prequalification Team (EMP/RHT/PQT)
Mr M. McDonald, Coordinator

Mr J.R.H. Kuwana

Mr D. Mubangizi, Group Lead, Inspections

Ms T. Muvirimi

Regulatory Systems Strengthening (RSS/RHT/RHT)
Dr M. Ward, Coordinator

Safety and Vigilance Team (EMP/RHT/SAV)
Miss P. Bourdillon-Esteve, Analyst

[10] Unable to attend: Regional Office for Africa; Regional Office for the Americas; Regional Office for the Eastern Mediterranean; Regional Office for Europe; Regional Office for South-East Asia.

[11] Unable to attend: Traditional and Complementary Medicine (HIS/Service Delivery and Safety (SDS)/TCM).

Global TB Programme (GTB)
Dr C. Gilpin, Laboratories, Diagnostics and Drug-Resistance (*LDR*)

Dr L. Nguyen, LDR

Prevention of Noncommunicable Diseases (PND)
Dr Dongbo Fu, Technical Officer, National Capacity

Ms M. Zweygarth (report writer)

Declarations of interest

Members of the WHO Expert Committee on Specifications for Pharmaceutical Preparations and temporary advisers reported the following:

Dr E. Adams, Dr M. Brits, Mr D. Churchward, Dr T. Dekker, Dr A. Garcia Arieta, Dr J. Gordon, Professor J. Hoogmartens, Professor Jin S., Dr O. Le Blaye, Dr J. Molzon, Dr A. Nicolas, Ms L. Paleshnuik, Dr J. Sabartova, Dr M. Da Luz Carvalho Soares and Mr S. Akbaralli Veljee reported no conflict of interest.

Professor S. Bawazir reported that he is in the process of establishing a new consultancy.

Professor H.G. Kristensen reported that he has provided testimonies as an independent expert in questions on validity and for infringement of patents at courts in Denmark, Norway and Sweden. In all cases testimony related to drug formulations. No items conflict with the subjects of the meeting.

Ms G.N. Mahlangu reported that she would receive an out-of-pocket allowance from her current employer, the Medicines Control Authority of Zimbabwe, in accordance with the travel allowances schedule for sponsored travel.

Dr J. Miller reported that he has acted as a consultant for national authorities.

Ms C. Munyiamba-Yeta reported that she was employed by the Zambian Regulatory Authority for seven years until 2014. For the moment she works as an independent consultant.

Mr J. Wilkinson reported that he was employed with the European Medical Devices Industry Association until December 2012.

The interests summarized above do not give rise to a conflict of interest such that the expert concerned should be partially or totally excluded from participation in the Expert Committee on Specifications for Pharmaceutical Preparations. However, following WHO's policy, they were disclosed within the Committee so that other members were aware of them. All other members of the Expert Committee declared no relevant interests.

Many of the Expert Committee Members have extensive governmental experience and expertise – including consulting with WHO – in the areas that are the subject of the Expert Committee agenda, and which were considered very relevant and important for the challenging tasks faced by the Committee. It was suggested that the Secretariat should provide more detail on the type of conflict to be reported in the declarations of interest for regulatory authorities. The Secretariat agreed to follow up this suggestion with the WHO Office of the Legal Counsel.

1. Introduction

The World Health Organization (WHO) Expert Committee on Specifications for Pharmaceutical Preparations met in Geneva from 12 to 16 October 2015. Mr Cornelius de Joncheere, Director of the Department of Essential Medicines and Health Products (EMP) at WHO, welcomed participants on behalf of the Director-General.

Mr de Joncheere welcomed the experts and advisers from all WHO regions, as well as observers and representatives from international organizations. He thanked them and their teams for their major contributions to the work of WHO in setting standards in the area of pharmaceuticals. He mentioned that this was the fiftieth anniversary of the Expert Committee's meetings. The Committee held its first meeting in 1947 under the name of Expert Committee on Unification of Pharmacopoeias to continue the work of technical experts of the League of Nations. The Committee's scope of work was extended from the maintenance of international pharmacopoeial standards to good manufacturing practices (GMP) and subsequently to other topics. Today it covers all aspects of medicines quality, with a strong focus on building quality assurance into the life cycle of products, from development to the supply to patients. A press event titled "Promoting quality medicines and saving lives – Commemorating the 50th anniversary of WHO programme to improve medicines quality worldwide" had been organized for 15 October 2015.

WHO's standard-setting work today is more important than ever, and is conducted under strengthened rules for selection of experts and for declarations of interests. The Expert Committee system is the backbone of WHO's normative function. The technical guidance is provided online and is widely used. The website, with the 75 medicines quality assurance-related guidelines adopted through the Committee and the online version of *The International Pharmacopoeia*, is at the top of the Organization's list for web queries.[1]

The Expert Committee has strong links with other WHO groups such as the Expert Committee on Biological Standardization (ECBS), the International Nonproprietary Names (INN) expert consultation, which met concurrently with this Committee, and the Expert Committee on the Selection and Use of Expert Medicines. Strong links also exist with global groups such as the world pharmacopoeias.

Health systems were a focus of the 2015 World Health Assembly. Besides the extensive work done to sustain the emergency response to the Ebola outbreak and to step up preparedness for future public health emergencies, other achievements included the adoption of a global action plan to combat antibiotic

[1] http://www.who.int/medicines/areas/quality_safety/quality_assurance/en/.

resistance, and the adoption of the Global Vaccine Action Plan. In the area of medicines, innovative ways of developing new medicines are an important topic, as is the work of the mechanism to combat substandard/spurious/falsely-labelled/falsified/counterfeit (SSFFC) products. Health has also been recognized as a central topic for global development in the Sustainable Development Goals (SDGs) launched in September 2015. The health-related goal – SDG 3, "Ensure healthy lives and promote well-being for all at all ages" – includes targets for improving access to good quality, affordable medicines and promoting research for needed medicines.

The Committee elected Ms G.N. Mahlangu as Chairperson, Professor J. Hoogmartens as Co-chairperson, and Professor S.A. Bawazir and Dr J. Sabartova as Rapporteurs. Ms Mahlangu then took the chair. Declarations of interest as shown on page 10 of this report were presented to the meeting participants in accordance with strengthened WHO rules for Expert Committees.

Open session

The Chairperson welcomed the members, technical advisers and observers to the open session of the Expert Committee. The open session had been arranged in response to earlier expressions of interest by the diplomatic missions. It was noted that there were no representatives from the missions.

The Secretary of the Expert Committee described the Committee's role in fulfilling WHO's normative mandate, and explained how WHO's Expert Committee system works. In its normative work the Committee sets rules for medicines quality assurance, and acts in response to global health emergencies and the needs of international organizations. An Expert Committee is the highest advisory body to the Director-General and is established in the constitution of the Organization. A set of strengthened rules and procedures, including new procedures for declaration of interests, govern invitations to and participation in an Expert Committee. The WHO Expert Committee on Specifications for Pharmaceutical Preparations maintains *The International Pharmacopoeia* and provides guidance on all topics relating to medicines quality assurance. The guidelines are developed in consultation with a wide range of international partners, including Collaborating Centres, international associations and organizations. Participants were reminded that they were acting in their personal capacity as experts.

The Secretary thanked all the partners for their major contributions to WHO's standard-setting work.

2. General policy

2.1 Cross-cutting pharmaceutical quality assurance issues

Expert Committee on the Selection and Use of Essential Medicines

The Expert Committee on the Selection and Use of Essential Medicines selects the medicines that satisfy the priority health-care needs of the population, taking into account disease prevalence, efficacy and safety, and comparative cost-effectiveness. However, the absolute cost of treatment will not constitute a reason to exclude a medicine that is shown to otherwise meet the established selection criteria. The WHO Model Lists of Essential Medicines (EML) for adults and for children are updated every two years.

The current EMLs include 416 medicines for adults and 289 medicines for children. Important additions in 2015 include 16 new medicines for treatment of cancer, four single-ingredient antivirals and two combination antivirals to treat hepatitis C, as well as four medicines to treat multidrug-resistant tuberculosis and one medicine to treat latent tuberculosis infection. Other additions included new contraceptive formulations, medicines affecting coagulation, medicines for hepatitis B, and some new formulations of existing medicines. Notably, it was decided not to recommend inclusion on the EML of ranibizumab for neovascular eye diseases, novel oral anticoagulants and so-called polypill therapy for cardiovascular disease.

The EML includes a number of biological medicines, and a process for adding biosimilars will need to be defined in the future. All applications and recommendations of this Expert Committee are published on the WHO website.

The Committee noted the report.

Regulatory support

An update was provided about WHO's regulatory support activities conducted on the basis of the Organization's normative guidance. WHO is one of the largest global providers of regulatory training, covering all aspects of regulation, including inspections, assessment of product data and post-marketing control of medicines. The wide implementation of a common basis of norms and standards has facilitated the creation of a number of successful harmonization initiatives and cooperative networks, such as the East African Community harmonization project and similar initiatives in the Southern African Development Community region and elsewhere. Joint assessment and inspection activities are also increasing. These developments are further supported by good practices (GXP) documents for regulatory authorities that are being developed through the Committee, such as the good review practice document developed under the leadership of the Asia-Pacific Economic Cooperation Regulatory Harmonization

Steering Committee and adopted by the Committee in 2014. A further overarching framework guidance document on good regulatory practices is being developed to promote regulatory consistency and collaboration.

The Committee noted the report.

Expert Committee on Biological Standardization (ECBS)

The ECBS met concurrently with the Expert Committee on Specifications for Pharmaceutical Preparations. Directions in biological standardization have been driven by three strategic aims that have shaped WHO's work in the past year, namely to:

1) ensure preparedness for public health emergencies;
2) step up access to biotherapeutic products; and
3) strengthen global regulatory systems.

With regard to public health emergencies, lessons learnt during the Ebola outbreak have led to thought being given to the development of rapid regulatory pathways to make needed products available to affected populations. WHO has played a critical role in accelerating clinical trials for candidate products in Ebola-affected countries. With unprecedented support from the global regulatory community, efficacy data for vaccines, diagnostic products and potential treatments were generated in record time. Based on the lessons learnt during the Ebola outbreak a blueprint has been prepared for a new research and development (R & D) framework, with appropriate prioritization of suitable candidate products, enabling a swift and concerted global response in case of future emergencies. The development of a road map on R & D for Middle East respiratory syndrome (MERS) coronavirus will serve as a pilot. The blueprint was intended to be presented to the World Health Assembly (WHA) in 2016.

The Committee noted the report.

2.2 International collaboration

United Nations Children's Fund (UNICEF)

UNICEF was established in 1946 to promote and protect children's rights. Health and nutrition and the fight against HIV/AIDS are among UNICEF's core commitments. The Supply Division in Copenhagen, Denmark, ensures that high-quality, good value medicines and other supplies reach children and their families quickly. In 2014, UNICEF supplied goods with a total value of US$ 3.38 billion, including US$ 1.48 billion worth of vaccines and US$ 251 million worth of pharmaceuticals. A web-based catalogue of products procured, including a wide range of medicines for all major health needs, is publicly available on the Internet.

UNICEF applies the WHO model quality assurance system for procurement agencies (MQAS) in inspections, assessment of product data and monitoring of supplier performance. The Committee was provided with a description of UNICEF's systems for qualifying products and suppliers, which is based on product assessment and inspections. Products are assessed using a product questionnaire as published in the MQAS guidance. Vaccines, antiretrovirals, antimalarials and medicines for treatment of tuberculosis must be WHO-prequalified, with measures in place to verify that the goods supplied do in fact meet prequalification standards. UNICEF inspects manufacturers to verify compliance with WHO GMP guidelines and participates in joint inspections with the WHO prequalification team (WHO/PQT) and other organizations. Since 2006 UNICEF has been a partner of the Pharmaceutical Inspection Co-operation Scheme (PIC/S).

Priority areas of UNICEF's work in 2015 included performance management to ensure timely delivery, measures to support sourcing and regulation in recipient countries, long-term arrangements with suppliers, participation in meetings on essential medicines and relevant WHO disease programmes, targeted activities to ensure the availability and quality of specific products or product groups for use in WHO Member States, and the implementation of the outputs of the Expert Committee on Specifications for Pharmaceutical Preparations. The Committee noted the report.

Pharmacopoeial Discussion Group (PDG)

The PDG – consisting of the European Pharmacopoeia, the United States Pharmacopeia (USP) and the Japanese Pharmacopoeia (JP) – met in Tokyo, Japan, from 30 June to 1 July 2015. It was reported that 29 of the 36 general chapters and 48 of the 62 excipient monographs on the current work programme had been harmonized and that in-depth discussions on a number of additional items currently on the PDG work programme had taken place. Significant progress had been made, for example, with the harmonization of chromatographic methods for certain products. Chapters on colour, conductivity and protein determination had reached PDG Stage 4 (public consultation phase); a chapter on uniformity of delivered dose was being harmonized between the European Pharmacopoeia and the Japanese Pharmacopoeia. Methods for biotechnology products were also being harmonized. Stage 4 documents are posted on the websites of all three participating pharmacopoeias. WHO is an observer to PDG.

To provide increased transparency on its activities, PDG will offer an easy way to access information on its work programme to its sister pharmacopoeias, including the possibility to provide comments on draft texts during the consultation period. Information with respect to increasing transparency was shared at the sixth WHO international meeting of world pharmacopoeias.

The Committee noted the report.

Model regulatory framework for medical devices

Over the past 20 years, medical devices have become an extremely diverse and complex product group, with a significant manufacturer base and large global sales. Resolution WHA 67.20 urges Member States to strengthen national regulatory systems for medical products, including medical devices. A survey on the current status of regulatory systems in Member States has shown that regulatory systems for medical devices are nonexistent in almost half of the countries and very limited in many others.

Medical devices differ in several important ways from pharmaceuticals, although they are often regulated by the same national authorities. Opportunities exist for collaboration between regulatory authorities. There is currently limited WHO guidance available for medical devices, aside from that originating from the WHO/PQT for in vitro diagnostics (IVDs). To support Member States in establishing systems to regulate medical devices, WHO has initiated the development of a model regulatory framework for use by national regulatory authorities.

It has been proposed that the Expert Committee on Specifications for Pharmaceutical Preparations oversees the development of a model regulatory framework for medical devices. The Expert Committee noted that it does not currently have sufficient expertise and resources to perform this additional work. It was therefore suggested that a subgroup of suitably qualified experts should be created. The Secretariat will follow up accordingly and seek to identify the required expertise from the existing WHO Expert Advisory Panels.

3. Quality control – specifications and tests

3.1 *The International Pharmacopoeia*

3.1.1 Updates

Fifth edition of *The International Pharmacopoeia*

The fifth edition of *The International Pharmacopoeia* was published on the WHO website in August 2015 and has been made available on CD. The new edition includes 32 new or revised monographs on pharmaceutical substances and dosage forms as listed in the preface. Other updates include two texts reproduced with the permission of the *European Pharmacopoeia*. A function has been added to the electronic interface enabling users to generate PDF documents for saving or printing. The Secretariat expressed its sincere thanks to all who had contributed to this fifth edition.

The Committee noted the report and congratulated the Secretariat on this achievement.

Trade names of stationary phases

The Secretariat has started publishing trade names of stationary phases found suitable during monograph elaboration, for the information of users of the monographs. The list is available on the WHO website[2] and will be updated continuously in accordance with new monographs included in *The International Pharmacopoeia*. It was agreed that a cross-reference to the list would be provided in *The International Pharmacopoeia* to direct users to this useful additional information.

3.1.2 Workplan 2015–2016

Priorities for new monographs

The International Pharmacopoeia specifies primarily the quality of essential medicines that are included on the WHO EML, on the invitations for expressions of interest for WHO prequalification, or in other United Nations (UN) and/or WHO documents recommending the use of medicines for treatment of specific diseases and/or for use by treatment programmes.

The Committee heard a description of the process used to establish a workplan for elaboration of monographs, which, while acknowledging limited resources, aimed to meet the expectations of the Member States, WHO

---

[2] http://www.who.int/entity/medicines/publications/pharmacopoeia/2015-08-26trade-names_stationary_phases-QAS15-640_04092015N.pdf?ua=1.

programmes and other partners. For future monograph elaboration, priority has been assigned to medicines belonging to the categories covered by the WHO/PQT and to medicines considered as life-saving commodities for women and children as identified by the UN Commission on Life-Saving Commodities for Women and Children (UNCoLSC) and for which public standards are not yet available. General texts will be developed as the need arises in connection with the prioritized monographs.

The Secretariat will follow up on an earlier collaboration between WHO/PQT and the *Chinese Pharmacopoeia* under the Global Fund project, during which some 50 monographs were developed, with a view to making these available to WHO for possible inclusion in *The International Pharmacopoeia.*

Monographs proposed for elaboration or suppression

In line with the above-mentioned priorities, a list of 31 high priority monographs for finished pharmaceutical products (FPPs) was proposed for elaboration (Table 1). Additional monographs for the corresponding active pharmaceutical ingredient (API) will be required. Ten monographs were identified for suppression (Table 2) following their deletion from the WHO EML. As the medicines concerned may still be part of national lists of essential medicines, it was agreed that suppressed monographs should be transferred to a publicly accessible "Archived" section of *The International Pharmacopoeia.*

Table 1
Dosage form monographs proposed for elaboration with high priority

abacavir, efavirenz and lamivudine tablets
abacavir, lamivudine and nevirapine dispersible tablets
artemether and lumefantrine dispersible tablets
artenimol and piperaquine phosphate dispersible tablets
artesunate and amodiaquine tablets
artesunate and mefloquine tablets
artesunate and pyronaridine tablets
artesunate rectal capsules
atazanavir and ritonavir tablets
dolutegravir tablets
efavirenz, lamivudine and tenofovir tablets
entecavir oral solution
entecavir scored tablets
estradiol valerate and norethisterone enantate injection

Table 1 *continued*

etravirine tablets
flucytosine slow release tablets
lamivudine and tenofovir tablets
linezolid oral suspension
moxifloxacin tablets
norethisterone enantate injection
p-aminosalicylic acid granules for oral solution
protionamide tablets
pyrazinamide dispersible tablets
raltegravir tablets
ribavirin syrup
ritonavir oral solution
simeprevir capsule
sofosbuvir tablet
terizidone capsules
terizidone tablets
zanamivir powder for inhalation

Table 2
Monographs proposed for suppression

ampicillin capsules
colchicine tablets
ergometrine hydrogen maleate tablets
indometacin tablets
pethidine hydrochloride tablets
piperazine adipate tablets
piperazine citrate tablets
prednisolone sodium phosphate injection
prednisolone sodium succinate powder for injections
probenecid tablets

The Committee endorsed the workplan as presented.

3.2 Specifications for medicines, including children's medicines and radiopharmaceuticals

3.2.1 Maternal, newborn, child and adolescent health medicines

Chlorhexidine digluconate solution and chlorhexidine digluconate topical solution/gel

The Committee was informed that work is ongoing to elaborate monographs for chlorhexidine digluconate solution and topical solution/gel for umbilical cord care. These medicines are listed in the 2010 report of the UNCoLSC as an important, low-cost intervention to reduce newborn mortality; the 7.1% chlorhexidine gluconate-containing solution or gel was added to the WHO EML for children in 2013. The Committee will be updated on the progress of the two monographs.

The Committee noted the report.

Estradiol cypionate

In accordance with the agreed workplan for *The International Pharmacopoeia* it was proposed to include a monograph on estradiol cypionate. A draft was received from a WHO Collaborating Centre in February 2015. The draft was discussed at the consultation on screening technology, sampling and specifications for medicines in April 2015 and circulated for comment in May 2015. Comments received were incorporated and the revised draft monograph was presented to the Committee.

The Committee adopted the monograph subject to the amendments agreed.

Levonorgestrel

Revision of the monograph on levonorgestrel in *The International Pharmacopoeia* was proposed in January 2015. A revised draft was discussed at the consultation on screening technology, sampling and specifications for medicines in April 2015 and sent out for public consultation in May 2015; comments were particularly sought on whether the monograph should include a limit test for dextronorgestrel. The revised monograph was presented to the Committee for discussion.

The monograph was adopted subject to the amendments agreed. The Committee also authorized the intended use of the reference substances Levonorgestrel for system suitability 1 CRS and Levonorgestrel for system suitability 2 CRS issued by the *European Pharmacopoeia* (see also 4.2.1).

Magnesium sulfate and magnesium sulfate injection

The Committee was informed that the suitability of the monographs on magnesium sulfate and magnesium sulfate injection had been re-evaluated by a

WHO Collaborating Centre, leading to the conclusion that the monographs are up to date and do not need revision.

The Committee endorsed this conclusion.

Misoprostol, misoprostol dispersion and misoprostol tablets

Access to monographs on misoprostol, misoprostol dispersion and misoprostol tablets is important for WHO Member States; misoprostol tablets have been identified as a life-saving product by the UNCoLSC. The first draft monograph on misoprostol was received from a WHO Collaborating Centre in 2014 and a preliminary version was presented to the Committee at its forty-ninth meeting. The draft was circulated for public consultation in January 2015, and was discussed and further revised at the informal consultation on screening technology, sampling and specifications for medicines in April 2015. At the same time, draft monographs for misoprostol tablets and dispersion were developed. All three drafts were presented to the Expert Committee at its fiftieth meeting, noting that it was proposed to send out all three texts again for public consultation after the Expert Committee meeting and to review the comments received with a subgroup of experts.

The Committee adopted the three monographs subject to amendments as agreed at the meeting and subject to the outcome of a further round of public consultation and subsequent review by a subgroup of experts as proposed. This will enable the Secretariat to publish the monographs in the next edition of *The International Pharmacopoeia*.

It was agreed that the monograph for misoprostol dispersion should be published in the section on monographs for pharmaceutical substances.

Norethisterone and norethisterone tablets

At the forty-ninth Expert Committee meeting in 2014 it was proposed to revise the monograph on norethisterone and to include a monograph on norethisterone tablets in *The International Pharmacopoeia*. Drafts were developed between October 2014 and June 2015 and were sent out for public consultation in July 2015. The drafts were revised according to comments received, and were presented to the Expert Committee.

The Committee accepted the two monographs and authorized the proposed intended use of the reference substance Norethisterone for system suitability issued by the *European Pharmacopoeia* (see also 4.2.1).

3.2.2 Antimalarial medicines

Artemether injection

The Committee was consulted regarding a proposed change that would widen the assay limits in the monograph on artemether injection in order to align them with limits specified in similar monographs. The Committee was further informed of a proposal received from a manufacturer for improvement of the related substances test. A WHO Collaborating Centre kindly agreed to perform further investigations in this regard, and the Committee will be informed of the results.

The Committee supported the proposed widening of the assay limits and endorsed their inclusion in the next edition of *The International Pharmacopoeia*.

3.2.3 Antituberculosis medicines

Cycloserine and cycloserine capsules

Following up on information received from a manufacturer it was proposed to revise the monographs on cycloserine and cycloserine capsules. Extensive additional tests were performed by a collaborating laboratory to evaluate the proposed changes. Revised drafts of the two monographs were received from the collaborating laboratory in July 2015 and circulated for public comment in August 2015. The revised monographs were presented to the Committee for discussion.

The Expert Committee adopted the monographs subject to the amendments agreed.

3.2.4 Medicines for tropical diseases

Mebendazole and mebendazole chewable tablets

The Committee was informed of a number of planned revisions to the monographs on mebendazole and mebendazole chewable tables. The Committee will be informed of progress.

The experts took note of this information.

3.2.5 Medicines for chronic diseases and for mental health

Carbamazepine, carbamazepine tablets, carbamazepine chewable tablets and carbamazepine oral suspension

Draft monographs on carbamazepine and related dosage forms were provided by a WHO Collaborating Centre in December 2014. The drafts were discussed at an informal consultation on screening technology, sampling and specifications for medicines held in April 2015. The text was published for comment in July 2015; comments were sought in particular as to whether the impurities listed under the section Impurities are degradation products or synthesis impurities.

The draft monograph on carbamazepine and the related dosage form monographs were presented to the Expert Committee. However, in light of new information about the nature of potential impurities, the Secretariat of *The International Pharmacopoeia* proposed to redesign the impurity specifications and to circulate the monographs again for public consultation after the meeting, with a subsequent review of comments by a subgroup of experts in early 2016.

The Committee adopted the monographs, subject to the amendments agreed and subject to a further round of consultation and revision as proposed.

3.2.6 Other anti-infective medicines

Clindamycin hydrochloride and clindamycin hydrochloride capsules

Initial draft monographs on clindamycin hydrochloride and clindamycin hydrochloride capsules were received from the responsible WHO Collaborating Centre in December 2014. The drafts were circulated for public comment in January 2015 and discussed at the informal consultation on screening technology, sampling and specifications for medicines in April 2015 before being presented to the Committee.

The Committee adopted the monographs subject to the amendments agreed.

Flucytosine and flucytosine intravenous infusion

Draft monographs on flucytosine and flucytosine intravenous infusion were circulated for comment in December 2014. The comments received were discussed at the consultation on screening technology, sampling and specifications for medicines in April 2015. The revised drafts were presented to the Committee.

The Committee adopted the proposed monographs.

3.2.7 Other medicines

Dextromethorphan hydrobromide and dextromethorphan oral solution

At the forty-ninth meeting of the Expert Committee it had been decided to revise the monograph on dextromethorphan hydrobromide in response to serious incidents that occurred after the consumption of dextromethorphan cough syrups contaminated with levomethorphan. As a result of these events, the Committee adopted a revised monograph on dextromethorphan hydrobromide, which included a statement that the substance must comply with a limit of not more than 0.1% levomethorphan hydrobromide using a suitable chiral method.

A suitable test for levomethorphan had been elaborated and was included in the draft revised monograph on dextromethorphan hydrobromide. The draft was sent out for public consultation in January 2015 and was revised further at an informal consultation in April 2015. At the same time, a monograph on dextromethorphan oral solution was developed, and was sent out for public consultation in August 2015.

The limit test for levomethorphan is not part of the routine release testing of the dosage form, and was therefore not included in the monograph itself. Instead, the monograph includes a statement that samples, if tested, must comply with a levomethorphan limit of not more than 0.1%, and provides a reference to the levomethorphan limit test to be published in the Supplementary information section of *The International Pharmacopoeia* (see below).

The Committee adopted both monographs subject to the amendments agreed.

Levomethorphan limit test for dextromethorphan-containing finished products

An additional limit test for levomethorphan in dextromethorphan-containing dosage forms is to be included in the Supplementary information section of *The International Pharmacopoeia*, enabling quality control laboratories to test suspicious finished product samples for levomethorphan. In 2014 the Expert Committee members reviewed a laboratory report describing the elaboration of suitable procedures. A reference substance containing a mixture of levomethorphan and dextromethorphan is still under establishment. The proposed test was further discussed at an informal consultation in April 2015 and was confirmed by a national quality control laboratory before the proposed text was sent out for comment in August 2015. No comments had been received by 25 September 2015.

The Committee adopted the proposed text.

3.2.8 Radiopharmaceuticals[3]

Review and update of radiopharmaceutical monographs by the International Atomic Energy Agency (IAEA) had been undertaken according to the update and submission process adopted by the Committee at its 2013 meeting. A coordination meeting was held at IAEA in 2014. In early 2015, the work priorities and time lines were aligned with the available expert time and resources. The final schedule for the updating of monographs was expected to be completed in October 2015.

A status update was provided on progress made in updating radiopharmaceutical monographs and associated documentation in *The International Pharmacopoeia*. A number of monographs had been submitted and circulated for comment in accordance with the Committee's consultation process, namely those for technetium (^{99m}Tc) exametazime, thallous (^{201}Tl) chloride and sodium iodine (^{131}I) solution, as well as a general monograph on radiopharmaceuticals. The following monographs had been reviewed by the experts and were ready for submission to WHO for consultation: technetium

[3] The representative from the IAEA was unable to attend the meeting; the WHO Secretariat presented a written report received from IAEA to the Committee.

(^{99m}Tc) bicitate, technetium (^{99m}Tc) succimer, technetium (^{99m}Tc) sulfur colloid and technetium (^{99m}Tc) mebrofenin. The following monographs were ready for final verification by designated experts and expected to be completed in January 2016: technetium (^{99m}Tc) sestamibi, technetium (^{99m}Tc) tin colloid, technetium (^{99m}Tc) pertechnate, technetium (^{99m}Tc) pyrophosphate, technetium (^{99m}Tc) pentetate, technetium (^{99m}Tc) tetrafosmin, technetium (^{99m}Tc) medronate and technetium (^{99m}Tc) mertiatide.

Based on the outcome of the recent IAEA Coordinated Research Project (CRP), the IAEA planned to arrange a review, with help from the CRP participants, of the monograph on cyclotron-produced ^{99m}Tc. Furthermore, a new monograph on extemporaneous preparation of radiopharmaceuticals would be drafted by the experts.

The Expert Committee noted the report.

3.3 General policy

Microbiological assay of antibiotics

There are currently five International Chemical Reference Substances (ICRS) which were established as secondary reference standards for tests according to Chapter 3.1, Microbiological assay of antibiotics, in *The International Pharmacopoeia*. To ensure the continuous fitness for purpose of these reference substances, their assigned potencies have to be monitored regularly in extensive, resource-consuming collaborative trials. In addition, a total of 21 monographs prescribe a microbiological assay for antibiotics, but no suitable reference substance has yet been established.

At its meeting in 2009 the Expert Committee had decided that in monographs for antibiotics which specify a microbiological assay, this test should be replaced by a chromatographic method where possible and appropriate.

Since 2009, significant progress has been achieved in developing physicochemical assay methods for pharmaceutical products. In view of the information provided above, the Secretariat of *The International Pharmacopoeia* proposed to:

(1) discontinue the use of five ICRS in microbiological assays of antibiotics and to delete the potency assignments in the ICRS leaflets;

(2) revise four monographs in order to replace the microbiological assay with liquid chromatography methods, considering methods already published in pharmacopoeias;

(3) revise four monographs in order to replace the ICRS by WHO International Standards for Antibiotics (ISA) or, preferably,

secondary standards derived from them and established by another pharmacopoeia for use in microbiological assay, which could foster work-sharing between pharmacopoeias;

(4) develop a concept document for the possible transition from microbiological to physicochemical assay in 14 monographs, considering in particular chromatographic methods published in the scientific domain, for discussion and possible endorsement by this Committee and the Expert Committee on Biological Standardization; and

(5) suppress the monographs for substances containing any of five active ingredients. Medicines containing these substances are no longer included in the WHO EML (19th edition) or in the relevant invitations for expression of interest to manufacturers.

The Committee agreed to the proposals described under points (1), (2), (4) and (5) above (see Table 3). With regard to the proposal outlined in point (3), the Committee agreed that the experts should be given more time to identify possible reference standards that can be referred to in each of the monographs. The relevant ICRS and monographs affected by these decisions are listed in Table 3.

Table 3
Recommendations relating to the use of microbiological assays for antibiotics

(1)	**ICRS no longer to be used for microbiological assays of antibiotics, and potency assignments to be deleted**
	nystatin (ICRS0369)
	framycetin sulfate (neomycin B) (ICRS0355)
	gentamicin sulfate (ICRS0319)
	spectinomycin hydrochloride (ICRS0415)
	streptomycin sulfate (ICRS0416)
(2)	**Monographs in which microbiological assay should be replaced by liquid chromatography methods**
	erythromycin ethylsuccinate
	erythromycin lactobionate
	erythromycin stearate
	tetracycline hydrochloride

Table 3 *continued*

(3) Monographs for which suitable standards other than ICRS should be identified[a]		
amphotericin B		
amphotericin B for injection		
bleomycin sulfate		
kanamycin for injection		
kanamycin monosulfate		
(4) Monographs for which a concept paper should be developed on the possible transition from microbiological to physicochemical methods		
amphotericin B	kanamycin acid sulfate	gentamicin sulfate
amphotericin B for injection	kanamycin for injection	streptomycin sulfate
bleomycin sulfate	kanamycin monosulfate	streptomycin for injection
erythromycin ethylsuccinate tablets	nystatin	paromomycin sulfate
erythromycin stearate tablets	nystatin tablets	
(5) Monographs that should be suppressed		
bacitracin	chlortetracycline hydrochloride	oxytetracycline dehydrate
bacitracin zinc	erythromycin (base)	oxytetracycline hydrochloride
bleomycin hydrochloride	neomycin sulfate	

[a] The Committee agreed that the experts should be given more time to identify possible reference standards that can be referred to in the monographs.

Replacement of mercuric acetate

The Secretariat of *The International Pharmacopoeia* is committed to eliminating the use of mercury salts in currently recommended methods in order to reduce the risk to analysts and the environment. In the past, mercuric acetate was used to titrate weak bases; however, such titrations are now obsolete and can be replaced with safer and better titration techniques, such as the direct titration with perchloric acid in anhydrous acetic acid. As a first step in phasing out mercury-based methods, a WHO Collaborating Centre has identified 47 monographs in which mercuric acetate is used as a reagent and has listed alternative methods used in other pharmacopoeias. As a possible next step, the Secretariat proposed that a concept should be developed to guide the replacement of obsolete titrations of pharmaceutical substances in *The International Pharmacopoeia* and the elaboration of the related assays.

The Committee took note of the update.

Draft note for guidance on organic impurities in active pharmaceutical ingredients and finished pharmaceutical products

Taking into account current practices in the use of *The International Pharmacopoeia* and available guidance on how to establish limits for impurities, a note for guidance on organic impurities in active pharmaceutical substances and FPPs was drafted.

The proposed note for guidance is intended to replace the text on "Related substances in finished pharmaceutical product monographs" in the Supplementary information section of *The International Pharmacopoeia*. The first draft was prepared by the Secretariat of *The International Pharmacopoeia* in January–March 2015 with input from a group of experts, and was discussed at the consultation on screening technology, sampling and specifications for medicines in April 2015. The draft was sent out for public consultation in April 2015, and the comments received were collated by the Secretariat. The revised proposed draft was presented to the Committee.

The Committee reviewed the proposed revised draft and provided further feedback. It was agreed to form a small working group to address a number of specific comments raised in the discussion. The working group met during the meeting and reported back to the Committee with a proposal for further revisions. The Committee agreed that the revised document should be discussed further within the small working group and with relevant experts. It should then be discussed at an informal consultation before being sent out again for public consultation, together with a brief explanatory note about the nature of the revisions. The Committee will review a revised draft at its next meeting.

4. Quality control – international reference materials (International Chemical Reference Substances and Infrared Reference Spectra)

4.1 Update on International Chemical Reference Substances (ICRS), including report of the ICRS Board

International Chemical Reference Substances (ICRS) are used as primary standards in physical and chemical tests that are described in *The International Pharmacopoeia*, as well as for setting official secondary standards. ICRS are used to identify and determine the purity or assay of pharmaceutical substances and preparations or to verify the performance of test methods. The standards are officially adopted by the Expert Committee.

The European Directorate for the Quality of Medicines & HealthCare (EDQM) is the custodian centre in charge of establishment, storage, distribution and monitoring of ICRS in *The International Pharmacopoeia*. Three steering committee telephone conferences were held in 2014, and two in 2015. In accordance with the work programme as agreed in March 2014, the ICRS listed below were established and released by the ICRS Board.

Routine monitoring of fitness for purpose was done on 17 ICRS in 2014, and no negative findings were reported; for 2015, 13 substances had been monitored with no negative findings. The EDQM welcomed the decisions to add dates and version numbers to monographs in *The International Pharmacopoeia*, as this facilitates quality assurance verification of ICRS batches in relation to their intended *International Pharmacopoeia* use.

Work is in progress to establish reference substances for capreomycin sulfate, enabling testing according to the recently adopted monographs on capreomycin, and for dextromethorphan for system suitability, enabling the performance of the limit test for levomethorphan adopted by the Committee at this meeting.

The Secretariat expressed its sincere thanks to EDQM for establishing, storing and distributing ICRS and providing related guidance, to the ICRS Board for reviewing establishment reports and releasing ICRS, and to the laboratories that participated in collaborative trials. The Expert Committee noted the report and joined the Secretariat in thanking the custodian centre for this major contribution. The Expert Committee noted the report and endorsed the release of the ICRS shown in Table 4.

Table 4
ICRS released by the ICRS Board

α-artemether ICRS 1
efavirenz ICRS 2
efavirenz impurity B ICRS 1
ritonavir ICRS 2
abacavir sulfate ICRS 2
paracetamol ICRS 3
artemether ICRS 2
rifampicin ICRS 3
stavudine impurity F ICRS 1

4.2 General policy

4.2.1 Chapter on reference substances and reference spectra

Following up on a recommendation made by the Expert Committee at its forty-ninth meeting to use in *The International Pharmacopoeia*, where appropriate, ultraviolet (UV) absorptivity values for assays and other quantification purposes with a view to limiting reference to ICRS, it was proposed to revise the chapter on reference substances and reference spectra.

Additional changes were proposed to reflect recent discussions within the ICRS Board and with the custodian centre for ICRS. A draft revised chapter was prepared by the Secretariat of *The International Pharmacopoeia* in January–March 2015 with feedback from a group of experts. The draft was discussed at the consultation on screening technology, sampling and specifications for medicines held from 13 to 15 April 2015 before being circulated for public consultation in May 2015. Comments received were duly collated before presentation of the draft to the Expert Committee at its meeting in October 2015.

Besides other changes, the revised chapter sets out the principles to be applied when reference substances are included in monographs that have been established by other pharmacopoeias for use according to *The International Pharmacopoeia*. A list of reference standards found suitable for such a use is included as an appendix to the draft revised chapter. The list includes the reference substances mentioned in the monographs on norethisterone and levonorgestrel (see 3.2.1). To facilitate continuous updating, the Committee recommended that the list should be maintained as a living document on the WHO website and referred to in the chapter on reference substances.

The Committee adopted the text subject to the amendments agreed.

5. Quality control – national laboratories

5.1 External quality assurance assessment scheme

The external quality assurance assessment scheme (EQAAS) is a proficiency testing scheme offered by WHO for the external evaluation of quality control management systems in chemical quality control laboratories. Since 2010 it has been organized with assistance from the EDQM.

The Committee was given an update on Phase 6 of the EQAAS studies. Unlike in Phase 5 studies, the samples sent out were used for two studies, reducing the burden of sending and receiving samples. Approximately 40 laboratories participated in Phase 6 studies. Analysis of samples was ongoing, with results expected at the end of 2015.

The Secretariat maintains close links with the WHO/PQT prequalifying quality control laboratories when carrying out the EQAAS studies. Preparations were beginning for Phase 7 of the EQAAS scheme.

The Committee noted the report.

5.2 Guidance on testing of "suspect" substandard/spurious/falsely-labelled/falsified/counterfeit medicines

In October 2014, the Committee had provided advice and endorsed a draft outline for Guidance on testing of "suspect" substandard/spurious/falsely-labelled/falsified/counterfeit (SSFFC) medicines.

Various related texts were reviewed at the informal consultation on screening technology, sampling and specifications for medicines held in April 2015, and work is in progress to draft concise guidelines on testing of "suspect" SSFFC medicines. A first draft was produced after the consultation and circulated for comment among the relevant experts.

The Committee noted the update and recommended that work on developing the guidelines be continued.

6. Prequalification of quality control laboratories

6.1 Update on the prequalification of quality control laboratories

The prequalification procedure for quality control laboratories was established in 2004. Participation is voluntary and is open to both public and private quality control laboratories. In October 2015 there were a total of 38 WHO-prequalified laboratories distributed among all six WHO regions. Two laboratories became prequalified in 2015, one in Uganda and one in India.

A peer audit scheme has been introduced as a capacity-building measure for laboratories involved in the prequalification procedure. Training has been conducted under this scheme in Armenia, Ghana and Nigeria and a further training programme is planned in Madagascar. Applications are currently also being received from manufacturer-linked laboratories, and in any future revision of the procedures consideration should be given to whether the prequalification procedure should be applicable to this type of laboratory.

The Committee noted the report.

6.2 Update on WHO quality monitoring projects

A quality monitoring survey of antiretrovirals started in the third quarter of 2015 and is ongoing, with samples being collected in five countries. A survey on antimalarials would start in the first quarter of 2016. It is planned that this survey will include artemisinin combination therapies in the initial phase of developing a spectral library for FPPs to support the use of screening methods for the detection of potential SSFFC products.

The Expert Committee expressed its appreciation for the report.

7. Quality assurance – collaboration initiatives

7.1 International meetings of world pharmacopoeias

In 2012, WHO brought together representatives from 23 national and regional pharmacopoeia authorities at the first meeting of world pharmacopoeias. The participants committed to working towards harmonization of pharmacopoeial standards in the global context by developing a guidance text on good pharmacopoeial practices (GPhP) aiming at convergence of approaches in defining pharmacopoeial standards (see 7.2). Harmonization of standards has become increasingly important for public health for several reasons. It will support the global fight against falsified and substandard medicines and will reduce the costs arising from meeting the different standards used in the production and testing of medicines, thus making good quality medicines accessible to more people.

The international meeting of world pharmacopoeias has become a recurring event which is co-hosted by WHO and a pharmacopoeia. Two meetings were held in 2015: the fifth International Meeting of World Pharmacopoeias co-hosted by the *United States Pharmacopeia* (USP) and WHO from 20 to 22 April 2015 in Rockville, USA, and the sixth International Meeting of World Pharmacopoeias co-hosted by the *Chinese Pharmacopoeia* (ChP) and WHO in Suzhou, China on 21–22 September 2015. Achieving global standards to expand access to medicines globally was key to the discussions at the September meeting, which was held in connection with the 2015 ChP Annual Scientific Symposium.

Representatives from 12 WHO Member States' pharmacopoeias attended, and more than 30 official pharmacopoeial authorities were represented. During this sixth international meeting the new guidelines on GPhP were prepared for finalization, based on feedback received during wide global consultation (see 7.2).

The representative of the *Japanese Pharmacopoeia* (JP) announced that the seventh WHO International Pharmacopoeia meeting would be co-hosted by the JP and WHO, and would be held in Tokyo from 13 to 15 September 2016 in conjunction with the 130th anniversary of the JP.

The Expert Committee noted the report and thanked the pharmacopoeias and the Secretariat for their major contributions to this achievement.

7.2 Good pharmacopoeial practices

The primary objective of the GPhP is to define approaches and policies on establishing pharmacopoeial standards with the ultimate goal of harmonization. The GPhP describe a set of guiding principles for national pharmacopoeial authorities and regional pharmacopoeial authorities, which facilitates the appropriate design, development and maintenance of pharmacopoeial standards.

A GPhP text has been drafted over the past three years at successive meetings of world pharmacopoeias (see 7.1). In view of the length of the third draft it was decided in 2014 to split it into a main text and a detailed technical annex to be developed by a separate drafting group. A technical annex was drafted on the basis of parts of the previous GPhP text with input from the JP, the *European Pharmacopoeia* and other pharmacopoeias. The significantly shortened fourth draft of the main text was then circulated for comments in September 2014, and was discussed at the fourth meeting of world pharmacopoeias held in Strasbourg, France, in October 2014. It was subject to further consultation with world pharmacopoeias from October 2014 to March 2015 and was discussed at the fifth international meeting of world pharmacopoeias, held in Washington, DC, USA in April 2015. Feedback received on the draft text at that meeting was discussed from 20 to 22 April 2015, leading to preparation of a fifth draft, which was circulated for further consultation among world pharmacopoeias. Comments were received from 15 parties, including five international associations, and were discussed at the sixth international meeting of world pharmacopoeias held in China in September 2015, leading to a sixth draft, which was subjected to the usual public consultation process.

At its forty-ninth meeting, the Expert Committee had been briefed on progress made on developing a GPhP text and had endorsed a concept paper on the purpose and benefits of GPhP. The final revised draft of the main guidance text and comments received during the public consultation process were presented to the Expert Committee at its fiftieth meeting.

The Committee provided its feedback in response to the comments received. The Committee adopted the guidance (Annex 1) with agreed amendments reflecting the comments received, subject to final concurrence being granted by the pharmacopoeias. Work will continue on drafting possible additional chapters and to develop the technical annex further, taking into account its complexity and the resources available. The Committee congratulated the Secretariat on facilitating the development of this document, which is a major step forward towards prospective harmonization of pharmacopoeial practices.

7.3 FIP–WHO technical guidelines: points to consider in the provision by health-care professionals of children-specific preparations that are not available as authorized products

The draft of a guidance document on extemporaneous preparation of medicines for children, which had been commissioned by WHO, was considered in 2011 by the WHO Expert Committee on the Selection and Use of Essential Medicines, which has a subcommittee on paediatric medicines. The Committee felt that extemporaneous preparation of medicines for children may be necessary in some situations but was concerned about the risks of inappropriate preparations.

Revisions of the document were submitted to the forty-sixth, forty-seventh, forty-eighth and forty-ninth meetings of the Expert Committee on Specifications for Pharmaceutical Preparations.

The draft was brought into balance with the contents of the WHO document *Development of paediatric medicines: points to consider in formulation* and includes parts from earlier drafts, e.g. the draft appendix on potential problems in compounding, a section on aspects of GMP and a glossary intended to facilitate a common interpretation of the guidance by a wide audience of practitioners. At its 2014 meeting the Expert Committee reviewed the draft and the comments received, and decided that a further meeting should be held between WHO, the International Pharmaceutical Federation (FIP) and other interested parties in order to discuss the text. The draft was then discussed at the informal consultation on paediatric formulations for medicines from 13 to 14 May 2015, and a revised draft was sent out for comment in June 2015. Feedback was received and collated and the draft was further revised in line with comments received. The proposed revised draft was presented to the Committee at its fiftieth meeting in October 2015, with a note that some points raised in the comments would require expert advice beyond the scope of advice from the Committee.

The Committee discussed the proposed draft and the comments, and adopted the guidance with amendments as agreed (Annex 2), subject to a future revision of remaining points with input from suitably qualified experts. The Committee thanked the main author and the experts who contributed to this very useful and relevant guidance. FIP expressed its appreciation to WHO for facilitating the preparation and adoption of this guidance through the Expert Committee.

8. Quality assurance – good manufacturing practices

8.1 Update of WHO good manufacturing practices for biologicals

The guidance on *Good manufacturing practices (GMP) for biological products* was first adopted by the Expert Committee on Biological Standardization (ECBS) as an annex to the GMP for pharmaceutical products, and was published in the WHO Technical Report Series in 1992. The guidance is widely used by regulators and is mandatory for prequalification of vaccines. To reflect the considerable developments since the adoption of the guidelines as well as current perspectives regarding GMP for manufacturers of biological products, a preliminary draft revision was prepared in 2008. A revised draft was prepared by a drafting group and was discussed at a consultation on GMP for biological products held in July 2014. The text was circulated for public consultation in 2015 before being presented to the ECBS at its October 2015 meeting, held concurrently with the meeting of the Expert Committee on Specifications for Pharmaceutical Preparations.

The proposed guidelines are intended to be an annex to *WHO Good manufacturing practices for pharmaceutical products: main principles* (WHO Technical Report Series, No. 986, 2014, Annex 2), and should be read in conjunction with other specific WHO guidelines and recommendations for specific classes of biological products (e.g. vaccines). An outline of the proposed revised guidelines and key changes and updates was presented to the Committee. The draft was also presented to the ECBS during its meeting.

The Expert Committee noted the report, and adopted the guidance text (Annex 3) following its adoption by the ECBS.

8.2 Update of questions and answers for WHO good manufacturing practices for active pharmaceutical ingredients

The *WHO good manufacturing practices for active pharmaceutical ingredients* (WHO Technical Report Series, No. 957, 2010, Annex 2), adopted by the Expert Committee in 2010, are in line with the International Conference on Harmonisation of Technical Requirements for Registration of Pharmaceuticals for Human Use (ICH) text adopted by numerous national and regional authorities. An Appendix 2 to this GMP text approved at the time was intended to eliminate ambiguities and uncertainties and help harmonize the inspections of both small molecules and biotech APIs.

To clarify technical issues and harmonize expectations during inspections, the Pharmaceutical Inspection Co-operation Scheme (PIC/S) through its Expert Circle on APIs and later the ICH, set up working groups to develop questions and answers (Q&As) on the API GMP guidance. WHO has been involved both as an observer and through technical advice in the PIC/S as well as the ICH-related working groups. The ICH Q&As were adopted on 10 June 2015.[4] During the consultation on data management, bioequivalence, GMP and medicines' inspection, held from 29 June to 1 July 2015, a draft working document titled *WHO good manufacturing practice guide for active pharmaceutical ingredients* (working document QAS/15.626) was discussed, and the participants unanimously recommended that the current Appendix 2 should be replaced by a cross-reference to the ICH website with the Q&As on *Q7: Good manufacturing practice guide for active pharmaceutical ingredients.*

The Expert Committee endorsed this proposal.

8.3 Update of WHO good manufacturing practices: validation

The need for revision of the published *Supplementary guidelines on good manufacturing practices: validation* (WHO Technical Report Series, No. 937, 2006, Annex 4) had been identified by PQT and a draft document was circulated for comment in early 2013. The focus of the revision was Appendix 7 (non-sterile process validation), which had been revised and was adopted by the Committee at its forty-ninth meeting in October 2014.

The Committee was informed that work is ongoing to revise the validation guidance and its appendices as relevant. The Committee noted the update and recommended that this work should be continued.

8.4 Update of model inspection report

A draft proposal for updating the *Guidance on GMP: inspection report* (WHO Technical Report Series, No. 908, 2002, Annex 5) and the *Model certificate of GMP* (WHO Technical Report Series, No. 908, 2002, Annex 6) in line with current trends and formats was first discussed at an informal consultation on inspection, GMP and risk management guidance in medicine manufacturing held in April 2014. The objectives of the revision were to promote consistency between formats used by inspectorates, thus facilitating collaborative activities and information-sharing, and to bring the document into line with current *WHO good manufacturing practices for pharmaceutical products: main principles* (WHO Technical Report Series, No. 986, 2014, Annex 2).

An outline of an update of the model inspection report prepared by PQT was submitted to the Expert Committee in October 2014; the Committee discussed the outline and endorsed the proposals of the informal consultation. A draft proposal for revision was prepared by the inspectors of the WHO/

[4] The ICH Q&As are available at: http://www.ich.org/fileadmin/Public_Web_Site/ICH_Products/Guidelines/Quality/Q7/ICH_Q7-IWG_QA_v5_0_14Apr2015_FINAL_for_publication_17June2015.pdf.

PQT, and was discussed at an informal consultation on data management, bioequivalence, GMP and medicines' inspection held in Geneva from 29 June to 1 July 2015. The revised draft guidance and model inspection report format were sent out for comment in August 2015. The comments received and a proposed revised draft were presented to the Committee at its fiftieth meeting.

The experts discussed the draft revised guidance and the model inspection report template and provided their input. It was agreed that the template should include subsections for inspection observations corresponding to the subsections of the WHO GMP text with cross-references to the set of six systems incorporating the general scheme of pharmaceutical manufacturing operations, as reflected, e.g. in the inspectional approach of the United States Food and Drug Authority.

The Committee adopted the guidance (Annex 4), subject to the amendments agreed.

8.5 Update and recommendations from the inspectors' meeting

8.5.1 Supplementary guidelines on good manufacturing practices for heating, ventilation and air-conditioning systems for non-sterile pharmaceutical dosage forms

The Committee was briefed about progress on updating the *Supplementary guidelines on good manufacturing practices for heating, ventilation and air-conditioning systems for non-sterile pharmaceutical dosage forms* (WHO Technical Report Series, No. 961, 2011, Annex 5). A revised draft of these guidelines was discussed at a consultation on data management, bioequivalence, GMP and medicines' inspection held from 29 June to 1 July 2015. The revision takes into account current trends in engineering as well as experience gained from the implementation of this guidance during inspections.

The guidelines were further revised by a consultant, based on the feedback received during the consultation and from the inspectors of PQT. On this occasion the text was also aligned with other relevant guidelines, notably the proposed revisions to *Supplementary guidelines on good manufacturing practices: validation* (WHO Technical Report Series, No. 937, 2006, Annex 4). The revised draft was circulated for public comment in September 2015. A large number of comments had been received, which will be discussed at a further technical consultation.

The Expert Committee noted the report.

8.5.2 Risk classification of inspection observations

Observations noted during inspections of manufacturing sites, contract research organizations and quality control laboratories need to be classified according to the risk to patients and level of compliance with relevant GXPs. Guidance on classification of observations will facilitate harmonization and increase the uniformity of approaches taken by inspectors, as well as the overall rating of GXP compliance by the site. During the consultation on data management, bioequivalence, GMP and medicines' inspection held on 29 June–1 July 2015, a draft working document on *Risk classification of inspection observations* was discussed. The draft was submitted to the Committee at its fiftieth meeting. Considering that other organizations were also drafting guidance in this area, the participants at the informal consultation recommended that WHO should join in with the ongoing activities in order to enable consistency between inspectorates, facilitating the sharing of information and inspection reports.

The Committee endorsed this proposal.

8.6 Guidance on good data and record management practices

In recent years the number of observations made regarding good data management practices during inspections of GMP, good clinical practice (GCP) and good laboratory practices (GLP) has been increasing. There is increased regulatory awareness of the need for integrity of data submitted as a basis for regulatory decisions. Good data management in line with scientific advances and regulatory developments is crucial for all stakeholders in regulation of health products, including patients, industry and regulators.

A proposal for a new guidance document on good data management was first discussed at an informal consultation held in April 2014. At its forty-ninth meeting the Committee discussed and endorsed a concept paper and the proposed structure of the guidance. A document was then drafted by the inspectors of PQT in close cooperation with a data management expert and national inspectors, and was discussed at the consultation on data management, bioequivalence, GMP and medicines' inspection held from 29 June to 1 July 2015. The draft was further revised on the basis of feedback received during the consultation, taking into account principles laid down in related WHO guidance as well as industry norms and regulatory requirements. The guidance promotes a risk-based approach and provides illustrative examples of good data management in practice. The draft was sent out for comments in September 2015 before being presented to the Committee at its fiftieth meeting. The Committee's view was sought on future collaboration with PIC/S to enable future revisions of the proposed guidance, aiming for convergence with PIC/S data management norms, which are at an early stage of development.

Recognizing the wide interest in and urgent need for this guidance, the Committee adopted the guidance (Annex 5), subject to the review of current and forthcoming comments by a subgroup and subject to circulation of the finalized document to the Expert Committee prior to publication.

9. Quality assurance – distribution and trade of pharmaceuticals

9.1 Good trade and distribution practices for starting materials

WHO guidance on good trade and distribution practices (GTDP) was developed in order to ensure the quality and integrity of starting materials and pharmaceutical products circulating in the global pharmaceutical market. The guidance was adopted in 2003. At the forty-seventh meeting of the Expert Committee in 2012 it was felt that there was a need to include new developments and concepts in both the WHO guidelines on GTDP for pharmaceutical starting materials and the good distribution practices (GDP) guide for pharmaceutical excipients issued by the International Pharmaceutical Excipients Council (IPEC), which is aligned with the WHO document. In July 2013 the IPEC Federation provided a proposed revision and update of the WHO guidelines, which then underwent several rounds of comments and was discussed at the forty-eighth and forty-ninth meetings of the Expert Committee. The draft document was revised in line with the experts' input and was circulated again for comment in March 2015. Comments were collated and reviewed by a subgroup of the Committee in July and August 2015. The revised draft was submitted to the Expert Committee at its fiftieth meeting.

It was agreed that a subgroup of experts should review the comments received and revise the guidance further. A revised draft was presented to the Committee members during the meeting. The Committee adopted the guidance subject to further review by a subgroup of experts. The final revised text is included in Annex 6.

9.2 WHO Certification scheme on the quality of pharmaceutical products moving in international commerce – questions and answers

The WHO Certification Scheme for finished pharmaceutical products is an international voluntary agreement, originally endorsed by the World Health Assembly in 1969, to provide information about the quality of pharmaceutical products moving in international commerce to countries which participate in the Scheme using model format templates provided by WHO, notably the Certificate of Pharmaceutical Product (CPP).

The Scheme has been revised several times, with each revision being endorsed by the World Health Assembly. A questions and answers (Q&A) document was developed as an interim measure in line with recommendations for revision of the Scheme. In 2010, WHO initiated a survey among its Member States about their use of the Scheme. The responses received indicated that the Scheme is appreciated as a valuable tool for exchange of regulatory information between Member States, but that it may need further adaptation and more active participation by a number of member countries to enable its useful application in the current regulatory and industry environment. At its forty-ninth meeting in 2014, the Expert Committee had therefore recommended that the Q&As should be updated. The CPP Network team of the International Federation of Pharmaceutical Manufacturers and Associations (IFPMA) proposed a revised document, which was circulated for comment in August 2015. The comments were reviewed by a small working group in September 2015, and the proposed revision was presented to the Committee in October 2015. The Committee reviewed the revised Q&As and heard from the WHO Regulatory Systems Strengthening Team and from a number of organizations represented at the meeting session about their experience with the use of the Scheme.

The Committee adopted the proposed revised Q&A document. Furthermore it was recommended that the 17th International Conference of Drug Regulatory Authorities (ICDRA) to be held in Cape Town, South Africa, from 27 November to 2 December 2016 should be used as an opportunity to advocate for active support of the effective functioning of the Scheme by Member States.

9.3 Guidance on medicines quality surveys

Following recommendations made by the Committee at its meetings in 2010 and 2011, two draft guidance documents were produced. These documents reflected the extensive experience of the WHO/PQT with the conduct of quality control testing surveys to monitor the quality of pharmaceutical products circulating in the markets of Member States. The *Proposal for a procedure on sampling and market surveillance* was drafted in 2012 in response to the Committee's recommendation to develop a sampling procedure. A second draft document entitled *Recommendations on the content of a survey protocol for surveys of the quality of medicines* was prepared in 2014. It describes the steps necessary for conducting quality surveys and proposes examples and standard operating procedures that can be adapted to different situations. This document was presented to the Expert Committee at its 2014 meeting. Noting its comprehensive nature the Committee had recommended in 2014 that it should be retained as a scientific background reference and that a shorter practical guide should be prepared.

A concise draft of the guidelines on the conduct of surveys of the quality of medicines was sent out for public consultation in July 2015. Comments received were consolidated and presented together with the revised draft text to the Committee in October 2015.

The Committee reviewed the document and the comments and provided its input. The Expert Committee adopted the proposed guidance, subject to amendments agreed (Annex 7).

9.4 Update on the monitoring and surveillance project

A pilot study of the WHO global monitoring and surveillance system was conducted between September 2012 and January 2013 and is now part of the workplan of the Member States mechanism on substandard/spurious/falsely-labelled/falsified/counterfeit (SSFFC) medical products established by the World Health Assembly Resolution WHA65.19. Participation has steadily increased and was reported to encompass 112 Member States in October 2015.

A rapid alert form with a minimum set of questions is used for reporting. Reports are submitted to WHO through focal points at national regulatory authorities (NRAs). Since 2012 there have been 900 reports of potential SSFFC products, leading to 12 International Drug Alerts being issued for SSFFC medical products presenting an immediate and significant threat to public health. Potential SSFFC products have been reported for all types of medicines. Frequently reported categories include antimalarials and antibiotics. This is a worrying finding in view of the emerging resistance to both.

Upon receipt of a report, WHO provides immediate technical support with a response time of 24–72 hours. The reports are uploaded to a database, and the data are analysed in order to detect patterns and to assess the scale, scope, extent and harm from SSFFC products. Detection and reporting are also used to prevent future harm. Evidence-driven action is taken to strengthen regulatory systems, raise awareness and engage stakeholders in combating SSFFC medical products. Future actions will involve strengthening the communication with focal points in participating NRAs and strengthening networks of NRAs globally.

The Expert Committee noted the report.

10. Prequalification of priority essential medicines and active pharmaceutical ingredients

10.1 Update on the Prequalification Team managed by WHO

The Prequalification Programme was launched by WHO in 2001 in partnership with the Joint United Nations Programme on HIV/AIDS (UNAIDS), UNICEF and the United Nations Population Fund (UNFPA).

The Committee was given an overview of the different workstreams and activities within PQT.

In terms of pharmaceutical products, medicines for hepatitis B and C have become eligible for prequalification, with two finished product applications undergoing screening and preparatory meetings having been held with several companies. Prequalification may also be opened up to other therapeutic areas if there is a need. WHO assessment times have decreased substantially in recent years. Additional guidance to applicants has been provided for specific product types and specific prequalification requirements. A total of 426 products were prequalified as of 12 October 2015. A collaborative registration procedure, which started in 2013, supports speedy registration of prequalified products in participating countries based on sharing of prequalification information.

Regarding prequalification of APIs, the Committee was informed that a total of 82 APIs have been prequalified to date. New API manufacturers had come forward in 2015 thus improving the prospects of continued access and competitiveness. Three applications for hepatitis C-related APIs are being processed. In general the number of applications for prequalification of both APIs and finished products has been stable, demonstrating continued interest.

PQT is involved in a wide range of collaborative initiatives. Within WHO, PQT maintains close links with many other programmes and units, including *The International Pharmacopoeia*. A standard text has been included in the API prequalification sign-off form to permit access by *The International Pharmacopoeia* to relevant data in the API master file. Monographs in *The International Pharmacopoeia* strongly support manufacturers working towards prequalification of their products; for example, the revised cycloserine monograph has been much appreciated by applicants. PQT offers a rotational fellowship programme, under which regulators from Member States spend three or six months working at WHO with the prequalification assessor team or inspectorate. This programme has greatly contributed to capacity-building and to the success of collaborative activities.

The Secretariat thanked PQT for its important input to, and feedback on, the guidance developed through the Expert Committee.

The Expert Committee noted the report.

10.2 Collaborative procedure between the World Health Organization (WHO) Prequalification Team and national regulatory authorities in the assessment and accelerated national registration of WHO-prequalified pharmaceutical products and vaccines

The *Collaborative procedure between the World Health Organization (WHO) Prequalification Team and national regulatory authorities in the assessment and accelerated national registration of WHO-prequalified pharmaceutical products* aims to make use of work done by the WHO/PQT to support efficient assessment for granting of marketing authorization by participating regulatory authorities. It is based on sharing of prequalification assessment and inspection reports with the consent of the prequalification holder. The procedure was first adopted in 2012 (WHO Technical Report Series, No. 981, 2013, Annex 4), and has been successfully implemented for medicines.

It was proposed to update the procedure and to extend it to vaccines. The revision was discussed with stakeholders and the Expert Committee was informed of the proposed revision at its 2014 meeting. A working document was sent out for public consultation in July 2015. The revised document, together with the comments received, was submitted to the Expert Committee in October 2015.

The Expert Committee adopted the proposed revision of the collaborative procedure, now titled *Collaborative procedure between the World Health Organization (WHO) Prequalification Team and national regulatory authorities in the assessment and accelerated national registration of WHO-prequalified pharmaceutical products and vaccines (revision)* (Annex 8), subject to the amendments agreed.

11. Regulatory guidance

11.1 Guidance for organizations performing in vivo bioequivalence studies

The performance of a bioequivalence study is usually a requirement for registration and prequalification of a multisource ("generic") product to ensure interchangeability of the product. Such studies should be undertaken in compliance with WHO GCP and considering relevant elements from WHO GLP and good practices for quality control laboratories.

An update of WHO's 2006 *Guidance for organizations performing in vivo bioequivalence studies* (WHO Technical Report Series, No. 937, 2006, Annex 9) in line with new developments was discussed at an informal consultation in April 2014. A working document was presented to the Expert Committee in October 2014, and the Committee supported the revision of the guidelines. The draft was then further revised by the inspectors of the WHO/PQT in collaboration with national inspectors and was circulated for public comment in May 2015. Comments received were discussed at an information consultation on data management, bioequivalence, GMP and medicines' inspection held from 29 June to 1 July 2015. A second draft was prepared taking into consideration the revised text on *Multisource (generic) pharmaceutical products: guidelines on registration requirements to establish interchangeability* (WHO Technical Report Series, No. 992, 2015, Annex 7), the new proposed guidelines on good data management (see 8.6), and PQT's experience of assessing and inspecting bioequivalence studies since 2006. Guidance was added on bioanalytical analysis, and areas with recurrent inspection findings were clarified. The updated draft was presented to the Committee in October 2015. The guidelines emphasize management responsibilities to ensure that adequate premises, equipment and quality systems are available to conduct good quality studies.

The Committee discussed the revised guidelines and agreed to the changes proposed in response to the comments. The revised guidelines (Annex 9) were adopted as presented.

11.2 WHO general guidance on variations to multisource pharmaceutical products

A marketing authorization holder is responsible for the quality, safety and efficacy of an FPP that is placed on the market throughout its life cycle. After the FPP has been authorized for marketing the manufacturer will often wish to make changes (variations) to the product for a number of reasons. Such changes may require the approval of the national medicines regulatory authority. The extent and nature of regulatory control of variations to registered pharmaceutical products varies considerably between WHO Member States.

In October 2013 the Expert Committee endorsed the development of *Guidelines for regulatory authorities on variations for multisource products.* A draft of the guidelines was developed between October 2013 and February 2014 and circulated for comment and feedback before being discussed by the Committee at its forty-ninth meeting. Based on feedback received, the guidance was revised to describe the main principles for variation procedures for implementation by regulatory authorities in accordance with risk–benefit and legal considerations specific to each authority. The guidance is intended to assist regulatory authorities to establish national requirements for the regulation of post-approval changes. It proposes categories of changes and reporting procedures for adaptation by regulatory authorities. The revised document was sent out for another round of comments in June 2015. Feedback was collated and the revised draft was presented to the Committee at its fiftieth meeting. The Committee discussed the proposal to revise the title of the guidance and to delete the term "multisource", as it was noted that a wider audience may use the document as written. However, it was concluded that the original name should be retained.

The Committee reviewed the guidance and the comments received, and adopted the guidance subject to the amendments agreed (Annex 10).

11.3 Update of biowaiver principles for assessment of interchangeable multisource (generic) products

Revised guidelines on interchangeability of multisource products were adopted by the Committee in 2014. The safety and efficacy of a multisource (generic) product is usually demonstrated through an in vivo bioequivalence study that establishes its therapeutic equivalence to a comparator product. A biowaiver is a regulatory approval process based on evidence of equivalence other than through in vivo bioequivalence testing. Existing guidance on whether a biowaiver can be granted – based on the permeability and solubility of the API according to the Biopharmaceutics Classification System (BCS) – is provided in the *Proposal to waive in vivo bioequivalence requirements for WHO Model List of Essential Medicines immediate-release, solid oral dosage forms* (WHO Technical Report Series, No. 937, 2006, Annex 8). The proposal includes a section describing the general biowaiver principles as well as three tables listing information on various categories of APIs included in the WHO EML.

In 2014 the Committee reviewed progress and endorsed the proposed approach to separate the guidance text from the tables, which will be maintained in a separate living document that can be updated in line with each new version of the EML (see 11.4). This is analogous to the approach suggested for the list of comparator products (see 11.5).

Following these discussions, the WHO Secretariat requested a WHO Collaborating Centre in Germany to provide a draft revised version of the guidance on the biowaiver principles. The draft text was presented to the Committee at its fiftieth meeting.

The Committee discussed the revised guidance and provided its feedback. The document will be further revised and sent out as a working document for comment.

11.4 Update of biowaiver list based on the WHO Model List of Essential Medicines

Following the forty-eighth meeting of the Expert Committee the Secretariat contacted a WHO Collaborating Centre in Germany to discuss the additional studies needed for the update of the currently published biowaiver list in line with successive updates of the WHO EML. A list of all APIs for which additional studies are necessary in view of the various updates of the EML, was collated and prioritized. The WHO Collaborating Centre submitted the proposed tables to be attached as separate, living documents to the revised guidance on biowaivers (see 11.3). The importance of providing well documented, reliable references and study data for the BCS classifications assigned in the list was noted. New references on the outcomes of existing studies have been added. The Collaborating Centre is continuing to carry out further studies and the list will be updated accordingly. The tables were presented to the Committee with a view to obtaining further feedback before the lists are circulated for comment.

The Committee recommended that the list should be further reviewed in line with comments made at the meeting and should be made available for public consultation. The list will be presented to the Committee for consideration at its next meeting.

11.5 Update of international comparator products list for equivalence assessment of interchangeable multisource (generic) products

A comparator product is a pharmaceutical product with which the multisource product is intended to be interchangeable in clinical practice. In 1999 the Expert Committee adopted a document containing a list of international comparator pharmaceutical products for bioequivalence testing and included a decision-tree for use in identifying comparator pharmaceutical products.

In 2014 the Expert Committee endorsed the decision that the guidance on general principles for selecting comparator products should be separated from the lists of comparator products and endorsed the revised *Guidance on the selection of comparator pharmaceutical products for equivalence assessment of interchangeable multisource (generic) products* (WHO Technical Report Series No. 992, 2015, Annex 8). The Committee further supported the proposal to seek the assistance of members of the International Generic Drug Regulators Pilot (IGDRP) – a collaborative network of medicines regulatory authorities aiming at work-sharing in approval of generic products – in validating the entries in the international comparator products list. Members of the Expert Committee were also invited to review the current international comparator products list and to submit comments and amendments to the Secretariat.

Based on these discussions and inputs, the experts prepared an updated draft list of comparator products, together with explanatory notes on the updating process and selection criteria for the products listed. The main difference from the existing approach is that there can be more than one acceptable market from which to source a comparator product, because many products are marketed in countries other than their countries of manufacture. The list and explanatory notes were presented to the Committee for discussion and feedback on the proposed updating approach.

The Committee recommended that the table should be reviewed and updated further to ensure its consistency and applicability before it is circulated for comment to all interested parties, and subsequently posted as a working document on the WHO website. The Committee will discuss maintenance of the list at its next meeting.

11.6 Good regulatory practices

Good governance principles and legal frameworks for health product regulation are critically needed in Member States. Following the recommendation made in 2010 at the 14th ICDRA to collect examples of best regulatory practice, and based on feedback gained from national regulatory authorities during WHO assessments, a project was initiated to develop WHO guidelines on good regulatory practices (GRP). WHO has facilitated collaborative activities between regulatory authorities and has reviewed feedback gathered from national regulatory authorities over more than a decade to identify the authorities' main needs.

The scope of the proposed GRP guidelines is intended to include all health products and health technologies, and set out high-level principles from which a series of companion documents – similar to the Good review practices document adopted by the Committee in 2014 – could be developed according to need, timing and available resources. The concept of leveraging the work of other authorities or good cooperation practices will be an important aspect of this work. The draft guidance will go through the usual consultation process and it is planned to present it for review to both the ECBS and the Expert Committee on Specifications for Pharmaceutical Preparations in 2016.

The Committee discussed the proposal and noted the importance of having such a framework. The Committee expressed its support for the plans to develop this guidance.

12. Nomenclature, terminology and databases

Quality assurance terminology

The Secretariat maintains a collection of terms and definitions included in the guidance documents adopted by the Committee, with references to the respective guidelines. The Secretariat reported that this database is being kept up to date. An updated version is in the process of being verified and finalized for publication on the WHO website.

The Committee took note of the update.

International Nonproprietary Names (INN) for pharmaceutical substances

The International Nonproprietary Name (INN) Programme assigns unique names to pharmaceutical substances to enable global consistency and identification. A record number of 239 requests for assignment of an INN had been received from manufacturers in 2015. A total of 196 INNs were published in 2015, 94 of which were for biological substances. The total number of requests, as well as the proportion of requests received for INNs for biologicals, has been increasing.

A biological qualifier (BQ) scheme is proposed by the INN Programme to identify a substance manufactured by a specific process under a specific quality system. The BQ would be assigned as a second qualifier in addition to the INN. The scheme is intended to apply to all biological substances, including both innovators and biosimilars. Discussion is ongoing among a wide range of partners. The BQ proposal, together with a Q&A document providing the detailed technical information, was to be presented to the INN Expert Group at its 61st Consultation in October 2015 for discussion.

Cell therapies are another complex and growing product group for which there is currently no global naming system. Names have been assigned to cell therapies in some regulatory systems. The INN Expert Group is discussing a naming scheme applicable to cell therapies.

The Expert Committee noted the report.

Revision of guidance on representation of graphic formulae

Guidance on how to represent graphic formulae in *The International Pharmacopoeia* and within the INN list was developed and adopted by the Expert Committee at its thirty-fourth meeting (TRS 863, Annex 1, 1996). A discussion took place on whether an update of this guidance would be useful to bring it into line with current practices. Such updated guidance could promote convergence in this area.

The Committee supported the proposal and recommended that work should start promptly to update WHO guidance on representation of graphic formulae.

13. Summary and recommendations

The World Health Organization (WHO) Expert Committee on Specifications for Pharmaceutical Preparations advises the Director-General of WHO on pharmaceutical quality assurance. Based on a wide consultation process, it provides independent expert recommendations and guidance to ensure that medicines meet identical standards of quality, safety and efficacy in all WHO Member States. The Committee held its first meeting in 1947 under the name of the Expert Committee on Unification of Pharmacopoeias. Over time, it expanded the scope of its standard-setting work from quality-control-testing specifications to all arrangements that must be made in the development, production, regulation and supply of medicines to ensure that the medicines reaching the patients are of the quality required for their intended use.

At its fiftieth meeting from 12 to 16 October 2015, the Expert Committee heard updates from the WHO Expert Committee on Biological Standardization, the WHO Expert Committee on the Selection and Use of Essential Medicines and the International Nonproprietary Names (INN) Expert Group, all of which met in Geneva. With respect to international collaboration, updates were presented by the United Nations Children's Fund (UNICEF) about the supply and quality assurance of health products in line with WHO guidance, and by the Pharmacopoeial Discussion Group (PDG) about progress achieved with the harmonization of pharmacopoeial standards.

In the area of quality control the Expert Committee adopted the proposed workplan for elaboration of monographs and reviewed new and revised specifications and general texts for quality control testing of medicines for inclusion in *The International Pharmacopoeia*. The Committee was informed that the fifth edition of *The International Pharmacopoeia* was published on the WHO website in August 2015 as well as being made available as a CD. A total of 22 texts, as listed below, were adopted. The Committee also endorsed nine International Chemical Reference Substances (ICRS) established by the custodian centre, the European Directorate for the Quality of Medicines & HealthCare (EDQM). The Expert Committee further noted the progress report of the external quality assurance assessment scheme (EQAAS), which has successfully completed six phases of proficiency testing studies and will begin Phase 7 in 2016. An update was given on the international meetings of world pharmacopoeias, which are co-hosted in turn by one of the participating pharmacopoeias together with WHO. These meetings had been instrumental in developing the good pharmacopoeial practices document adopted by the Committee at its fiftieth meeting, subject to concurrence of the world pharmacopoeias. This text provides guidance on the appropriate design, development and maintenance of pharmacopoeial standards and will facilitate prospective harmonization of standards among pharmacopoeias globally.

In the various quality assurance-related areas, the Expert Committee adopted new guidance on good data and record management, on establishing national requirements for the regulation of post-approval changes to pharmaceutical products and on the conduct of surveys of the quality of medicines, as well as a guidance text developed in collaboration with the International Pharmaceutical Federation (FIP) on the provision of children-specific preparations that are not available as authorized products. The Expert Committee was briefed on WHO prequalification of medicines, which has continued to attract the interest of applicants, including additional manufacturers of APIs. Additional medicines have become eligible for prequalification, notably treatments for hepatitis B and C. A collaborative procedure for speedy registration of medicines that have been fully assessed and prequalified by WHO is currently offered by 26 regulatory authorities in collaboration with WHO, and a revision of this procedure to extend it to prequalified vaccines was discussed and adopted at the meeting. Prequalification of quality control laboratories is also ongoing and two quality monitoring surveys – one on HIV/AIDS medicines and one on antimalarials – are under way. The Committee also heard updates from the WHO regulatory support unit, which offers a modular assessment tool and capacity-building advice for regulatory systems, and from the WHO monitoring and surveillance project for reporting of medicines quality problems by Member States. Acknowledging the need for a model regulatory framework for medical devices the Committee discussed possibilities for WHO to oversee this work through its Expert Committee structure.

A list of decisions and recommendations made by the Expert Committee at its fiftieth meeting is given below.

The following guidelines were adopted and recommended for use:

- Good pharmacopoeial practices (Annex 1)
- FIP–WHO technical guidelines: Points to consider in the provision by health-care professionals of children-specific preparations that are not available as authorized products (Annex 2)
- Guidance on good manufacturing practices: inspection report, including Appendix 1: Model certificate of good manufacturing practices (revision) (Annex 4)
- Guidance on good data and record management practices (Annex 5)
- Good trade and distribution practices for pharmaceutical starting materials (revision) (Annex 6)
- WHO Certification scheme on the quality of pharmaceutical products moving in international commerce: questions and answers (Q&A) (revision)

- Guidelines on the conduct of surveys of the quality of medicines (Annex 7)
- Collaborative procedure between the World Health Organization (WHO) prequalification team and national regulatory authorities in the assessment and accelerated national registration of WHO-prequalified pharmaceutical products and vaccines (revision) (Annex 8)
- Guidance for organizations performing in vivo bioequivalence studies (revision) (Annex 9)
- WHO general guidance on variations to multisource pharmaceutical products (Annex 10)

The Committee also adopted the revised guidance on good manufacturing practices for biological products (Annex 3), following its adoption by the Expert Committee on Biological Standardization on 16 October 2015.

The following monographs were adopted for inclusion in *The International Pharmacopoeia*:

For maternal, newborn, child and adolescent health medicines

- estradiol cypionate
- levonorgestrel (revision), including the use of the reference substances Levonorgestrel for system suitability 1 CRS and Levonorgestrel for system suitability 2 CRS issued by the *European Pharmacopoeia*
- misoprostol
- misoprostol dispersion
- misoprostol tablets
- norethisterone (revision), including the use of the reference substance Norethisterone for system suitability issued by the *European Pharmacopoeia*
- norethisterone tablets, including the use of the reference substance Norethisterone for system suitability issued by the *European Pharmacopoeia*

For antimalarial medicines

- artemether injection (revision)

For antituberculosis medicines

- cycloserine (revision)
- cycloserine capsules (revision)

For medicines for chronic diseases and for mental health

- carbamazepine
- carbamazepine tablets
- carbamazepine chewable tablets
- carbamazepine oral suspension

For other anti-infective medicines

- clindamycin hydrochloride
- clindamycin hydrochloride capsules
- flucytosine
- flucytosine intravenous infusion

For other medicines

- dextromethorphan hydrobromide
- dextromethorphan oral solution

For the Supplementary section of *The International Pharmacopoeia*:

- levomethorphan limit tests for dextromethorphan-containing finished products

General policy

- Chapter on *Reference substances and reference spectra*

The Committee also agreed to proposals to discontinue the use of certain ICRS for the purpose of microbiological assays, to replace microbiological assays by physicochemical methods in certain monographs, to suppress a number of monographs that currently prescribe microbiological assays but pertain to medicines no longer included in the WHO Model List of Essential Medicines (19th edition) or in the relevant invitations for expression of interest from manufacturers.

International Chemical Reference Substances (ICRS)

The Committee endorsed the release of the following ICRS newly characterized by the custodian centre, the European Directorate for the Quality of Medicines & HealthCare (EDQM) and released by the ICRS Board:

- α-Artemether ICRS 1
- Efavirenz ICRS 2
- Efavirenz impurity B ICRS 1
- Ritonavir ICRS 2

- Abacavir sulfate ICRS 2
- Paracetamol ICRS 3
- Artemether ICRS 2
- Rifampicin ICRS 3
- Stavudine impurity F ICRS 1.

Recommendations

The Expert Committee made the recommendations listed below in the various quality assurance-related areas. Progress on the suggested actions will be reported to the Committee at its next meeting. The Committee recommended that the Secretariat, in collaboration with experts as appropriate, should carry out the following activities.

The International Pharmacopoeia

- Continue the development of monographs, general methods and texts and general supplementary information, including radiopharmaceutical monographs elaborated by the International Atomic Energy Agency (IAEA), in accordance with the workplan.
- Identify possible reference standards that can be referred to in five specific monographs which currently prescribe microbiological assays using ICRS, and for which no suitable alternative reference standard or physicochemical assay method has yet been identified.
- Proceed with the revision of the draft *Note for guidance on organic impurities in active pharmaceutical ingredients and finished pharmaceutical products*, intended to replace the text on *Related substances in finished pharmaceutical product monographs* in the Supplementary information section of *The International Pharmacopoeia*.

Quality control – national laboratories

- Continue with the development of guidelines on testing of "suspect" substandard/spurious/falsely-labelled/falsified/counterfeit medicines.

Quality assurance – good manufacturing practices

- Add a cross-reference to the *WHO good manufacturing practices for active pharmaceutical ingredients* to the *ICH Q7 Guideline: Good manufacturing practice guide for active pharmaceutical ingredients – questions and answers*.

- Proceed with revising the *Supplementary guidelines on good manufacturing practices: validation* including the appendices as relevant.
- Continue with the revision of the *Supplementary guidelines on good manufacturing practices for heating, ventilation and air-conditioning systems for non-sterile pharmaceutical dosage forms.*
- Pursue the revision of the draft working document on *Risk classification of inspection observations* in collaboration with the Brazilian Health Surveillance Agency (ANVISA), the European Medicines Agency (EMA), the Pharmaceutical Inspection Co-operation Scheme (PIC/S) and other organizations currently drafting guidance in this area.

Regulation and regulatory collaboration

- Continue revising the proposed *Prerequisites for waiver of in vivo bioequivalence requirements for the WHO Model List of Essential Medicines immediate-release, solid oral dosage forms*
- Further review the biowaiver list and make the draft updated list available for public consultation.
- Further review the proposed updated international comparator products list to ensure its consistency and applicability before circulating it for comment to all interested parties and subsequently posting it as a working document on the WHO website.
- Pursue the ongoing initiative to develop a high-level guidance document on good regulatory practices for health products and health technologies, for adoption through both the Expert Committee on Specifications for Pharmaceutical Preparations and the Expert Committee on Biological Standardization.
- Investigate possibilities to set up an expert group on regulation of medical devices, composed of suitably qualified experts appointed to existing Expert Advisory Panels.

Nomenclature, terminology and databases

- Continue to provide the database of terms and definitions covered by this Expert Committee on the WHO website.
- Proceed with the proposed update of guidance on graphic representation of chemical formulae used, for example, in *The International Pharmacopoeia.*

Acknowledgements

Special acknowledgement was made by the Committee to:
Mrs W. Bonny, Medicines Quality Assurance (MQA), Technologies Standards and Norms (TSN), Mr H. Chen, MQA, Ms M. Gaspard, MQA, Dr S. Kopp, Group Lead, MQA, Dr H. Schmidt, MQA; Dr D.J. Wood, Coordinator, TSN; Mr D. Mubangizi, Group Lead, Inspection Services, Prequalification Team (PQT), Ms J.K. Sawyer, Liaison Officer, PQT, Dr M.M. Stahl, Group Lead, Medicines Assessment, PQT, Mr I.R. Thrussell, Expert Inspector, PQT; Dr L. Rägo, Head, Regulation of Medicines and other Health Technologies; Mr C. de Joncheere, Director, Department of Essential Medicines and Health Products, WHO, Geneva, Switzerland; and Ms M. Zweygarth, Geneva, Switzerland, who were instrumental in the preparation and proceedings of the meeting.

Technical guidance included in this report has been produced with the financial assistance of the European Union, the Bill & Melinda Gates Foundation, the Reproductive, Maternal, Newborn and Child Health Fund and UNITAID.

The Committee also acknowledged with thanks the valuable contributions made to its work by the following agencies, institutions, organizations, pharmacopoeias, WHO Collaborating Centres, WHO Programmes, especially PQT, and persons:

Active Pharmaceutical Ingredients Committee, European Chemical Industry Council, Brussels, Belgium; Belgian Association of the Pharmacists of the Pharmaceutical Industry, Meerbeke, Belgium; Asia-Pacific Economic Cooperation, Singapore; Brazilian Health Surveillance Agency/ANVISA, Brasilia, DF, Brazil; Commonwealth Pharmacists Association, London, England; European Commission, Brussels, Belgium; European Directorate for the Quality of Medicines & HealthCare on behalf of the European Pharmacopoeia, Council of Europe, Strasbourg, France; European Federation of Pharmaceutical Industries and Associations, Brussels, Belgium; European Generic and Biosimilars Medicines Association, Brussels, Belgium; European Generic Medicines Association, Brussels, Belgium; European Medicines Agency, London, England; The Global Fund to Fight AIDS, Tuberculosis and Malaria, Vernier, Switzerland; International Atomic Energy Agency, Vienna, Austria; International Federation of Pharmaceutical Manufacturers and Associations, Geneva, Switzerland; International Generic Pharmaceutical Alliance, Brussels, Belgium; International Pharmaceutical Excipients Council – Americas, Arlington, VA, USA; International Pharmaceutical Excipients Council Europe, Brussels, Belgium; International Pharmaceutical Federation, The Hague, Netherlands; International Society for Pharmaceutical Engineering, Tampa, Florida, USA; International Society for Pharmaceutical Engineering, Thousand Oaks, CA, USA; Latin American Association of Pharmaceutical Industries (ALIFAR), Buenos Aires, Argentina; Medicines and Healthcare Products

Regulatory Agency, Inspection, Enforcement and Standards Division, London, England; Pan-American Network for Drug Regulatory Harmonization, Washington, DC, USA; Parenteral Drug Association, Bethesda, Maryland, USA; Pharmaceutical Inspection Co-operation Scheme, Geneva, Switzerland; The Stop TB Partnership, Geneva, Switzerland; Swissmedic, Swiss Agency for Therapeutic Products, Berne, Switzerland; Therapeutic Goods Administration, Woden, ACT, Australia; United Nations Children's Fund, Supply Division, Copenhagen, Denmark; United Nations Children's Fund, New York, USA; United Nations Development Programme, New York, USA; United Nations Industrial Development Organization, Vienna, Austria; The World Bank, Washington, DC, USA; World Intellectual Property Organization, Geneva, Switzerland; World Self-Medication Industry, Ferney-Voltaire, France; World Trade Organization, Geneva, Switzerland.

Laboratoire National de Contrôle des Produits Pharmaceutiques, Chéraga, Alger, Algeria; Instituto Nacional de Medicamentos, Buenos Aires, Argentina; Expert Analytic Laboratory, Centre of Drug and Medical Technology Expertise, Yerevan, Armenia; Laboratoire national de contrôle de qualité des médicaments et consommables médicaux, Cotonou, Benin; Agency for Medicinal Products and Medical Devices, Control Laboratory, Sarajevo, Bosnia and Herzegovina; Instituto Nacional de Controle de Qualidade em Saúde, Rio de Janeiro, Brazil; Laboratoire National de Santé Publique, Ouagadougou, Burkina Faso; National Product Quality Control Centre, Ministry of Health, Phnom Penh, Cambodia; Laboratoire National de Contrôle de Qualité des Médicaments et d'Expertise, Yaoundé, Cameroon; Departamento de Control Nacional, Unidad de Control de Calidad de Medicamentos comercializados, Institutu de Salud Pública, Santiago de Chile, Chile; National Institutes for Food and Drug Control, Beijing, People's Republic of China; Medicamentos y Productos Biológicos del INVIMA, Bogotá, Colombia; Laboratorio de Análisis y Asesoría Farmacéutica, Facultad de Farmacia, Universidad de Costa Rica, San José, Costa Rica; Laboratorio de Normas y Calidad de Medicamentos, Caja Costarricense de Seguro Social, Universidad de Costa Rica, Alajuela, Costa Rica; Laboratoire National de la Santé Publique, Abidjan, Côte d'Ivoire; Oficina Sanitaria Panamericana, OPS/OMS, Havana, Cuba; National Organization for Drug Control and Research, Cairo, Egypt; Drug Quality Control and Toxicology Laboratory, Drug Administration and Control Authority, Addis Ababa, Ethiopia; Centrale Humanitaire Médico-Pharmaceutique, Clermont-Ferrand, France; Food and Drugs Board, Quality Control Laboratory, Accra, Ghana; Laboratoire national de contrôle de qualité des medicaments, Conakry, Guinea; Laboratory for Quality Evaluation and Control, National Institute of Pharmacy, Budapest, Hungary; Central Drugs Laboratory, Kolkata, India; Provincial Drug and Food Quality Control Laboratory, Yogyakarta, Indonesia; Food and Drugs Control Laboratories, Ministry of Health and Medical Education, Tehran, Islamic Republic of Iran; Caribbean Regional

Drug Testing Laboratory, Kingston, Jamaica; Mission for Essential Drugs and Supplies, Nairobi, Kenya; National Quality Control Laboratory for Drugs and Medical Devices, Nairobi, Kenya; Food and Drug Quality Control Center, Ministry of Health, Vientiane, Lao People's Democratic Republic; Laboratoire de Contrôle de Qualité des Médicaments, Agence du Médicament de Madagascar, Antananarivo, Madagascar; Centre for Quality Control, National Pharmaceutical Control Bureau, Petaling Jaya, Selangor, Malaysia; Laboratoire National de la Santé du Mali, Bamako, Mali; Laboratoire National de Contrôle des Médicaments, Rabat, Morocco; Quality Surveillance Laboratory, Windhoek, Namibia; National Medicines Laboratory, Department of Drug Administration, Kathmandu, Nepal; Laboratoire National de Santé Publique et d'Expertise, Niamey, Niger; Central Quality Control Laboratory, Directorate General of Pharmaceutical Affairs and Drug Control, Ministry of Health, Muscat, Oman; Drug Control and Traditional Medicine Division, National Institute of Health, Islamabad, Pakistan; Instituto Especializado de Análisis, Universidad de Panamá, Panama; Centro Nacional de Control de Calidad, Instituto Nacional de Salud, Lima, Peru; Bureau of Food and Drugs, Department of Health, Muntinlupa City, Philippines; Laboratory for Quality Control of Medicines, Medicines Agency, Ministry of Health, Chisinau, Republic of Moldova; National Drug and Cosmetic Control Laboratories, Drug Sector, Saudi Food and Drug Authority, Riyadh, Saudi Arabia; Laboratoire National de Contrôle des Médicaments, Dakar Etoile, Senegal; Pharmaceutical Division, Applied Sciences Group, Health Sciences Authority, Singapore; Centre for Quality Assurance of Medicines, Faculty of Pharmacy, North-West University, Potchefstroom, South Africa; Research Institute for Industrial Pharmacy, North-West University, Potchefstroom, South Africa; National Drug Quality Assurance Laboratory, Ministry of Health, Colombo, Sri Lanka; National Drug Quality Control Laboratory, Directorate General of Pharmacy, Federal Ministry of Health, Khartoum, Sudan; Pharmaceutical Analysis Laboratory, R&D, The School of Pharmacy, Muhimbili University of Health and Allied Sciences, Dar-es-Salaam, United Republic of Tanzania; Tanzania Food and Drug Authority, Dar-es-Salaam, United Republic of Tanzania; Bureau of Drug and Narcotic, Department of Medical Sciences, Ministry of Public Health, Nonthaburi, Thailand; Laboratoire National de Contrôle des Médicaments, Tunis, Tunisia; National Drug Quality Control Laboratory, National Drug Authority, Kampala, Uganda; Central Laboratory for Quality Control of Medicines of the Ministry of Health of Ukraine, Kiev, Ukraine; Laboratory of Pharmaceutical Analysis, State Pharmacological Centre, Ministry of Health of Ukraine, Kiev, Ukraine; Laboratorio Control de Productos MSP, Comisión Para El Control de Calidad de Medicamentos, Montevideo, Uruguay; Instituto Nacional de Higiene "Rafael Rangel", Caracas, Venezuela; National Institute of Drug Quality Control, Hanoi, Viet Nam; Medicines Control Authority, Control Laboratory of Zimbabwe, Harare, Zimbabwe.

Farmacopea Argentina, Buenos Aires, Argentina; Farmacopeia Brasileira, Brasilia, DF, Brazil; British Pharmacopoeia Commission, Medicines and Healthcare Products Regulatory Agency, London, England; *Farmacopea Chilena, Valparaíso, Chile*; Pharmacopoeia of the People's Republic of China, Beijing, People's Republic of China; Croatian Pharmacopoeia, Zagreb, Croatia; Czech Pharmacopoeia, Prague, Czech Republic; Danish Pharmacopoeia Commission, Copenhagen, Denmark; European Pharmacopoeia, European Directorate for the Quality of Medicines & HealthCare, Council of Europe, Strasbourg, France; Finnish Medicines Agency, Helsinki, Finland; Pharmacopée française, Agence nationale de sécurité sanitaire des produits de santé, Saint-Denis, France; German Pharmacopoeia Commission, Bonn, Germany; Indian Pharmacopoeia Commission, Raj Nagar, Ghaziabad, India; Indonesian Pharmacopoeia Commission, Jakarta, Indonesia; Iranian Pharmacopoeia, Iranian Association of Pharmaceutical Scientists, Tehran, Islamic Republic of Iran; Committee of the Japanese Pharmacopoeia, Tokyo, Japan; Kazakhstan Pharmacopoeia, Pharmacopoeia Centre of the Republic of Kazakhastan, Almaty, Kazakhstan; Pharmacopoeia of the Republic of Korea, Cheongwon-gun, Chungcheongbuk-do, Republic of Korea; Lithunian Pharmacopoeia Commission, Vilnius, Lithuania; Mexican Pharmacopoeia, México DF, Mexico; Philippines Pharmacopoeia, Manila, Philippines; Polish Pharmacopoeia Commission, Warsaw, Poland, Portuguese Pharmacopoeia, Lisbon, Portugal; State Pharmacopoeia of the Russian Federation, Moscow, Russian Federation; Serbian Pharmacopoeia, Belgrade, Serbia; Slovakian Pharmacopoeia Commission, Bratislava, Slovakia; Spanish Pharmacopoeia, Royal, Madrid, Spain; Swedish Pharmacopoeia, Uppsala, Sweden; Swiss Pharmacopoeia, Berne, Switzerland; Thai Pharmacopoeia, Nonthaburi, Thailand; Pharmacopoeia of Ukraine, Ukrainian Scientific Pharmacopoeial Center for Quality of Medicines, Kharkov, Ukraine; United States Pharmacopeia, Rockville, MD, USA; Vietnamese Pharmacopoeia, Hanoi, Viet Nam.

WHO Centre Collaborateur pour la Conformité des Médicaments, Laboratoire national de Contrôle des Produits Pharmaceutiques, Alger, Algeria; WHO Collaborating Centre for Drug Quality Assurance, Therapeutic Goods Administration Laboratories, Woden, ACT, Australia; WHO Collaborating Centre for Drug Quality Assurance, National Institute for the Control of Pharmaceutical and Biological Products, Beijing, People's Republic of China; WHO Collaborating Centre for Research on Bioequivalence Testing of Medicines, Frankfurt am Main, Germany; WHO Collaborating Centre for Drug Information and Quality Assurance, National Institute of Pharmacy, Budapest, Hungary; WHO Collaborating Centre for Quality Assurance of Essential Drugs, Central Drugs Laboratory, Calcutta, India; WHO Collaborating Centre for Regulatory Control of Pharmaceuticals, National Pharmaceutical Control Bureau, Jalan University, Ministry of Health, Petaling Jaya, Malaysia; WHO Collaborating

Centre for Drug Quality Assurance, Pharmaceutical Laboratory, Centre for Analytical Science, Health Sciences Authority, Singapore; WHO Collaborating Centre for Quality Assurance of Drugs, North-West University, Potchefstroom, South Africa; WHO Collaborating Centre for Quality Assurance of Essential Drugs, Bureau of Drug and Narcotic, Department of Medical Sciences, Ministry of Public Health, Nonthaburi, Thailand.

Health Systems and Innovation Cluster, WHO, Geneva, Switzerland; Department of Essential Medicines and Health Products, WHO, Geneva, Switzerland; Regulation of Medicines and other Health Technologies, WHO, Geneva, Switzerland; Prequalification Team, WHO, Geneva, Switzerland; International Nonproprietary Names, WHO, Geneva, Switzerland; Policy Access and Use, WHO, Geneva, Switzerland; Regulatory Systems Strengthening, WHO, Geneva, Switzerland; Safety and Vigilance Team, WHO, Geneva, Switzerland; Technologies Standards and Norms, WHO, Geneva, Switzerland; Traditional and Complementary Medicine, WHO, Geneva, Switzerland; Office of the Legal Counsel, WHO, Geneva, Switzerland; Control of Neglected Tropical Diseases, WHO, Geneva, Switzerland; Global Malaria Programme, WHO, Geneva, Switzerland; Global TB Programme, WHO, Geneva, Switzerland; HIV/AIDS Programme, WHO, Geneva, Switzerland; Prevention of Noncommunicable Diseases, WHO, Geneva, Switzerland; WHO Regional Office for Africa, Brazzaville, Congo; WHO Regional Office for the Americas/Pan American Health Organization, Washington, DC, USA; WHO Regional Office for the Eastern Mediterranean, Cairo, Egypt; WHO Regional Office for Europe, Copenhagen, Denmark; WHO Regional Office for South-East Asia, New Delhi, India; WHO Regional Office for the Western Pacific, Manila, Philippines.

Abbott, Allschwil, Switzerland; Abbott Laboratories, Abbott Quality & Regulatory, Dept. 03QY, Abbott Park, IL, USA; Dr F. Abiodun, Benin City, Nigeria; Professor E. Adams, Laboratorium voor Farmaceutische Chemie en Analyse van Geneesmiddelen, Leuven, Belgium; Dr M. Adarkwah-Yiadom, Standard Officer, Ghana Standards Board, Drugs, Cosmetics and Forensic Laboratory Testing Division, Accra, Ghana; Professor I. Addae-Mensah, Department of Chemistry, University of Ghana, Legon, Ghana; Divisiốn de Química y Tecnología Farmacéutica, AEMPS. Madrid, Spain; Dr K. Agravat, Regulatory Affairs, Unimark Remedies Limited, Ahmedabad, India; Ms R. Ahmad, Centre for Product Registration, National Pharmaceutical Control Bureau, Ministry of Health, Petaling Jaya, Malaysia; Ajanta Pharma Ltd, Kandivli (West), Mumbai, India; Apotex Inc., Toronto, Ontario, Canada; Amgen Inc., Thousand Oaks, CA, USA; Amgen Inc., Engineering, West Greenwich, RI, USA; Dr P. Aprea, Director, Directorate of Evaluation and Control of Biologicals and Radiopharmaceuticals, National Administration of Medicines, Food and Medical Technology, Buenos Aires, Argentina; Dr N. Aquino, Inspector and Specialist in GMP and Risk Management, Brazilian Health Surveillance Agency, Brasilia, DF,

Brazil; Dr A.C. Moreira Marino Araujo, Health Expert, Drugs Office, Post Approval Changes of Synthetic Drugs, Brazilian Health Surveillance Agency, Brasilia, DF, Brazil; Dr H. Arentsen, Regulatory Intelligence and Policy Specialist, Regulatory Development Strategy, H. Lundbeck A/S, Copenhagen-Valby, Denmark; Astellas Pharma Europe BV, Leiderdorp, Netherlands; AstraZeneca Pharmaceuticals (China) Co., Ltd, Taizhou City, Jiangsu Province, China; AstraZeneca, Alderley Park, Cheshire, England; Dr C. Athlan, Quality Reviewer, Swissmedic, Swiss Agency for Therapeutic Products, Berne, Switzerland; Dr A. Ba, Directeur, Qualité et Développement, Centrale Humanitaire Medico-Pharmaceutique, Clermont-Ferrand, France; Dr H. Baião, Infarmed, Portugal; Dr P. Baker, United States of America Food and Drug Administration, China Office, USA; Dr J.R. Ballinger, Guy's and St Thomas Hospital, London, England; Dr E. Bamanyekanye, Départment de la Pharmacie, du Médicament et des Laboratoires (DPML), Burundi; Mr N. Banerjee, Cipla Limited, Goa, India; Dr H. Batista, US Food and Drug Administration, Silver Spring, MD, USA; Mr B. Baudrand, OTECI, Paris, France; Dr R. Bauer, Head of Institute, Institute Surveillance, Austrian Federal Office for Safety in Health Care, Austrian Agency for Health and Food Safety, Vienna, Austria; Dr O.P. Baula, Deputy Director, State Pharmacological Center, Ministry of Health, Kiev, Ukraine; Professor S.A. Bawazir, Advisor to the Executive President, Saudi Food and Drug Authority, Riyadh, Saudi Arabia; Bayer Health Care Pharmaceuticals, Bayer Pharma AG, Berlin, Germany; Dr M.G. Beatrice, Vice President, Corporate Regulatory and Quality Science, Abbott, Abbott Park, IL, USA; Dr T.L. Bedane, Drug Administration and Control, Addis Ababa, Ethiopia; Ms T.J. Bell, WHO Focal Point, US Food and Drug Administration, Silver Spring, MD, USA; Dr M. Silvana Bellini, EDQM Laboratory, Strasbourg, France; Dr I.B.G. Bernstein, Director, Pharmacy Affairs, Office of the Commissioner/Office of Policy, US Food and Drug Administration, Silver Spring, MD, USA; Mr L. Besançon, General Secretary and CEO, International Pharmaceutical Federation, The Hague, Netherlands; Dr R.P. Best, President and CEO, International Society for Pharmaceutical Engineering, Tampa, FL, USA; Dr A. Bevilacqua, US Pharmacopeia, Bedford, MA, USA; Dr J. Bishop III, Review Management Staff, Office of the Director, Center for Biologics Evaluation and Research, United States Food and Drug Administration,, Silver Spring, MD, USA; Dr L. Bonthuys, Pretoria, South Africa; Mr M.H. Boon, Deputy Director, Overseas Audit Unit – Audit Branch, Audit & Licensing Division, Health Products Regulation Group, Singapore; Dr G. Born, Institute of Pharmaceutical Technology, Johann Wolfgang Goethe-University, Frankfurt, Germany; Professor R. Boudet-Dalbin, Paris, France; Dr B. Blum, Sandoz, France; Dr G. Bourdeau, Méréville, France; Dr S.K. Branch, Acting Group Manager, Special Populations Group, Medicines and Healthcare Products Regulatory Agency, London, England; Dr E. Brendel, Bayer HealthCare AG, Elberfeld, Germany; Dr M. Brits, Director, WHO Collaborating

Centre for the Quality Assurance of Medicines, North-West University, Potchefstroom Campus, Potchefstroom, South Africa; Mr C. Brown, Inspections Enforcement and Standards Division, Medicines and Healthcare Products Regulatory Agency, London, England; Dr W. Bukachi, Project Coordinator, International Affairs, US Pharmacopeia, Rockville, MD, USA; Ms A. Bukirwa, National (Food and) Drug Authority, Kampala, Uganda; Bureau of Drug and Narcotic, Department of Medical Sciences, Ministry of Public Health, Nonthaburi, Thailand; Dr F. Burnett, Managing Director, Pharmaceutical Procurement Service, Organization of Eastern Caribbean States, Casties, St Lucia; Dr W. Cabri, Research and Development, Director, Chemistry and Analytical Development, Sigma-tau Industrie Farmaceutiche Riunite SpA, Pomezia, Italy; Dr M.Cahilly, Warren, Vermont, USA; Dr. D. Calam, Wiltshire, England; Dr N. Cappuccino, Lambertville, NJ, USA; Dr L. Cargill, Director, Caribbean Regional Drug Testing Laboratory, Kingston, Jamaica; Professor (Madame) R. Jiménez-Castellanos, Department of Pharmaceutics and Pharmaceutical Technology, Faculty of Pharmacy, Seville, Spain; Dr A. Castro, Regulatory Affairs Director and Senior Pharmacist, Roche Servicios SA, Heredia, Costa Rica; Dr D. Catsoulacos, Scientific Administrator, Manufacturing and Quality Compliance, Compliance and Inspection, European Medicines Agency, London, England; European Medicines Agency, London, England; Mr J.-M. Caudron, Braine-le-Château, Belgium; Mr P. Cenizo, Southern African Pharmaceutical Regulatory Affairs Association (SAPRAA), Randburg, South Africa; Dr A.N.K. Chali, Chemical and Pharmaceutical Assessor, Uppsala, Sweden; Dr B. Chapart, Pharma Review Manager, Global Analytical Development, Sanofi-Aventis Pharma, Anthony, France; Ms Cheah Nuan Ping, Director, Cosmetics & Cigarette Testing Laboratory, Pharmaceutical Division, Applied Sciences Group, Health Sciences Authority, Singapore; Dr X. Chen, Director, Division of Drug Distribution Supervision, State Food and Drug Administration, Beijing, People's Republic of China; Professor Y. Cherrah, Faculté de Médecine et Pharmacie, Rabat, Morocco; Dr B.K. Choi, Director, Pharmaceutical Standardization, Osong Health Technology Administration Complex, Research and Testing Division of the Ministry of Food and Drug Safety, Cheongwon-gun, Chungbuk, Republic of Korea; Dr Y.H. Choi, Scientific Officer, Korea Food & Drug Administration, Cheongwon-gun, Chungbuk, Republic of Korea; Dr D. Churchward, Expert GMPD Inspector, Inspection Enforcement and Standards, Medicines & Healthcare products Regulatory Agency, London, England; Cipla Limited, Mumbai, India; Ms I. Clamou, Assistant Manager, Scientific,Technical and Regulatory Affairs, European Federation of Pharmaceutical Industries and Associations, Brussels, Belgium; Dr M. Cooke, Senior Manager, Global Quality, Operations, AstraZeneca, Macclesfield, Cheshire, England; Dr C. Craft, Member, United States Pharmacopeia International Health Expert Committee, Rockville, MD, USA; Ms J. Crawford, Inpatients Pharmacy, Waitakere Hospital, Auckland,

New Zealand; Ms T. Crescenzi, United States of America Food and Drug Administration, Silver Spring, MD, USA; Critical Paths to TB Regimens (CPTR), Global Regulatory Pathways Work Group, Tucson, AZ, USA; Dr R.L. Dana, Senior Vice President, Regulatory Affairs and Parenteral Drug Association Training and Research Institute, Parenteral Drug Association, Bethesda, MD, USA; Mr M.M. Das, Barisha, Kolkata, India; Dr V. Davoust, Quality & Regulatory Policy, Pharmaceutical Sciences, Pfizer Global Research & Development, Paris, France; Dr D. de Kaste, National Institute for Public Health and the Environment, Bilthoven, Netherlands; Professor T. Dekker, Research Institute for Industrial Pharmacy, North-West University, Potchefstroom, South Africa; Dr M. Derecque-Pois, Director General, European Association of Pharmaceutical Full-line Wholesalers, Brussels, Belgium; Directorate General of Pharmaceutical Affairs and Drug Control, Ministry of Health, Muscat, Oman; Dr R. Diyana, Senior Bioavailability/Bioequivalence Evaluator, National Authority for Food and Drug Control, Indonesia; DMB (French association of data management professionals), Suresnes, France; Professor E. Doelker, University of Geneva, Geneva, Switzerland; Professor J.B. Dressman, Director, Institut für Pharmazeutische Technologie, Biozentrum, Johann Wolfgang Goethe-Universität, Frankfurt am Main, Germany; Mrs S. Dube-Mwedzi, Consultant Regulatory Officer, Medicines Control Authority of Zimbabwe, Harare, Zimbabwe; Dr A.T. Ducca, Senior Director, Regulatory Affairs, Healthcare Distribution Management Association, Arlington, VA, USA; Dr T.D. Duffy, Lowden International, Tunstall, Richmond, N. Yorks, England; Dr P. Ellis, Director, External Advocacy, Quality Centre of Excellence, GlaxoSmithKline, Brentford, Middlesex, England; European Compliance Academy Foundation, Heidelberg, Germany; European Medicines Agency, London, England; Fedefarma, Ciudad, Guatemala; F. Hoffman-La Roche Ltd, Basel, Switzerland; Dr A. Falodun, Department of Pharmaceutical Chemistry, Faculty of Pharmacy, University of Benin, Benin City, Nigeria; Federal Ministry of Health, Berlin, Germany; Dr R. Fendt, Head, Global Regulatory & GMP Compliance Pharma, Care Chemicals Division, BASF, Limburgerhof, Germany; Mr A. Ferreira do Nascimento, Agência Nacional de Vigilância, Brasília, Brazil; Mr M. FitzGerald, European Association of Pharmaceutical Full-line Wholesalers, Brussels, Belgium; Dr A. Flueckiger, Head, Corporate Health Protection, Corporate Safety, Health & Environmental Protection, F. Hoffmann-La Roche, Basel, Switzerland; Dr G.L. France, Head, Q&A Compliance, EU Region, Novartis Consumer Health Services SA, Nyon, Switzerland; Dr B. Fritschel, Johnson & Johnson, New Brunswick, NJ, USA; Dr A. Fuglsang, Haderslev, Denmark; Mr T. Fujino, Director, International Affairs, Japan Generic Medicines Association, Tokyo, Japan; Mr A. García Arieta, Head, Service on Pharmacokinetics and Generic Medicines, Division of Pharmacology and Clinical Evaluation, Department of Human Use Medicines, Spanish Agency of Medicines and Medical Devices, Madrid, Spain; Miss Y. Gao, Project Manager, Chinese Pharmacopoeia

Commission, Beijing, People's Republic of China; Dr M. Garvin, Senior Director, Scientific and Regulatory Affairs, Pharmaceutical Research and Manufacturers of America, Washington, DC, USA; Dr A. Gayot, Faculté de Pharmacie de Lille, Lille, France; Dr X. Ge, Senior Analytical Scientist, Pharmaceutical Laboratory, Pharmaceutical Division, Applied Sciences Group, Health Sciences Authority, Singapore; German Expert Group on Computerized, Darmstadt, Germany; Dr L. Gibril, Compliance Coordinator, Novartis Pharma SAE, Amiria, Cairo, Egypt; Gilead Sciences International Ltd, Abington, Cambridge, England; Dr F. Giorgi, Research and Development, Analytical Development Manager, Sigma-tau Industrie Farmaceutiche Riunite SpA, Pomezia, Italy; Dr L. Girard, Head, Global Pharmacopoeial Affairs, Novartis Group Quality, Quality Systems and Standards, Basel, Switzerland; GlaxoSmithKline, Brentford, Middlesex, England; GlaxoSmithKline Biologicals SA, Wavre, Belgium; GlaxoSmithKline, Sales Training Centre, Research Triangle Park, NC, USA; Dr C. Sánchez González, Coordinator of Policies and Regulatory Affairs Centro para el Control de Medicamentos, Equipos y Dispositivos Médicos, La Habana, Cuba; Dr J. Gordon, Nova Scotia, Canada; Dr T. Gould, Brighton East, Victoria, Australia; Ms J. Gouws, Department of Health, Medicines Control Council, Pretoria, South Africa; Dr M. Goverde, QC Expert Microbiology, Novartis Pharma AG, Basel, Switzerland; Ms R.Govithavatangaphong, Director, Bureau of Drug and Narcotics, Department of Medical Sciences, Ministry of Public Health, Nonthaburi, Thailand; Dr L. Graham, Medicines & Healthcare products Regulatory Agency, London, England; Dr J. Grande, Manager, Regulatory Affairs, McNeil Consumer Healthcare, Markham, England; Dr A. Gray, Senior Lecturer, Department of Therapeutics and Medicines Management and Consultant Pharmacist, Centre for the AIDS Programme of Research in South Africa (CAPRISA), Nelson R Mandela School of Medicine, University of KwaZulu-Natal, Congella, South Africa; Dr M. Guazzaroni Jacobs, Director, Quality and Regulatory Policy, Pfizer Inc., New York, NY, USA; Ms N.M. Guerrero Rivas, Radiofarmacia de Centroamérica, SA, Ciudad del Saber, Panamá, Panama; Guilin Pharmaceutical Company Ltd, Guilin, People's Republic of China; Dr R. Guinet, Agence nationale de sécurité du médicament et des produits de santé, Saint-Denis, France; Dr S. Gupta, Mankind Pharma Limited, Unit-II, Vill. Kishanpura, Paonta Sahib, Disst. Sirmour, India; Professor R. Guy, Professor of Pharmaceutical Sciences, Department of Pharmacy & Pharmacology, University of Bath, Bath, England; Mr L. Gwaza, Medicines Regulation, Evaluations & Registration Division, Medicines Control Authority of Zimbabwe, Harare, Zimbabwe; Dr N. Habib, Director General of Medical Supplies, Ministry of Health, Oman; Dr S. Haidar, Acting Director, Division of Generic Drug Bioequivalence Evaluation, Office of Study Integrity and Surveillance, Center for Drug Evaluation and Research, Food and Drug Administration, Silver Spring, MD, USA; Mr B.J. Hamid, Jakarta, Indonesia; Dr N. Hamilton, Industrial Quality and Compliance,

Industrial Affairs, Sanofi Aventis, West Malling, Kent, England; Ms J. Hantzinikolas, Therapeutic Goods Administration, Department of Health, Woden, ACT, Australia; Dr S. Harada, International Affairs Division, Minister's Secretariat, Ministry of Health, Labour and Welfare, Tokyo, Japan; Dr B. Hasselbalch, Acting Associate Director, Policy and Communications, and Director, Division of Policy, Collaboration & Data Operations, Office of Compliance, Center for Drug Evaluation and Research, United States Food and Drug Administration, Silver Spring, MD, USA; Dr A. Hawwa, Lecturer in Pharmacy (Medicines in Children), Medical Biology Centre, Queen's University Belfast, Belfast, Northern Ireland; Dr M. Hayes-Bachmeyer, Technical Regulatory Affairs, Pharmaceuticals Division, F. Hoffmann-la Roche, Basel, Switzerland; Mr Y. Hebron, Manager, Medicines and Cosmetics Analysis Department, Tanzania Food and Drugs Authority, Dar-es-Salaam, United Republic of Tanzania; Dr G.W. Heddell, Director, Inspection Enforcement & Standards Division, Medicines and Healthcare Products Regulatory Agency, London, England; Dr D. Hege-Voelksen, Swissmedic, Swiss Agency for Therapeutic Products, Berne, Switzerland; Ms J. Hiep, QA Pharmacist and Auditor, Adcock Ingram, Bryanston, South Africa; Ms M. Hirschhorn, Head, Quality and Chemistry Sector, Comisión para el Control de Calidad de Medicamentos (Drug and Control Commission), Montevideo, Uruguay; Mrs Hong J., Senior Pharmacist and Director of Hubei Provincial Institutes for Food and Drug Control, Wuhan Hubei, China; Mrs Hong L., Senior Pharmacist and Director of Zhejiang Provincial Institutes for Food and Drug Control, Hangzhou, China; Professor J. Hoogmartens, Leuven, Belgium; Dr K. Horn, Managing Director, Institute for Pharmaceutical and Applied Analytics, Official Medicines Control Laboratory, Bremen, Germany; F. Hoffmann-La Roche Ltd, Basel, Switzerland; Dr K. Hoppu, Director, Poison Information Centre, Helsinki University Central Hospital, Helsinki, Finland; Dr H. Hoseh, Head of Registration Unit, Drug Directorate, Jordan Food and Drug Administration, Jordan; Dr X. Hou, Chemical & Materials, Singapore; Dr N. Ibrahim, National Pharmaceutical Control Bureau, Ministry of Health, Jalan University, Petaling Jaya, Indonesia; Indian Drug Manufacturers' Association, Mumbai, India; Infarmed, Lisbon, Portugal; Ipsen Pharma, Dreux, France; Dr J. Isasi Rocas, Pharmaceutical Chemist, Lima, Peru; Professor R. Jachowicz, Head, Department of Pharmaceutical Technology and Biopharmaceutics, Jagiellonian University Medical College, Faculty of Pharmacy, Kraków, Poland; Mr I. Jackson, Operations Manager, GMDP Inspections, Inspection, Enforcement & Standards Division, Medicines and Healthcare Products Regulatory Agency, London, England; Dr S.A. Jaffar, Director General, Directorate General of Pharmaceutical Affairs and Drug Control, Ministry of Health, Muscat, Oman; Johnson & Johnson, Latina, Italy; Dr R. Jähnke, Global Pharma Health Fund e.V., Frankfurt, Germany; Dr M. James, GlaxoSmithKline, Brentford, Middlesex, England; Dr A. Janssen, Manager, Regulatory Affairs,

DMV Fonterra Excipients, FrieslandCampina Ingredients Innovation, Goch, Germany; Professor S. Jin, Chief Expert for Pharmaceutical Products, National Institutes for Food and Drug Control, Beijing, People's Republic of China; Dr P. Jones, Director, Analytical Control, Pharmaceutical Sciences, Pfizer Global R&D, Sandwich, England; Dr H. de Jong, International Pharmaceutical Federation, The Hague, Netherlands; Dr Y. Juillet, Consultant, Paris, France; Mr D. Jünemann, Teaching Assistant; Institut für Pharmazeutische Technologie, Biozentrum, Johann Wolfgang Goethe-Universität, Frankfurt am Main, Germany; Ms A. Junttonen, Senior Pharmaceutical Inspector, National Agency for Medicines, Helsinki, Finland; Dr S. Kafkala, Analytical Development Director, Genepharm S.A., Pallini, Greece; Dr V. Kamde, Quality Management, Oman Pharmaceuticals, Oman; Dr M. Kaplan, Director, Institute for Standardization and Control of Pharmaceuticals, Jerusalem, Israel; Dr M. Karga-Hinds, Director, Barbados Drug Service, Christchurch, Barbados; Dr A.M. Kaukonen, National Agency for Medicines, Helsinki, Finland; Ms H. Kavale, Cipla, Mumbai, India; Dr T. Kawanishi, Director General, National Institute of Health Sciences, Tokyo, Japan; Dr S. Keitel, Director, European Directorate for the Quality of Medicines and Healthcare, Strasbourg, France; Dr K. Keller, Director and Professor, Federal Ministry of Health, Bonn, Germany; Dr M. Keller, Inspector, Division of Certificates and Licencing, Swissmedic, Swiss Agency for Therapeutic Products, Berne, Switzerland; Dr L. Kerr, Scientific Operations Adviser, Office of Laboratories and Scientific Services, Therapeutic Goods Administration, Woden, ACT, Australia; Mr M. Khan, United States of America Food and Drug Administration, Silver Spring, MD, USA; Dr M. Khan, Director, Federal Research Center Life Sciences, US Food and Drug Administration, Silver Spring, MD, USA; Dr S. Khoja, Vapi, Gujarat, India; Professor K. Kimura, Drug Management and Policy, Institute of Medical, Pharmaceutical and Health Sciences, Kanazawa University, Kanazawa-city, Japan; Dr W. Kongsuk, Bureau of Drug and Narcotic, Department of Medical Sciences, Nonthaburi, Thailand; Dr H. Köszegi-Szalai, Head, Department for Quality Assessment and Control, National Institute of Pharmacy, Budapest, Hungary; Dr S. Kouakap, Ministère de la Santé, Cameroon; Dr A. Kovacs, Secretariat, Pharmaceutical Inspection Co-operation Scheme, Geneva, Switzerland; Ms S. Kox, Senior Director Scientific Affairs, European Generic Medicines Association, Brussels, Belgium; Dr P. Kozarewicz, Scientific Administrator, Quality of Medicines Sector, Human Unit Pre-Authorization, European Medicines Agency, London, England; Dr A. Krauss, Principal Chemist, Office of Laboratories and Scientific Services, Therapeutic Goods Administration, Woden, ACT, Australia; Professor H.G. Kristensen, Vedbaek, Denmark; Dr J. Kumar, HLL Lifecare Ltd., Kanagala, Belgaum, India; Mr A. Kupferman, Bangkok, Thailand; Dr S. Kumar, Assistant Drugs Controller, Central Drugs Standard Control Organization, Food and Drug Administration Bhawan, New Delhi, India; Professor S. Läer, Institut für Klinische Pharmazie und Pharmakotherapie,

Heinrich-Heine-Universität, Düsseldorf, Germany; Dr O. Le Blaye, Inspector, Trials and Vigilance Inspection Department, Agence nationale de sécurité du médicament et des produits de santé, Saint-Denis, France; Dr L. Lee, Compendial Compliance Lead, Amgen Inc., Newbury Park, California, USA; LFB Biomédicaments, Lille Cedex, France; Dr B. Li, Deputy Director General, National Institutes for Food and Drug Control, Ministry of Public Health, Beijing, People's Republic of China; Dr H. Li, Head, Chemical Products Division, Chinese Pharmacopoeia Commission, Beijing, People's Republic of China; Dr R. Lichtenstein, Head of Business Analytics and Master Data, Galderma SA, Lausanne, Switzerland; Dr C.M. Limoli, International Programs, Center for Drug Evaluation and Research, United States Food and Drug Administration, Silver Spring, MD, USA; Dr A. Lodi, Head, Laboratory Department, European Directorate for the Quality of Medicines and HealthCare, Strasbourg, France; Mr M. Lok, Head of Office, Office of Manufacturing Quality, Therapeutic Goods Administration, Woden, ACT, Australia; Ms M.Y. Low, Director, Pharmaceutical Division, Applied Sciences Group, Health Sciences Authority, Singapore; Lupin Ltd, Mumbai, Maharashtra, India; Dr J.C. Lyda, Senior Director, Regulatory Affairs, Parenteral Drug Association Europe, Glienicke/ Berlin, Germany; Agence du Médicament, Madagascar; Mr D. Mader, Compliance Auditor, GlaxoSmithKline, Cape Town, South Africa; Dr C. Makokha, Kikuyu, Kenya; Ms G.N. Mahlangu, Director-General, Medicines Control Authority of Zimbabwe, Harare, Zimbabwe; Mangalam Drugs and Organics Limited, Mumbai, India; Dr M.A. Mantri, Bicholim, Goa, India; Martindale Pharma, Brentwood, Essex, England; Dr J.Y. Martey, Accra, Ghana; Dr B. Matthews, Alcon, Hemel Hempstead, England; Dr Y. Matthews, Regulatory Operations Executive, GE Healthcare, Amersham, Bucks, England; Dr S.V.M. Mattos, Especialista em Regulação de Vigilância Sanitária, Coordenação da Farmacopeia Brasileira, Brazilian Health Surveillance Agency, Brasília, Brazil; Dr J.L. Mazert, France; Dr G. McGurk, Executive Inspector, Irish Medicines Board, Dublin, Ireland; Dr A. Mechkovski, Moscow, Russian Federation; Medicines and Healthcare Products Regulatory Agency, London, England; Medopharm, Chennai, Tamilnadu, India; Dr M. Mehmandoust, Agence nationale de sécurité du médicament et des produits de santé, Saint-Denis, France; Dr D. Mehta, Vigilance and Risk Management of Medicines, Medicines and Healthcare Products Regulatory Agency, London, England; Dr C. Mendy, Manager, Regulatory Policy, International Federation of Pharmaceutical Manufacturers and Associations, Geneva, Switzerland; Dr K. Mettke, GCP Inspector, Federal Institute for Drugs and Medical Devices, Bonn, Germany; Micro Labs Ltd, Kilpauk, Chennai, India; Dr M. Mikhail, Fresenius Kabi, Bad-Homburg, Germany; Dr J.H.McB. Miller, Ayr, Scotland; Dr O. Milling, Medicines Inspector, Medicines Control Division, Danish Medicines Agency, Copenhagen, Denmark; Dr S. Mills, Pharmaceutical Consultant, Ware, England; Ministry of Health,

Government of Pakistan, Islamabad, Pakistan; Ministry of Health and Welfare, Tokyo, Japan; Dr J. Mitchell, GlaxoSmithKline, Belgium; Dr S. Moglate, United Nations Population Fund, UN City, Copenhagen, Denmark; Dr N.H. Mohd, Director General of Medical Supplies, Ministry of Health, Muscat, Oman; Ms N.H. Mohd Potri, Senior Assistant, Director, GMP and Licensing Division, Centre for Compliance and Licensing, National Pharmaceutical Control Bureau, Ministry of Health Malaysia, Petaling Jaya, Malaysia; Dr J.A. Molzon, Bethesda, MD, USA; Dr I. Moore, Product and Quality Assurance Manager, Croda Europe, Snaith, England; Dr J. Morénas, Assistant Director, Inspection and Companies Department, Agence nationale de sécurité du médicament et des produits de santé, Saint Denis, France; Dr K. Morimoto, Expert, Office of Review Management, Review Planning Division, Pharmaceutical and Medical Devices Agency, Tokyo, Japan; Direction of Medicine and Pharmacy, Ministry of Health, Rabat, Morocco; Dr J.M. Morris, Irish Medicines Board, Dublin, Ireland; Mr T. Moser, Galenica, Berne, Switzerland; Dr M. Mugad, HLL Lifecare Ltd, Kanagala, Belgaum, Karnataka, India; Dr A.E. Muhairwe, Executive Secretary and Registrar, National Drug Authority, Kampala, Uganda; Dr. S. Mülbach, Director, Senior Regulatory Counsellor, Vifor Pharma, Glattbrugg, Switzerland; Ms C. Munyimba-Yeta, Director, Inspectorate and Licensing, Pharmaceutical Regulatory Authority, Lusaka, Zambia; Dr Murthi, Accutest Research Laboratory Ltd, Navi Mumbai, Maharashtra, India; Mylan, Allschwil, Switzerland; Mylan Laboratories Limited, Drug Regulatory Affairs, Jinnaram Mandal, Andhra Pradesh, India; Dr D.A. van Riet-Nales, Member Quality Working Party, European Medicines Agency, Senior Assessor, Department of Chemical Pharmaceutical Assessments, College ter Beoordeling van Geneesmiddelen, Utrecht, Netherlands; Ms N. Nan, Chief Pharmacist, National Institutes for Food and Drug Control, Beijing, People's Republic of China; Miss X. Nan, Project Officer, China Center for Pharmaceutical International Exchange, Beijing, People's Republic of China; Mr N. Nanerjee, Cipla Ltd, Goa, India; Dr E. Narciandi, Head, Technology Transfer Department, Center for Genetic Engineering & Biotechnology, Havana, Cuba; National Agency of Drug and Food Control, Jakarta Pusat, Indonesia; National Authority of Medicines and Health Products (INFARMED), Directorate for the Evaluation of Medicinal Products, Lisbon, Portugal; National Institute of Drug Quality Control of Vietnam, Hanoi, Viet Nam; NBCD Working Group, Leiden, Netherlands; Starship Hospital, New Zealand; Dr R. Neri, Sanofi, Antony, France; Dr E. Nickličková, Inspector, State Institute for Drug Control, Prague, Czech Republic; Professor A. Nicolas, Radiopharmacist, Expert analyse, Pharmacie, Hôpital Brabois Adultes, Vandoeuvre, France; Dr H.K. Nielsen, Technical Specialist, Essential Medicines, Medicines and Nutrition Centre, UNICEF Supply Division, Copenhagen, Denmark; Professor B. Ning, Deputy Director, Division of Chemical Drugs, National Institutes for Food and Drug Control, Beijing, People's Republic of China; Dr P. Njaria, Head, Quality Assurance Unit and

Instrumentation, National Quality Control Laboratory, Nairobi, Kenya; Dr C. dos Santos Nogueira, Especialista em Regulação e Vigilância Sanitária, ANVISA, Brasilia, Brazil; Dr K. Nodop, Inspections, European Medicines Agency, London, England; Novartis Group Quality, Novartis, Basel, Switzerland; Professor A. Nunn, Formby, Liverpool, England; Dr A. Ojoo, Technical Specialist, Paediatric Formulations, United Nations Children's Fund Supply Division, Nordhavn, Copenhagen, Denmark; Mr S. O'Neill, Managing Director, The Compliance Group, Dublin, Ireland; Dr L. Oresic, Head, Quality Assurance Department, Croatian Agency for Medicinal Products and Medical Devices, Zagreb, Croatia; Dr P.B. Orhii, Director-General, National Agency for Food and Drug Administration and Control, Abuja, Nigeria; Dr N. Orphanos, International Programs Division, Bureau of Policy, Science, and International Programs, Therapeutic Products Directorate, Health Products & Food Branch, Health Canada, Ottawa, Canada; Professor T.L. Paál, Director-General, National Institute of Pharmacy, Budapest, Hungary; Dr P.R. Pabrai, New Delhi, India; Dr R. Pai, Johannesburg, South Africa; Mrs L. Paleshnuik, Arnprior, Ontario, Canada; Dr S. Parra, Manager, Generic Drugs Quality Division 1, Bureau of Pharmaceutical Sciences, Therapeutic Products Directorate, Health Canada, Ottawa, Ontario, Canada; Mr B. Passek, BMG, Germany; Dr D.B. Patel, Secretary-General, Indian Drug Manufacturers' Association, Mumbai, India; Dr P.S. Patil, Umedica Laboratories Pvt Ltd, Vapi, Gujarat, India; Dr S.R. Srinivas Patnala, Grahamstown, South Africa; Dr S. Patnala, Professor, Pharmaceutical Analysis and Coordinator, University Instrumentation Facility, KLE University, Belgaum, India; Paul-Ehrlich-Institut, Langen, Germany; Dr A. Pazhayattil, Apotex Inc., Toronto, Ontario, Canada; Mr C. Perrin, Pharmacist, International Union Against Tuberculosis and Lung Disease, Paris, France; Dr M. Phadke, Senior Manager, Analytical Research, IPCA Laboratories, Mumbai, India; Pharmaceutical Inspection Co-operation Scheme, Geneva, Switzerland; Pharmaceuticals and Medical Devices Agency (PMDA), Tokyo, Japan; Dr B. Phillips, Medicines and Healthcare Products Regulatory Agency, London, England; Dr R.D. Pickett, Supanet, Bucks, England; Dr B. Pimentel, European Chemical Industry Council, Brussels, Belgium; Polychromix, Inc., Wilmington, MA, USA; Dr A. Pontén-Engelhardt, Head of Stability Management, Global Quality, Operations, AstraZeneca, Södertälje, Sweden; Ms A. Poompanich, Bangkok, Thailand; Dr H. Potthast, Federal Institute for Drugs and Medical Devices, Berlin, Germany; Dr R. Prabhu, Regulatory Affairs Department, Cipla, Mumbai, India; Dr J. Prakash, Principal Scientific Officer, Indian Pharmacopoeia Commission, Raj Najar, Ghaziabad, India; Dr P.B.N. Prasad, Deputy Drugs Controller (India), Central Drugs Standard Control Organisation, Bhavan, S.R.Nagr, Hyderabad, India; Dr R.P. Prasad, Director, Department of Drug Administration, Kathmandu, Nepal; Ms S.J. Putter, Walmer, Port Elizabeth, South Africa; Quality Systems and Standards – Group Quality, Novartis Pharma AG, Basel, Switzerland;

Ms M.-L. Rabouhans, Chiswick, London, England; Dr M. Rafi, Assistant Manager (Regulatory Affairs), HLL Lifecare Limited, Belgaum, Karnataka, India; Dr A. Rajan, Director, Celogen Lifescience & Technologies, Mumbai, India; Mr T.L. Rauber, Specialist in Health Surveillance, Agência Nacional de Vigilância Sanitária Agency, Brasilia, Brazil; Mr N. Raw, Inspection, Enforcement and Standards Division, Medicines and Healthcare Products Regulatory Agency, London, England; Mr N. Rech, Brazilian Pharmacopoeia, Brazilian Health Surveillance Agency, Brasilia, DF, Brazil; Dr J.-L. Robert, Luxembourg; Dr S. Rönninger, Global Quality Manager, F. Hoffmann-La Roche, Basel, Switzerland; Dr J. Isasi Rosas, CNCC, Chorrillos, Lima, Peru; Dr N. Ruangrittinon, Bureau of Drug and Narcotic Department of Medical Sciences, Ministry of Public Health, Nonthaburi, Thailand; Dr J. Sabartova, Prague, Czech Republic; Dr L.A. Sotelo Ruiz, Comisión de Control Analítico y Ampliación de Cobertura, Tlalpan, Distrito Federal, Mexico; Rusan Pharma Ltd, Selaqui, Dehradun, India; Dr P.L. Sahu, Indian Pharmacopoeia Commission, Raj Nagar, Ghaziabad, Uttar Pradesh, India; Dr E.I. Sakanyan, Director, Centre of the Pharmacopoeia and International Collaboration, Federal State Budgetary Institution, Scientific Centre for Expert Evaluation of Medicinal Products, Moscow, Russian Federation; Dr C. Sánchez González, Adviser, Centre para el Control de Medicamentos, Equipos y Dispositivos Médicos, Havana, Cuba; Dr E. Moya Sánchez, Radiofarmaceutica-Evaluadora de Calidad, División de Química y Tecnología Farmacéutica, Departamento de Medicamentos de Uso Umano, Agencia Española de Medicamentos y Productos Sanitarios, Madrid, Spain; Sanofi Aventis, Antony, France; Sanofi, Bridgewater, NJ, USA; Dr G. Mendes Lima Santos, Coordinator of Therapeutic Equivalence, Brazilian Health Surveillance Agency, Brasilia, DF, Brazil; Dr B. Santoso, Sleman, Yogyakarta, Indonesia; Dr T. Sasaki, Pharmaceutical and Medical Devices Agency, Tokyo, Japan; Dr J. Satanarayana, Matrix Laboratories, Secunderabad, India; Dr B. Schmauser, Bundesinstitut für Arzneimittel und Medizinprodukte, Bonn, Germany; Dr A. Schuchmann, Brazil; Dr I. Seekkuarachchi, Project Manager, Takeda Pharmaceutical Co., Osaka, Japan; Dr A. Seiter, Member, United States Pharmacopeia International Health Expert Committee, Rockville, MD, USA; Ms K. Sempf, Teaching Assistant, Institut für Pharmazeutische Technologie, Biozentrum, Johann Wolfgang Goethe-Universität, Frankfurt am Main, Germany; Dr U. Shah, Formulation Research Fellow, Cheshire, Merseyside & North Wales LRN, Medicines for Children Research Network, Royal Liverpool Children's NHS Trust, Liverpool, England; Dr R. Shaikh, Pakistan; Shasun Research Centre, Chennai, Tamil Nadu, India; Dr P.D. Sheth, Vice-President, International Pharmaceutical Federation, New Delhi, India; Ms R. Shimonovitz, Head of Inspectorates, Institute for Standardization and Control of Pharmaceuticals, Ministry of Health, Israel; Shin Poong Pharmaceutical Co. Ltd, Seoul, Republic of Korea: Dr P.G. Shrotriya, Ambli, Ahmedabad, India; Dr M. Sigonda, Director-General, Tanzania Food and

Drugs Authority, Dar-es-Salaam, United Republic of Tanzania; Dr G.L. Singal, Drugs Controller of Haryana, Department of Health Services, Civil Dispensary, Panchkula, Haryana, India; Dr A.K. Singh, Daman, India; Dr G.N. Singh, Secretary-cum-Scientific Director, Government of India, Central Indian Pharmacopoeia Laboratory, Ministry of Health and Family Welfare, Raj Nagar, Ghaziabad, India; Dr S. Singh, Professor and Head, Department of Pharmaceutical Analysis, National Institute of Pharmaceutical Education and Research, Nagar, Punjab, India; Ms K. Sinivuo, Senior Researcher and Secretary, National Agency for Medicines, Helsinki, Finland; Dr L. Slamet, Jakarta Selatan, Indonesia; Mr D. Smith, Faerie Glen, Pretoria, South Africa; Dr R. Smith, Wolfson Brain Imaging Centre, University of Cambridge, Cambridge, England; Dr N. Kumar Soam, Mankind Pharma Limited, Unit-II, Vill. Kishanpura, Paonta Sahib, Disst. Sirmour, India; Dr M. Da Luz Carvalho Soares, Expert Health Regulation, Brazilian Health Surveillance Agency, Brasilia, Brazil; Dr C. Sokhan, Deputy Director, Department of Drug and Food, Phnom Penh, Cambodia; Dr A. Spreitzhofer, AGES PharmMed, Vienna, Austria; Mr K. Srinivas, Group Legal Counsel, Trimulgherry, Secunderabad, Andhra Pradesh, India; State Regulatory Agency for Medical Activities, Ministry of Labour, Health and Social Affairs, Tbilisi, Georgia; Dr J.A. Steichen, Manager, Regulatory and Quality Compliance Services, Safis Solutions, LLC, Indianapolis, IN, USA; Dr Y. Stewart, Scientific, Technical and Regulatory Affairs, European Federation of Pharmaceutical Industries and Associations, Brussels, Belgium; Dr L. Stoppa, Inspections & Certifications Department, Manufacturing Authorisation Office, Italian Medicines Agency, Rome, Italy; Dr R.W. Stringham, Scientific Director, Drug Access Team, Clinton Health Access Initiative, Boston, MA, USA; Dr N. Sullivan, Director, Sensapharm, Sunderland, England; Mr Philip Sumner, Pfizer Global Engineering, New York, NY, USA; Dr Sun Cuilain D., Senior Analytical Scientist, Pharmaceutical Laboratory, Pharmaceutical Division, Applied Sciences Group, Health Sciences Authority, Singapore; Dr V. Suvarna, Medical Director, Boehringer Ingelheim India Private Limited, India; Dr E. Swanepoel, Head, Operations, Research Institute for Industrial Pharmacy, North-West University, Potchefstroom, South Africa; Professor M. Sznitowska, Department of Pharmaceutical Technology, Medical University of Gdansk, Gdansk, Poland; Dr K. Tadano, Committee of the Japanese Pharmacopoeia, Tokyo, Japan; Dr K. Takahashi, Senior Policy Advisor, Division of Regulations, Guidance and Standards, Office of Policy for Pharmaceutical Quality, Center for Drug Evaluation and Research, Food and Drug Administration, Silver Spring, MD, USA; Tanzania Food and Drugs Authority, Dar-es-Salaam, United Republic of Tanzania; Dr D. Teitz, Manager, Bristol-Myers Squibb Company, New Brunswick, NJ, USA; Teva API Division, Petah Tiqva, Israel; Dr N. Thao, National Institute of Drug Quality Control, Hanoi, Viet Nam; Dr B.B. Thapa, Chief Drug Administrator, Department of Drug Administration, Ministry of Health and Population, Kathmandu, Nepal;

The Danish Medicines Agency, Denmark; Dr R. Torano, Pharmacopoeial Technical Expert, GlaxoSmithKline, Co. Durham, England; Dr P. Travis, Team Leader – Compendial Affairs Group, Pfizer Inc., Parsippany, NJ, USA; Ms M. Treebamroong, Senior Pharmacist, Drug Quality and Safety, Department of Medical Sciences, Bureau of Drug and Narcotic, Ministry of Public Health, Nonthaburi, Thailand; Mr R. Tribe, Holder, ACT, Australia; Associate Professor Trinh Van Lau, Director, National Institute of Drug Quality Control, Hanoi, Viet Nam; Professor Tu Guoshi, National Institute for the Control of Pharmaceutical and Biological Products, Ministry of Public Health, Beijing, People's Republic of China; Dr C. Tuleu, Senior Lecturer and Deputy Director, Department of Pharmaceutics and Centre for Paediatric Pharmacy Research, School of Pharmacy, University of London, London, England; Dr Richard Turner, British Pharmacopoeia Commission, Medicines and Healthcare Products Regulatory Agency, London, England; United States of America Food and Drug Administration, Center for Drug Evaluation and Research, Silver Spring, MD, USA; United States of America Food and Drug Administration, Office of Pediatric Therapeutics, Office of the Commissioner, Rockville, MD, USA; Ms E. Uramis, GMP Advisor, Oficina Central Polo Científico, Havana, Cuba; Dr A.R.T. Utami, National Agency for Drugs and Food Control, Jakarta Pusat, Indonesia; Dr R. Vaillancourt, International Pharmaceutical Federation, The Hague, Netherlands; Validation and Qualification Department, Pharmaceutical Laboratory, Esteve, Spain; Mrs M. Vallender, Editor-in-Chief, British Pharmacopoeia Commission Secretariat, London, England; Mr M. van Bruggen, EU Liaison – Regulatory Intelligence, F. Hoffmann-La Roche, Basel, Switzerland; Mr F. Vandendriessche, Merck, Sharp and Dohme Europe, Brussels, Belgium; Mr P. van der Hoeven, APIC, Brussels, Belgium; Dr J.E. van Oudtshoorn, Pretoria, South Africa; Dr A.J. van Zyl, Sea Point, Cape Town, South Africa; Dr G. Vedoya, CABA, Instituto Nacional de Medicamentos (INAME/ANMAT), Argentina; Mr S. Akbaralli Veljee, Director, Food and Drugs Administration, Directorate of Food and Drugs Administration, Government of Goa, Dhanwantari, Bambolim, Goa, India; Dr A. Kumar Velumury, Cipla Ltd, New Delhi, India; Mr A. Vezali Montai, Specialist in Regulation and GMP, Agência Nacional de Vigilância, Brasília, Brazil; Mrs L. Vignoli, Regulatory Affairs, Pharmaceuticals and Cosmetics, Roquette Cie, Lestren, France; Dr O. del Rosario Villalva Rojas, Executive Director, Quality Control Laboratories, National Quality Control Center, National Institute of Health, Lima, Peru; Mr L. Viornery, Agence nationale de sécurité du médicament et des produits de santé, Saint Denis, France; Dr L. Virgili, USA; Mr J. Wang, Deputy Commissioner, Dalian Food and Drug Administration, Dalian, Liaoning, People's Republic of China; Mr P. Wang, Deputy Secretary-General, Chinese Pharmacopoeia Commission, Beijing, People's Republic of China; Mrs T. Wang, Deputy Director, Shenzhen Municipal Institute for Drug Control, Shenzhen, People's Republic of China;

Dr G. Wang'ang'a, Head, Microbiological and Medical Devices Units, National Quality Control Laboratory, Nairobi, Kenya; Dr A. Ward, Regulatory Affairs, Avecia Vaccines, Billingham, England; Dr D. Waters, Acting Scientific Operations Advisor, Office of Laboratories and Scientific Services, Therapeutic Goods Administration, Woden, ACT, Australia; Dr W. Watson, Associate Manager, CMC Regulatory Affairs, Gilead Sciences International, Cambridge, England; Dr J. Welink, Medicines Evaluation Board, Utrecht, Netherlands; Ms Wei N., Associate Researcher, Division of Chemical Drugs, National Institutes for Food and Drug Control, Beijing, China; Professor W. Wieniawski, Polish Pharmaceutical Society, Warsaw, Poland; Mr J. Wilkinson, Director, Devices, Medicines and Healthcare products Regulatory Agency, London, England; Dr J. Skutnik Wilkinson, Biogen, Oneco, CT, USA; Dr M. Jiwo Winanti, Senior GMP Inspector, National Authority for Food and Drug Control, Indonesia; Dr S. Wolfgang, US Food and Drug Administration, Silver Spring, MD, USA; Mr E. Wondemagegnehu Biwota, Addis Ababa, Ethiopia; World Self-Medication Industry, Ferney-Voltaire, France; Dr B. Wright, Group Manager, GMP/GDP, North East Region, Medicines Inspectorate, Medicines and Healthcare Products Regulatory Agency, York, England; Professor Z.-Y. Yang, Guangzhou Municipal Institute for Drug Control, Guangzhou, People's Republic of China; Professor Z.-Y. Yang, Member, United States Pharmacopeia International Health Expert Committee, Rockville, MD, USA; Ms C. Munyimba-Yeta, Director Operations (Plant), NRB Pharma Zambia Limited, Lusaka South Multi Facility Economic Zone, Lusaka, Zambia; Dr D. Yi, Scientist, US Pharmacopeia, Rockville, MD, USA; Dr H. Yusufu, National Agency for Food and Drug Administration and Control, Abuja, Nigeria; Dr M. Zahn, Keltern, Germany; Dr H. Zhang, GMP Department Head, Center for Certification & Evaluation, Shanghai Food and Drug Administration, Shanghai, People's Republic of China; Dr G. Zenhäusern, Senior Case Manager, Sector Authorisation, Swissmedic, Berne, Switzerland; Professor (Mrs) Zhang M., Deputy Director, Institutes for Food and Drug Control, and Vice Chairman, Antiobiotic Subcommittee, Chinese Pharmacopoeia Commission, China; Dr T. Zimmer, CD Safety, Quality & Environmental Protection, Boehringer Ingelheim, Ingelheim, Germany; Dr N. Zvolinska, Deputy Director, Pharmaceutical Department, State Pharmacological Centre, Ministry of Health, Kiev, Ukraine.

Annex 1

Good pharmacopoeial practices

1. Background

A pharmacopoeia's core mission is to protect public health by creating and making available public standards to help ensure the quality of medicines. Pharmacopoeia standards support regulatory authorities in controlling the quality of pharmaceutical substances, their finished pharmaceutical products (FPPs) and related materials and will provide a tool with which the user or procurer can make an independent judgement regarding quality, thus safeguarding the health of the public.

Today there are 49 pharmacopoeias in the world (according to the World Health Organization (WHO) list of pharmacopoeias, 2015). There are differences between these pharmacopoeias, including the use of technology reflected in each pharmacopoeia as well as the breadth of medicines and other articles included. Pharmacopoeias are embedded in their respective national or regional regulatory environment and reflect specifications approved by the regulatory body.

Efforts towards pharmacopoeial harmonization started more than a century ago. When WHO was created in 1948, this was included in its mandate. This led to the creation of *The International Pharmacopoeia*, which was the first global pharmacopoeial activity. Many others followed.

Pharmacopoeial harmonization has been defined by the Pharmacopoeial Discussion Group (PDG) as "when a pharmaceutical substance or product tested by the document's harmonized procedure yields the same results and the same accept/reject decision is reached".

Developments in science and medical practice, globalization and the presence of spurious/falsified/falsely labelled/counterfeit (SFFC) products require pharmacopoeias to continuously revise their monographs and other text. Harmonization and reinforced collaboration among pharmacopoeial committees and regulators, supported by adequate interaction with industry, will assist in facing new challenges and resource constraints.

The first initiative to reopen the discussion on international harmonization of quality control specifications on a global scale was taken in a side meeting of the 10th International Conference of Drug Regulatory Authorities (ICDRA) entitled: "Pharmacopoeial Specifications – Need for a Worldwide Approach?" in Hong Kong on 24 June 2002. This led to further discussions among regulators during the 11th ICDRA meeting held in Madrid in 2004. Other international events during the following years enabled discussions with and among pharmacopoeias on this topic.

The main suggestion emerging from all these events was the development of good pharmacopoeial practices (GPhP) to encourage harmonization, facilitated by WHO.

It was agreed to develop the GPhP under the auspices of the WHO Expert Committee on Specifications for Pharmaceutical Preparations, benefiting from its well-established international standard-setting processes and procedures. These processes include an international consultation process, which enables the participation of all stakeholders and users in the development process. The final guidance would then be presented, in line with the procedure, to WHO's 194 Member States and pharmacopoeial authorities.

2. Purpose and scope of good pharmacopoeial practices

The primary objective of the GPhP guidance is to define approaches and policies in establishing pharmacopoeial standards with the ultimate goal of harmonization.

These GPhP describe a set of principles that provide guidance for national pharmacopoeial authorities (NPAs) and regional pharmacopoeial authorities (RPAs) that facilitates the appropriate design, development and maintenance of pharmacopoeial standards.

Although the principles may also apply to other products, the focus of these good practices is pharmaceutical substances and FPPs.

3. Glossary

Terms in this document are used in accordance with WHO terminology, while recognizing that individual pharmacopoeias may apply their own nomenclature policies.

active pharmaceutical ingredient. Any substance or mixture of substances intended to be used in the manufacture of a pharmaceutical dosage form and that, when so used, becomes an active ingredient of that pharmaceutical dosage form. Such substances are intended to furnish pharmacological activity or other direct effect in the diagnosis, cure, mitigation, treatment, or prevention of disease or to affect the structure and function of the body.

dosage form. The form of the completed pharmaceutical product, e.g. tablet, capsule, elixir, suppository or injection.

excipient. A substance or compound, other than the active pharmaceutical ingredient and packaging materials, that is intended or designated to be used in the manufacture of a pharmaceutical product.

finished pharmaceutical product. A finished dosage form of a pharmaceutical product that has undergone all stages of manufacture, including packaging in its final container and labelling.

period of use. Utilization period of multidose products after opening, reconstitution or dilution of a solution.

pharmaceutical substance. Any substance of a defined quality used in the production of a pharmaceutical product, but excluding packaging materials. This includes active pharmaceutical ingredients and pharmaceutical excipients.

shelf life. The period of time during which a pharmaceutical product, if stored as indicated on the label, is expected to comply with the specification as determined by stability studies on a number of batches of the product. The shelf life is used to establish the expiry date of each batch.

4. Benefits of good pharmacopoeial practices

GPhP are designed to facilitate collaboration among pharmacopoeias, leading to possibilities for work-sharing, harmonization of standards and the recognition of published standards between NPAs and RPAs.

In addition to the above, the establishment of GPhP may result in the following:

1) strengthening of global pharmacopoeial cooperation;
2) providing stakeholders with a better understanding of how pharmacopoeial standards are developed and maintained in a transparent manner;
3) improving cooperation between NPAs/RPAs and stakeholders (e.g. regulators, pharmaceutical industry) with a view to facilitating the harmonization of pharmacopoeial standards and reducing duplication of work;
4) increasing access to and the availability of affordable, quality medicines.

By establishing common practices, GPhP can facilitate adoption or adaptation of the standards from one pharmacopoeia by another pharmacopoeia, proactively harmonizing the requirements with considerably less effort than is currently needed.

GPhP should ultimately enable harmonization of pharmacopoeial standards.

5. Implementation

While the implementation of the GPhP by NPAs and RPAs is voluntary, it is recommended and encouraged, as a high level of participation will result in greater benefit to the stakeholders and ultimately to patients.

6. Monograph development

Development of a monograph requires consideration of information and candidate materials. This information may come from donors, literature, various publicly available sources, from other pharmacopoeias, or may be generated within the laboratory resources of a pharmacopoeia and/or of a competent authority (such as an official medicines control laboratory). The draft text should be displayed for public comments with sufficient time allowed for review and input by stakeholders.

Pharmacopoeias are encouraged to conform, where possible, to the work of harmonization initiatives (e.g. WHO, International Conference on Harmonisation of Technical Requirements for Registration of Pharmaceuticals for Human Use (ICH) and the PDG)).

6.1 General considerations

Pharmacopoeial monographs provide an important tool for assurance of the quality of marketed pharmaceutical ingredients and products through testing of their quality. They generally cover chemical, biological and herbal FPPs and their ingredients, which have either been approved by national regulatory authorities or are otherwise legally marketed. Some pharmacopoeias also include standards for items such as natural products, nutritional products and medical devices. The principles of GPhP apply equally to substances and products used in both human and veterinary medicine. It is recognized that different requirements may be applied to human and veterinary medicines, such as those included in the ICH and the corresponding Veterinary International Conference on Harmonization (VICH) requirements.

Specifications in pharmacopoeias are one facet of the overall control of the quality of FPPs and their ingredients (active pharmaceutical ingredients (APIs) and excipients). Monographs provide publicly available standards that a product or a component of a product is expected to meet during its shelf life. Thus, a substance should be able to demonstrate compliance with a pharmacopoeial monograph up to the point at which it is used to prepare an FPP. An FPP should demonstrate compliance with a monograph, if available, throughout its shelf life. Pharmacopoeial specifications are used within pharmaceutical product marketing authorization systems and by manufacturers, suppliers, purchasers and those acting on behalf of patients.

Before developing a monograph it is important to consider the specifications (tests and acceptance criteria) needed to assure the quality of a given pharmaceutical substance or FPP. Specifications that limit market access by, for example, favouring one manufacturer to the exclusion of others should be avoided.

The ICH guideline Q6A (*Specifications: test procedures and acceptance criteria for new drug substances and new drug products: chemical substances*), for example, could be used as a basis. Whenever possible, specifications should be applied consistently in monographs across all participating pharmacopoeias, regardless of whether the requirements are specified in the specific monograph or are incorporated in general monographs. However, there may be situations where different acceptance criteria are required depending on the national or regional regulatory authorities. Additional tests might be added by NPAs and RPAs, depending on national or regional regulations.

Pharmacopoeial standards allow independent testing and are a critical part of the "safety net" of standards that help ensure the quality, safety and efficacy of FPPs. They are closely allied with good manufacturing practice (GMP) standards.

Pharmacopoeial standards should be available for FPPs and their APIs and associated materials at an appropriate time to support and benefit patients through the availability of medicines with consistent quality. They are usually based on the shelf-life specifications approved by regulatory authorities[1] or on the specifications of unlicensed products (e.g. compounded and other preparations, as defined by national or regional regulations).

The monographs may employ various validated analytical procedures for the tests that are designed to be suitable for a competent analyst to perform using established technologies and facilities.

Pharmacopoeial standards are public standards that are science-based and data-driven and based on sound analytical measurement and accompanying validation data.

Pharmacopoeias respect the intellectual property of donors and recognize the importance of maintaining the confidentiality of proprietary third-party information. Pharmacopoeias endeavour to work collaboratively with regulators (including medicines regulatory authorities, official medicines control laboratories and inspectorates), the pharmaceutical industries (including manufacturers and trade associations), academia, health-care professionals and patient advocacy groups (as appropriate), and other stakeholders in the development of public standards.

6.1.1 Adoption of pharmacopoeial standards

(a) Text in a pharmacopoeial monograph or general chapter is approved by an expert body of the pharmacopoeia, following publicly available rules and procedures. This includes public consultation and the application of conflict of interest and confidentiality rules.

(b) Reference standards cited in a pharmacopoeia are also approved by a pharmacopoeial expert body.

[1] In the case of *The International Pharmacopoeia* this relates to the shelf-life specifications evaluated by the WHO Prequalification Team.

6.1.2 Open and transparent process

Pharmacopoeial standards are based on current scientific knowledge and reflect the quality of pharmaceutical substances and FPPs available.

Pharmacopoeias ensure openness and transparency throughout the development and revision of monographs and other texts, which includes:

i. engaging stakeholders in the routine development and revision of pharmacopoeial standards through adequate and timely public notice and comment;
ii. engaging stakeholders in the timely development and revision of standards to address major public health concerns;
iii. general transparency of the pharmacopoeial approaches, including making work programmes publicly available;
iv. good communication with stakeholders through forums, workshops and other interactions;
v. timely response to user enquiries;
vi. opportunities for user training and education on the pharmacopoeial process and finalized standards;
vii. rapid correction of errors published in compendial text, when necessary;
viii. timely and appropriate revision and/or withdrawal of compendial standards, when necessary. (The legal status of monographs that have been withdrawn will depend on the national regulatory framework.)

6.1.3 Harmonization

Pharmacopoeias should harmonize standards wherever possible through monographs and general chapters. Harmonization may occur through several processes including, but not limited to: adoption or adaptation[2] of existing standards; development of a new standard through coordinated consideration (prospective harmonization); revision of a standard between two or more pharmacopoeias (bilateral or multilateral harmonization); and creation or revision of standards through a harmonization initiative (e.g. PDG).

6.1.4 Legal recognition

Pharmacopoeial monographs may acquire legal status and then provide a basis for enforcement depending on applicable national or regional requirements.

[2] The source of the text should be indicated.

6.1.5 Compliance with a pharmacopoeial monograph

Any pharmaceutical substance or FPP subject to a monograph must comply with all of the mandatory requirements within the pharmacopoeia, throughout its period of use or shelf life.

The assays and tests described are the official methods upon which the standards of the pharmacopoeia depend. The analyst may not be precluded from employing alternative methods depending on national and regional legislation. A validation of the alternative analytical procedure should be done to show at least an equivalent performance to the analytical procedure described in the monograph. Subject to regulatory approval an alternative method of analysis may be used for routine analytical purposes. In this case it is necessary to provide a rationale for its inclusion, validation data and data comparing results obtained using the pharmacopoeial method and the alternative method.

In case of doubt or dispute, the official pharmacopoeial methods prevail and are alone authoritative.

6.1.6 Analytical requirements

Pharmacopoeial procedures and acceptance criteria are set with the intention that they should be used as compliance requirements and not as requirements to guarantee total quality assurance.

To achieve maximum benefit from the examination of a product, the recommended approach is that, wherever possible, a variety of different analytical techniques should be employed, considering the feasibility and affordability of the methods.

6.1.7 Acceptance criteria

Acceptance criteria are numerical limits, ranges or other suitable measures for acceptance of the results of analytical testing to allow determination of pass/fail criteria. Acceptance criteria indicated in a pharmacopoeial monograph allow for analytical error, for unavoidable variations in manufacturing processes and for deviations to an extent considered acceptable under practical storage conditions. They provide standards with which pharmaceutical substances or FPPs must comply throughout their shelf life or period of use.

6.2 Technical guidance

The technical guidance provided in this section shall be considered as the minimum requirements agreed between the participating pharmacopoeias. They do not preclude national or regional pharmacopoeias from supplementing such requirements in their monographs in accordance with national or regional regulations.

6.2.1 Monographs for pharmaceutical substances

Prior to the preparation of any monograph it is essential to gather as much information as possible on the substance in question.

In particular it is necessary to ascertain:

- the origin of the substance;
- the method(s) of preparation of the substance, if needed;
- whether the substance is a mixture or a single entity;
- whether different entities (e.g. acid, base or salt) are available;
- the physicochemical characteristics of the substance that contribute to its identity and classification, for example, solubility or optical rotation;
- whether there are differences in physical form, for example, crystallinity or polymorphism, since these properties may affect the behaviour of the substance;
- whether a single optical isomer (e.g. enantiomer) as well as mixtures of isomers (e.g. racemate) are available;
- whether anhydrous or different hydrates or solvates are available.

Substances that are to be described in a monograph may be members of a group of very similar substances. A general monograph may be drafted stating the attributes common to all members of the group and that can be used to identify single members of the group.

6.2.1.1 Monograph title

The International Nonproprietary Name (INN) or modified INN (INNM) established by WHO should be considered for use wherever it is available, while recognizing that individual pharmacopoeias may apply their own nomenclature policies.

6.2.1.2 General information to define the pharmaceutical substance

A pharmacopoeial monograph includes information regarding the pharmaceutical substance, such as:

- graphic formula;
- empirical/molecular formula and relative molecular mass (the latter is calculated based on the figures of the International Table of Relative Atomic Masses considering, where appropriate, the degree of hydration);
- Chemical Abstracts Service (CAS) registry number, if available;

- chemical name;
- the possible existence of isomers, so as to be able to specify either which isomer is present or to state that the substance is a mixture of isomers;
- in the case of an optical isomer, the absolute configuration is given by the R/S system at the asymmetrical centre(s) or any other appropriate system (e.g. for carbohydrates and amino acids);
- state of hydration or solvation, where relevant, ascertaining the state of hydration or solvation by an appropriate technique in order to distinguish clearly between substances which are well-defined hydrates and solvates and those that contain variable quantities of water or solvent(s):
  - for well-defined hydrates or solvates, water or solvent content ranges are specified;
  - for substances containing variable amounts of water or solvents, only a maximum content is given;
  - where substances exist as both non-hydrated (or non-solvated) and hydrated (or solvated) forms, and if all these forms are used and can be clearly distinguished, they may be treated as individual substances depending on the regulatory approach prevailing in the country or region.

In therapeutics, well-defined chemical combinations or even mixtures are sometimes used. In such cases it is necessary to specify precisely each component of the combination or mixture, with its chemical structure and the proportion in which it is present.

6.2.1.3 Content

Assay limits are specified between which the content must fall. In certain instances the content may be given only as a lower limit. The assay limits take account of the precision of the method as well as the acceptable purity of the substance. Assay limits are normally expressed with reference to the dried, anhydrous and/or solvent-free substance.

In setting limits for the API content, account is taken of:

- the method of preparation, which determines the degree of purity that may be reasonably required;
- the precision and accuracy of the analytical method;
- where a separation technique is employed both for the test for related substances and the assay, content limits are set taking into account the maximum permitted amount of impurities and the analytical error;

- the evaluation of the extent of degradation during storage (since the limits are intended to apply throughout the shelf life of the substance and not just at the time of release testing);
- a sufficient number of experimental results obtained on several batches (at least three), if possible, of different origins and ages.

6.2.1.4 Qualitative properties of the pharmaceutical substance

The statements under this heading are not to be interpreted in a strict sense and are not to be regarded as analytical requirements. Caution statements may be included here.

The principal characteristics that may be referred to are:

- appearance;
- solubility;
- stability factors;
- hygroscopicity;
- solid-state properties;
- other characteristics, as necessary.

6.2.1.5 Identification

The tests given in the identification section are not designed to give a full confirmation of the chemical structure or composition of the substance. They are intended to give confirmation, with an acceptable degree of assurance, that the substance is the one stated on the label. The specificity of the identification should be such that pharmaceutical substances exhibiting similar structures can be distinguished. When an identification series is being investigated it is desirable that other similar substances, whether or not they are the subject of monographs of the pharmacopoeia, are examined at the same time to ensure that a particular combination of tests within a series will successfully distinguish one similar substance from another. False-positive reactions caused by the presence of known impurities should be avoided.

Some of the purity tests in a monograph may also be suitable for identification purposes, possibly in a modified form. A system of cross-references to the section(s) can be exploited. This is particularly relevant in cases where distinction between closely related materials depends on properties that are also parameters in purity or composition control. In some cases an organic impurity procedure may be introduced to differentiate the analyte from similar, common, dangerous adulterants.

In the case of monographs for similar pharmaceutical substances, identification of the type of substances may be supplemented by selective but discriminating tests to identify individual members of the group.

6.2.1.6 Impurities and other tests

Certain tests may apply to special grades (e.g. parenteral preparations, dialysis solutions) or a test may have a special limit for a particular use: the particular application of a test/limit is indicated within the test.

6.2.1.6.1 *Organic impurities*

This section is principally directed at limiting impurities in chemical substances.

In the interests of transparency, information may be included on the impurities controlled by a test and the approximate equivalent (e.g. percentage or parts per million) of the prescribed limit in terms of the defined impurities or class of impurities.

Monographs should include tests and acceptance criteria for impurities that are likely to occur in substances used in approved medicinal products, insofar as the necessary information and samples (substance and impurities) are available from the producers.

Monographs on organic chemicals usually have a test entitled "Related substances" (or a test with equivalent purpose under a different title), designed to control related organic impurities. Impurities to be controlled include intermediates and by-products of synthesis, co-extracted substances in products of natural origin and degradation products.

Monographs on pharmaceutical substances should take account of the principles defined in ICH guideline Q3A (R2) (*Impurities in new drug substances*), or comparable guidelines, and follow regulatory decision-making. Products of fermentation and semi-synthetic products derived therefrom should be limited applying the same principles, but should be covered by thresholds considered appropriate for these substances. The same principle applies to excipients.

Unusually potent or toxic impurities. In addition to the above-mentioned requirements, impurities that are unusually potent or produce toxic or unexpected pharmacological effects need to be specifically considered. In this context, requirements for genotoxic impurities may be followed.

Monographs frequently have to be designed to cover different impurity profiles because of the use of different synthetic routes and purification procedures.

For pharmacopoeial purposes the objective of a purity test using a separation method will usually be the control of impurities derived from one or more known manufacturing processes and decomposition routes. However, the experimental conditions, especially the detection system, are chosen for the test so as not to make it unnecessarily narrow in scope.

Where monographs include a chromatographic method, this should provide a reliable means of locating all specified impurities on the chromatogram.

6.2.1.6.2 *Inorganic impurities*

Inorganic impurities include reagents, ligands and catalysts, elemental impurities, inorganic salts and other materials such as filter aids (where relevant).

Where known impurities are present, these are typically covered by specific tests.

6.2.1.6.3 *Residual solvents*

When applicable, residual solvents need to be controlled, for example, as outlined in the ICH guideline Q3C (Impurities: guideline for residual solvents).

6.2.1.6.4 *Other tests*

The following tests should be considered, but are not limited to:

- foreign anions and/or cations;
- loss on drying;
- semi-micro determination of water (Karl Fischer);
- micro determination of water (colorimetric titration);
- sulfated ash/residue on ignition;
- residue on evaporation;
- sterility;
- microbiological quality;
- bacterial endotoxins.

6.2.1.7 Assay

Assays are included in monographs unless, for example:

- all the foreseeable impurities can be detected and limited with sufficient precision;
- certain quantitative tests, similar to assays, are carried out with sufficient precision;
- the tests performed are sufficient to establish the quality of the substance (usually a non-active ingredient, for example, ethanol and water).

In certain cases more than one assay may be necessary, for example, when the substance to be examined consists of a combination of two parts that are not necessarily present in absolutely fixed proportions, so that the assay of only one of the two constituents does not make it possible to determine correctly the content of the substance as a whole.

In the case of well-defined salts, the assay of only one of the components, preferably the pharmacologically active component, is generally considered sufficient.

6.2.2 Monographs for finished pharmaceutical products

General tests and acceptance criteria that are applied to a specific pharmaceutical dosage form (and are not specific to a particular formulation) may be grouped together, for example, uniformity of mass/content, friability and disintegration as applied to tablet testing. These tests may be included in a general monograph for a pharmaceutical dosage form, in this example, tablets, as the test procedures are the same for all tablets.

Specific tests group together those procedures that are required to provide evidence that an FPP is of a suitable quality, and are specific to a particular pharmaceutical dosage form. As an example, tests described in tablet monographs may include identification, related substances, assay and dissolution. Specific tests are designed to control the purity, composition and release; these tests are dependent on the pharmaceutical substance.

Prior to the preparation of any monograph it is essential to gather as much information as possible on the product in question. In particular it is necessary to ascertain:

- if the FPP contains a mixture or a single pharmaceutical substance;
- if the FPP can be prepared from different entities (e.g. acid, base or salt);
- in cases where the pharmaceutical substance exhibits polymorphism, if the crystallographic form of the entity should be identified in the FPP monograph;
- if the FPP is available in different strengths, whether all strengths can be controlled under one monograph.

6.2.2.1 Monograph title

The titles of monographs for FPPs combine the name of the pharmaceutical substance and the pharmaceutical dosage form.

The pharmaceutical substance name should be based on the INN or national name, wherever it is available (the common name should be used where an INN or national name is not available). It is supplemented, when required, by the INNM. The name is followed by the nationally or regionally accepted pharmaceutical dosage form taxonomy (or published standard term).

For FPPs containing more than one pharmaceutical substance ("combination products"), the individual INNs should be used where possible.

Combination Names (Co-names) may exist in national pharmacopoeias for prescribing purposes.

6.2.2.2 General information to define the finished pharmaceutical product

Such information may include elements relating to the API, an expression of the content and other essential features of the dosage form. An appropriate reference to the relevant general monographs may be included.

The following should be observed:

- the pharmaceutical substance will be referred to in this section; it is not necessary to reproduce the defining information found in the pharmaceutical substance monograph within this section of the FPP monograph (e.g. the chemical name);
- any reference to producing a salt of the active moiety *in situ* during the manufacture of the FPP should be made in this section;
- the definition only refers to the name of the pharmaceutical substance; where the content is expressed in terms other than those described in the title of the monograph, the limits stated under "Content" (see 6.2.2.3) should reflect the label claim.

6.2.2.3 Content

Assay limits are specified between which the content of the pharmaceutical substance in the FPP must fall. Limits for each pharmaceutical substance (if more than one) or individual component are included. The assay limits must take account of the precision of the method as well as the strength of the FPP. Assay limits are normally expressed with reference to the active moiety or the label claim in accordance with the national or regional requirements.

Limits should be justified and account should be taken of:

- the strength of the FPP;
- the stability of the pharmaceutical substance in a specific FPP.

In the case of antibiotics determined by microbiological assay, the content limit is expressed in International Units (IU); where these exist a content limit is given in terms of a range, for example:

> "The precision of the assay is such that the fiducial limits of error are not less than 95% and not more than 105% of the estimated potency. The upper fiducial limit of error is not less than 97.0% and the lower fiducial limit of error is not more than 110.0% of the stated number of IU".

6.2.2.4 Identification

The tests given in the identification section are not designed to give a full confirmation of the chemical structure or composition of the API in the product. They are intended to give confirmation, with an acceptable degree of assurance, that the API(s) in the product is/are the one(s) stated on the label. Special attention must be given to the sample preparation to ensure that the API is adequately extracted from the sample matrix.

The minimum number of tests should be included, commensurate with providing adequate assurance of identity. For example, the monograph may contain at least two procedures to identify the API(s) in a pharmaceutical dosage form; one test per API may be sufficient if the technique used is considered to be a fingerprint of the active moiety (e.g. infrared absorption spectrophotometry).

6.2.2.5 Impurities and other tests

This section should include all of the specific tests that are required to prove the quality of the specific FPP.

The "Tests" section is intended to:

- limit the impurities within the FPP. This includes degradation impurities throughout the shelf life of the FPP and impurities that occur due to the manufacturing process. In certain circumstances it is necessary to control FPP impurities resulting from the synthesis of the pharmaceutical substance;
- ensure the homogeneity of the API(s) from dose to dose within the FPP;
- take account of the potential for the sample matrix to restrict the release of the active moiety in the FPP (i.e. a dissolution test in a monograph for tablets);
- limit the pyrogenic content of a parenteral FPP (i.e. a test for bacterial endotoxins or a monocyte activation test).

6.2.2.5.1 *Impurities: title of test(s)*

Where the test is intended to control specified and unspecified impurities, the title of the test should be "related substances" or "related compounds", or similar, in line with national or regional practices.

Where the test is intended to control one or a limited number of specified impurities the title of the test should indicate the impurity or impurities controlled.

6.2.2.5.2 *Related substances (or related compounds)*

Further to the section on pharmaceutical substance monographs, the following should be considered for related substances tests specified in FPP monographs:

- specific, quantitative techniques (i.e. high performance liquid chromatography (HPLC)) are preferred;
- non-specific or non-quantitative techniques should be used only if a specific method is not available or is unsuitable;
- methods should be developed with the aim of controlling degradation products and impurities. In certain circumstances it is necessary to control impurities from synthesis of the pharmaceutical substance in the FPP (for example, when they are detected in the test for related substances at a level greater than the limit for unspecified impurities);
- impurities being controlled at a level above the limit for unspecified impurities should be identified using a reference standard or other suitable techniques.

The principles outlined in, for example, ICH guideline Q3B (R2) (*Impurities in new drug products*) could be used as a starting point.

6.2.2.6 Performance testing

Depending on the dosage form, adequate performance testing may need to be included in the monograph. Such tests may include, but are not limited to, dissolution or deposition of the emitted dose.

6.2.2.7 Uniformity

Pharmaceutical preparations presented in single-dose units should comply with the test(s) as prescribed in the specific dosage form monograph.

Acceptance criteria will be specified regionally for a specific product or pharmaceutical form.

6.2.2.8 Other tests

The following tests should be considered, but are not limited to:

- sterility;
- bacterial endotoxins;
- microbiological quality;
- if necessary, tests for excipients such as antioxidants and antimicrobial agents.

6.2.2.9 Products of natural origin

Attention needs to be paid to the requirements in the different regions for minimizing the risk of transmitting animal spongiform encephalopathy agents via human and veterinary medicinal products.

6.2.2.10 Assay

The assay quantifies the amount of API in the FPP. It may also quantify certain excipients, such as preservatives, depending on national and regional legislation. Where possible the method used should be harmonized with that in the pharmaceutical substance monograph, but this may not be possible because of the sample matrix.

Assays are included in all FPP monographs unless certain quantitative tests, similar to assays, are carried out with sufficient precision (for example, uniformity of content, where a mean of individual results could be considered an accurate assay).

In certain cases more than one assay may be necessary, for example, where the FPP contains two or more APIs.

For products such as antibiotics, the results of the quantitative tests may not fully represent the therapeutic activity, in which case a microbiological assay and a test for composition are included.

Specific assays should be used where possible, for example, liquid or gas chromatography. Specific assays remove interference from excipients (formulation matrix) which could lead to significant errors when using non-specific assays.

Whenever possible, a stability-indicating procedure should be used for the assay. Generally, chromatographic procedures are preferred. When a non-stability-indicating assay is proposed, a separate stability-indicating impurity procedure should be provided.

7. Analytical test procedures and methods

Analytical test procedures and methods are employed to establish quality aspects such as identity, purity and content of pharmaceutical substances and FPPs. An analytical method and/or technique specified in a pharmacopoeia should be robust, reliable, accurate, precise, sensitive, specific and use readily available materials and equipment.

A pharmacopoeia provides different types of methods, mainly physical, physicochemical or chemical methods and microbiological tests, for the analysis of pharmaceutical substances and FPPs. The type of method applied for analysis depends on the nature of the substance or product.

The principles of method validation apply to all types of analytical procedures in a pharmacopoeia. However, it is the responsibility of the user to verify that a particular method is valid for the particular pharmaceutical substance or FPP being tested.

The validation of analytical procedures described in monographs should comply with the requirements as laid down, for example, in the *WHO*

Supplementary guidelines on good manufacturing practices: validation, Appendix 4 on Analytical method validation, in WHO Technical Report Series, No. 937, 2006, Annex 4, and ICH guideline Q2 (R1) (*Validation of analytical procedures: text and methodology*).

Annex 2

FIP–WHO technical guidelines: Points to consider in the provision by health-care professionals of children-specific preparations that are not available as authorized products

1. Introduction and scope

1.1 Background

Paediatric patients should have access to authorized, age-appropriate preparations of medicines that can be administered safely and effectively. Nothing in this document should detract from this objective. However, it is recognized that such preparations are not always available and in such cases a safe and effective alternative must be sought.

In the context of paediatric pharmacy practice, and for the purpose of this document, compounding is the technique applied by pharmacists to produce medicines from active pharmaceutical ingredients (APIs) or using authorized medicines when no commercially available, authorized, age-appropriate or adequate dosage form exists. Unless stated explicitly in this document, the compounded medicine is assumed to be dispensed immediately after preparation and not kept in stock. Compounding does not apply to reconstitution of authorized medicines prior to dispensing. A clarification of the terminology of preparation of medicines for children has been proposed by Ernest et al. 2012 (*1*).

The risks and benefits of compounding and of the alternatives should be fully understood by practitioners. Practitioners who do not have appropriate knowledge should seek advice.

Compared to the use of authorized medicines there are significant risks associated with compounding; quality, safety and efficacy can rarely all be assured, and many errors have been reported in the preparation of such medicines. In some situations compounding of a medicine for a child may be the only option, which may be supported by evidence of quality and occasionally evidence of bioavailability by industry or other parties, such as academia. There may be alternatives to compounding, which should also be considered, for example, use of a commercially available therapeutic alternative or manipulation of authorized dosage forms.

This points-to-consider document is supported by a literature review of the evidence available (*2*). An annex to the report contains an update on the abstracts and papers published in 2010–2015.

This document is to be considered as a time-limited document that addresses current needs for advice in the search for an alternative to an authorized, age-appropriate dosage form. Wherever possible the guidance is informed by the relevant evidence. However, the evidence base is weak or non-existent in most situations. Consequently, the guidance is predominantly informed by best practice, based on sound scientific and therapeutic principles and expert consensus. Although the guidance takes the form of a working practical document it is important to invite comment and input from interested practitioners so that the guidance can be developed further in response to feedback. The document addresses mainly paediatric medicines for oral administration; comments and proposals concerning other routes of administration are invited as well.

1.2 Purpose

The purpose of the document is to:

- provide evidence-based or best practice advice about alternatives to compounding of medicines for paediatric patients;
- describe the main potential problems of compounding and educate practitioners on how to avoid them;
- provide brief advice on compounding;
- reduce the risk of providing children-specific preparations without informed knowledge.

The document will not reproduce guidance and standards that already exist (e.g. good manufacturing practices (GMP) standards for facilities and documentation). Where appropriate, reference is made to the relevant resources and publications.

1.3 Target audience and health-care settings

The document is intended for a wide audience of health-care stakeholders including:

- all practitioners involved in health care of the paediatric population but mainly pharmacists, physicians, paediatricians and nursing staff;
- national medicines regulatory authorities and professional bodies, e.g. national paediatric organizations and national pharmacy associations;
- general hospitals and health clinics;
- specialized paediatric hospitals and primary care clinics;
- the pharmaceutical industry, given its role in providing information.

Pharmaceutical manufacturers can often provide useful information on validated compounded formulas and other information relating to the manipulations and specific characteristics of formulations.

2. Glossary

The definitions given below apply to the terms used in these guidelines. They may have different meanings in other contexts.

active pharmaceutical ingredient (API). Any substance or mixture of substances intended to be used in the manufacture or compounding of a pharmaceutical dosage form and that, when so used, becomes an active ingredient of that pharmaceutical dosage form. Such substances are intended to furnish pharmacological activity or other direct effect in the diagnosis, cure, mitigation, treatment or prevention of disease, or to affect the structure and function of the body.

authorized dosage form. A pharmaceutical dosage form that has been authorized by the competent authority to be marketed for the treatment of specific indications.

beyond-use date. The date after which a compounded preparation should not be stored, transported or used; the date is determined from the date or time the preparation is compounded. It is also known as the *expiry date*.

compounding. Preparation under the supervision of a pharmacist following national legislation of an unlicensed medicine to meet the specific needs of a patient when no suitable authorized dosage form is available. This may involve preparation from the authorized dosage form or from the active pharmaceutical ingredient and usually involves addition of excipients to produce an acceptable product.

dispensing pharmacy. The pharmacy receiving the prescription for a patient and providing the pharmaceutical preparation to the patient. For compounded medicines, the dispensing pharmacy is not necessarily the compounding pharmacy.

dose rounding. Amending a dose that has been calculated accurately on the basis of body weight or surface area to correspond with an amount of the dosage form that is easy to measure and administer. Account of therapeutic index should be taken before rounding the dose.

excipient. A substance or compound, other than the active pharmaceutical ingredient and packaging materials, that is intended or designated to be used in the manufacture or compounding of a pharmaceutical product.

expiry date. The date after which a compounded preparation should not be stored, transported or used; the date is determined from the date or time the preparation is compounded. It is also known as *beyond-use date*.

good manufacturing practices. A system of practice and processes to assure the quality and safety of manufactured pharmaceutical products, specified in, for example, WHO guidelines.

labelling information. Information to the user provided on the container or package label or in the patient information leaflet.

manipulation of a dosage form. Authorized dosage forms may be manipulated (or modified), often at the point of administration, to provide the appropriate dose (e.g. by segmenting tablets) or to facilitate administration (e.g. by crushing a tablet and adding to food).

pharmaceutical dosage form. The physical form in which a medicine is presented; the name of a dosage form combines its physical form and the intended route of administration, e.g. a tablet (to be swallowed), oral suspension (liquid suspension of solid particles intended for oral intake and swallowing).

route of administration. The way in which a medicine is given to a patient, e.g. oral administration (administration via the oral route), rectal administration (administration to the rectum), parenteral administration (administration via the blood, muscular or subcutaneous routes).

summary of product characteristics. Summary of product characteristics approved by the competent authority. The information may alternatively be presented in the container or package label.

verification. A process of providing any type of adequate evidence, e.g. new (bio)analytical data, from the literature or by referencing to existing practices to support that the proposed modification will not change the pharmaceutical characteristics of the original preparation in a way that will negatively impact the safety and/or efficacy of the medicine.

3. Alternatives to compounding

Before deciding to compound, consider possible alternatives that will give the greatest assurance of clinical effectiveness and safety.

The main alternatives to compounding are described below.

3.1 Sourcing of a commercially-available (marketed) or manufactured product[1] if available

A marketed, authorized, age-appropriate finished pharmaceutical preparation should always be sourced when available. Where appropriate and in accordance with the national regulations, this could include:

- off-label use of a medicine authorized in the country where the medicine is to be dispensed;
- (off-label) use of an imported product authorized in the country of origin;
- use of a manufactured product made in authorized facilities in the country where the medicine is to be dispensed.

[1] This includes products prepared to GMP standards, for example, at an accredited hospital manufacturing unit.

The logistics of supply, costs and access are obvious factors that might present obstacles, but practitioners should liaise with suppliers, importers and regulatory authorities to access these products if possible.

Importation of products may be expensive, and reputable suppliers should be used to avoid spurious/falsely-labelled/falsified/counterfeit (SFFC) medicines. Quality assurance systems should be in place, for example, to ensure that recall systems are available and that information is provided in the local language.

The use of compounded products for children should not be justified on the grounds that they are cheaper than marketed products. Other options, including local manufacture in accordance with GMP standards, should be investigated.

3.2 Dose rounding

If the dose prescribed does not correspond to a dosage form that is commercially available, consider whether the dose can be suitably amended while maintaining safety and efficacy.

The therapeutic index of the medicine and patient characteristics need to be considered before making a decision.

Some medicine doses are calculated accurately on the basis of body weight, yet the therapeutic index is such that one dose can be used for a broad age and weight band. Consult the WHO Model formulary for children.[2]

3.3 Therapeutic alternatives

If a medicine is prescribed in a formulation that is not available, e.g. in an age-appropriate form, consider the possibility of using a commercially available medicine with a similar therapeutic action, which is available in a more suitable form. Examples are presented in Appendix 1.

3.4 Manipulation of dosage forms

In situations where the prescribed dose is different from what is marketed, or there are administration-related difficulties, the possibilities for manipulation of a dosage form as outlined below can be considered. Formularies or manufacturer's information, if available, and the labelling or the summary of product characteristics (SmPC) should be consulted.

A report with evidence-based guidelines on the manipulation of medicines to obtain the required dose for children was published by the

[2] Available from: http://apps.who.int/medicinedocs/en/m/abstract/Js17151e/.

Manipulation of Drugs Required in Children (MODRIC) research group in 2013 (*3*).

The practitioner should bear in mind that manipulation, such as tablet splitting, tablet/capsule dispersion, or tablet crushing and mixing with food or drink, may increase the potential for inaccurate dosing and may affect the efficacy, stability and bioavailability of the dosage form, in particular when mixed with food or drink. Excipients that are safe for adults may not necessarily be so for children.

When medicines are mixed with food or drink, including breast milk for very young children, an unpleasant tasting mixture may cause aversion in the child. In addition, the compatibility of the product with the food, drink or breast milk will need to be taken into account. Where a child shows signs of refusal or aversion other options should be considered.

3.4.1 Tablet splitting

Not all tablets should be split. In general, those with a sustained-release or enteric coating should not be split, but it may be possible to split tablets with a sustained-release matrix. Formularies or manufacturer's information, if available, and the product label or SmPC should be consulted.

Some tablets allow splitting, either by breaking, if scored, or by using a tablet cutter designed for the purpose. If the child is able to take solid dosage forms safely, a tablet segment can be given; otherwise it can be dispersed or mixed with food or drink as described below in section 3.4.3.

Tablets without a score line cannot, in general, be split into uniform segments meeting relevant uniformity requirements. Information about possible splitting of such tablets may however be provided in the SmPC or on the label. Tablet splitting was reviewed by Freeman et al. (2012) (*4*).

Consider on a case-by-case basis whether splitting of tablets might lead to toxicity or reduced effect as a result of inaccurate dosing or an effect on the release profile. This is especially important in situations where the API is potent or has a narrow therapeutic index, if there is a lack of appropriate information, or if an accurate dose cannot be assured.

Consideration should be given to splitting tablets with an appropriate commercial tablet splitter in the pharmacy. If possible, tablets with score lines and uniform distribution of the API should be sourced and information sought on the stability of segments. If carers are cutting segments, they should be given a suitable tablet splitter and receive adequate instruction on the method for preparing and storing tablet segments.

3.4.2 Tablet/capsule dispersion for oral administration

It may be possible to disperse immediate-release tablets or the contents of capsules in water or another liquid. If the tablet disperses, the tablet or a fraction of it can be dispersed in a small volume appropriate for the child concerned and the whole dose given when a suspension is formed, or mixed with a flavoured vehicle if required. To ensure that the whole dose is administered the measuring device should be rinsed and the resulting solution or suspension administered. It is necessary to consider the impact of dispersion and the risk of interactions with the vehicle on the bioavailability.

Conventional tablets do not disperse readily but some form a suspension within a short time. Soluble tablets and dispersible tablets disintegrate and dissolve or disperse within a short time in water at room temperature.

If the tablet disperses in a known volume of water to form a stable suspension, a fractional dose can be appropriately measured with a syringe. As extraction of soluble API from the tablet may be incomplete, the suspension should be shaken or stirred before measuring the dose and not filtered unless it has been established that the API is fully dissolved. Dose uniformity of the prepared suspension cannot be assured and the risk of overdosing or underdosing must be considered. This may depend on the volume of prepared suspension that is to be extracted for administration. Any such tablet (whether a dispersible or conventional-release tablet) compounded to a dispersion or solution should be administered immediately after preparation and the remainder should be discarded.

When the dispersion is intended for tube feeding, parameters such as particle size, viscosity, dosing volume and compatibility of the oral preparation with the tube material should be considered. Dispersions may be too viscous or may contain large particles that can mean that administration by feeding tube is not feasible. Adsorption of API to the tube material results in inappropriate dosing; this concern is most relevant for lipophilic and low-dose potent APIs.

WHO is promoting the use of flexible solid oral dosage forms such as dispersible tablets (*5*). Custom-made dispersible tablets for paediatric dosing should be used wherever possible but it is still necessary to ensure that carers understand how they are to be administered.

3.4.3 Crushing tablets/opening capsules and mixing powder with food or drink

The practice of crushing tablets or opening capsules and adding the powder to a palatable drink or sprinkling it onto solid food has been reviewed (*6*). Although common, there may be little evidence to support the efficacy and safety of this practice since stability and bioavailability may be altered. With the exception of multiple-unit preparations, which can be opened and administered without affecting efficacy and safety, modified-release tablets and capsules cannot be crushed or opened without affecting bioavailability and/or stability, and this should therefore not be done. Insoluble tablet excipients are in suspension and may compromise product appearance, whereas soluble excipients may alter stability, for example, by changing the pH of the preparation.

In the case of potent APIs, consider the risks associated with handling of powdered material to parents or carers.

In general, the decision on whether to crush tablets should be based on bioavailability and acceptability studies. Information should be sought from manufacturers (e.g. the label or SmPC and website) and formularies whenever possible. The process is acceptable only if bioavailability is not affected by food or drink, and the product has to be used immediately to minimize stability problems.

It is difficult to ensure that a complete dose has been taken and the practice of nurses and carers handling powdered medicines may present health concerns. Tablet dispersion may be a simpler, more reliable and potentially safer method.

Liquid-filled capsules should generally not be opened since it is difficult to remove and measure the total contents.

3.4.4 Giving the injectable form by the oral route

Oral administration is possible for some injections. If the injectable form of the API is the same as the oral form (for example, labetalol hydrochloride, ondansetron hydrochloride) it can be assumed that the API will be absorbed enterally from the injectable formulation. However, as the API is in solution, more rapid absorption and higher peak levels may occur than would result from the slower absorption from a solid oral dosage form. When evaluating whether an injection is suitable for oral use, specialist advice, e.g. consultation with a medicines information centre in the region, should be sought because there are important factors which must be considered, e.g. first-pass effect, oral bioavailability, gastric acidity (e.g. effect on stability), pH effects (e.g. precipitation of soluble salts of weak acids) and palatability.

Injections may contain excipients that may have undesirable effects in some patients, e.g. propylene glycol and ethanol. The pH of some injections may be high or low and they should therefore not be given orally, or alternatively should be diluted before administration to avoid irritation. The taste of the injectable form may not be known and may not be acceptable. Advice should be sought from the manufacturer and from experts to assist in deciding whether the injectable form can be administered orally.

3.4.5 Splitting suppositories

There is little information available on the accuracy with which suppositories can be split. Splitting is usually associated with major problems with regard to accurate dosing and is therefore generally discouraged. Most commercially available suppositories are formulated as suspensions, which means that sedimentation of the solid API particles may occur during solidification of the suppository; therefore, if suppositories need to be split, this should be done lengthwise.

Therapeutic index and the consequences of over- or underdosing should be taken into account when determining whether it is safe to split suppositories. If possible, this should be done in the pharmacy.

3.4.6 Rectal administration

There may be opportunities to give oral or injectable dosage forms by rectal administration (*7*).

3.4.7 General advice when changing the route of administration

Whenever a change of the route of administration for an authorized medicine is considered, advice should be sought from formularies and the literature and even from specialists. In general, altering the route of administration results in a different pharmacokinetic profile introducing a high risk of dosing errors and may compromise safety and efficacy. Hence, this practice is generally discouraged.

4. Compounding

4.1 Good manufacturing practices aspects

The dispensing pharmacy receives the prescription for a patient and provides the pharmaceutical preparation to the patient. For compounded medicines the dispensing pharmacy is not necessarily the compounding pharmacy. Regardless of where the product is compounded the dispensing pharmacy is responsible for ensuring the safety and quality of the product.

When a batch of non-authorized medicine is prepared, including for stock, the preparing pharmacy or hospital unit should meet – depending on a risk assessment – the GMP or good pharmacopoeial practices (GPhP) requirements pertaining to personnel, premises and equipment, quality assurance system, documentation and product dossier. Further, an authorization by the competent authority to carry out operations may be needed, in accordance with the national legislation. In this respect, one should refer to the relevant international and national guidance and to other guidelines, including WHO guidelines on GMP (*8*, *9*), the Pharmaceutical Inspection Co-operation Scheme (PIC/S) GPP *Guide to good practices for the preparation of medicinal products in healthcare establishments* (*10*) and corresponding national guidelines.

When compounding is a one-off event, the intended prescription should be prepared for an identified individual patient for immediate dispensing. In such cases requirements may be less strict. Nevertheless, certain requirements need to be met:

- the preparing pharmacy should have appropriate premises and equipment;
- the pharmacist and staff, or entitled persons, must have sufficient training and background for compounding;
- access to relevant literature (e.g. pharmacopoeias, formularies, handbooks and scientific journals) and the Internet must be available;
- general instructions for the preparation of each dosage form should be available;
- a record on each preparation should be retained showing the calculations, key processing and packaging steps, and also including the name of the person responsible for each step.

4.2 Some potential problems

In some situations, for example, if the method of preparation and the stability of an oral liquid are well documented, e.g. if compounding has been supported by evidence of quality, stability data and occasionally evidence of bioavailability by industry or other parties, such as academia, and all facilities and ingredients are available, it may be less pressing to seek an alternative to compounding. On the other hand, if there are no stability data and, for example, the API forms a caking suspension in the only available excipients (e.g. a syrup), an alternative must be considered to ensure safe and effective treatment.

In any case, the decision on how to prepare and/or provide an unlicensed preparation should be based on an assessment of risks and benefits of the dosing strategy. On a case-by-case basis, potential benefits from their use should be weighed against all possible risks arising from preparation and administration of such medicines. Even in cases where the compounded preparation can be considered a verified formulation, the impact of compounding on bioavailability may not be known.

Formulation of a compounded medicine is associated with a number of potential problems that may impact on its safety and effectiveness. Awareness of the relative complexity of the formulation and of the things that can go wrong will help to avoid such problems. Guidance on compounding has been published (e.g. *11*). A review of extemporaneous compounding is also available (*12*).

Consideration must be given to the properties of the API (e.g. aqueous solubility, pH effect on solubility, particle size, polymorphism) and stability of both API and the compounded formulation, i.e. chemical, physical and microbiological instability.

Care must also be taken in the selection of excipients and their safety in relation to the age of the child as well as any possible adverse effects of the "inactive" components of the preparation should be considered. The use of preservatives, ethanol and sugars must be carefully considered. Some guidance and literature references on the formulation can be found in *Development of paediatric medicines: points to consider in formulation* (*5*).

4.2.1 Oral liquids

Deterioration of an oral liquid may be a result of chemical, physical or microbiological instability which can lead to a subtherapeutic dose of the medicine, exposure to toxic degradation products or ingestion of unacceptable numbers of microorganisms. It is important for pharmacists, clinicians and nursing staff to be aware of potential problems caused by instability and microbial contamination to ensure that any medicine used is effective and safe.

APIs in compounded liquids may be susceptible to chemical reactions leading to degradation. Publications reporting the stability of compounded paediatric preparations include a review by Glass and Haywood 2013 (*13*). The most common reactions are *hydrolysis*, oxidation and reduction. Usually the reaction rate or type is influenced by pH. Other factors that may increase the rate of reaction include the presence of trace metals which catalyse the oxidation of captopril, methyldopa or exposure to light, which catalyses the oxidative degradation of 6-mercaptopurine. The rate of chemical degradation usually increases with temperature.

The API in the preparation may be totally or partially in solution or predominantly in the solid state as a suspension. APIs in solution are more susceptible to chemical degradation than APIs in the solid state (i.e. suspensions); thus suspensions of acetazolamide and chlorothiazide are more stable than solutions. However, it cannot be assumed that a compounded suspension is always more stable than a solution. In a suspension, an equilibrium exists between the API in the solid state and an API in solution, and even though the amount of API dissolved may be minimal, the conditions could be optimal for degradation. Furosemide is a notable example: it undergoes hydrolysis in acidic conditions where the solid state is predominant, but is much more stable at alkaline pH where it is totally in solution.

Preparations made from tablets contain excipients such as binders and disintegrating agents in addition to the API. These excipients may reduce chemical stability by changing the pH to a value at which more rapid degradation occurs. This probably explains why amiloride solution prepared from pure API is more stable than an oral liquid prepared from tablets.

Hygroscopicity and/or moisture-sensitivity of the API also play a key role in degradation. These characteristics of the API(s) should be understood before compounding from a tablet to a liquid form. A common example of such an API is tenofovir disoproxil fumurate.

Dispersions and suspensions of medicine with low therapeutic index require special consideration with regard to efficient resuspension to avoid medication error.

4.2.2 Microbial contamination

Microbial growth in an oral liquid may cause a foul odour and turbidity and adversely affect palatability and appearance. High titres of microorganisms may be hazardous to health especially in very young or immunocompromised patients. By-products of microbial metabolism may cause a change in the pH of the preparation and reduce the chemical stability or solubility of the API. Microbial contamination during preparation must be minimized by using clean equipment, water of adequate quality and by avoiding contaminated raw materials and containers. If sodium benzoate or benzoic acid are used as antimicrobial preservatives, the final pH must be less than 5 so that the active unionized form is predominant. Consequently the API must also be stable at this pH.

Many factors can reduce the effectiveness of the preservative, including use of contaminated materials, chemical degradation, binding of preservative to suspending agents or tablet excipients, incorrect storage or unhygienic use of the final product.

4.3 Basic considerations

- *Quality of API and excipients*

  It is important to ensure that the API and the excipients meet pharmacopoeial standards with regard to both identity and purity. The choice of excipients should be restricted to those that have been used in authorized medicines intended for the same route of administration and at similar concentrations.

- *Consider use of an authorized dosage form as a starting point*

  It may be safer and more effective to crush tablets or use the contents of hard capsules with an appropriate suspending vehicle than to prepare medicines from an API and excipients. There are many formulations available with a validated shelf life but sourcing of suspending agents may be difficult and/or expensive.

  There might be instances when a pharmacist crushes a number of tablets or opens a number of capsules, dilutes the powder with a suitable excipient and doses the powder in ready-to-use single-dose sachets. Before doing so, consider the stability of the preparation, including stability with respect to humidity and exposure to air.

- *Consult literature and guidelines if available*

  Use a validated formulation whenever possible (i.e. based on literature, stability studies and guidelines). Consult product information and the latest national and international guidelines and/or a specialist information centre if possible.

- *Potential medication error*

  Medication errors in preparing compounded medicines occur often, and some have resulted in serious harm to patients or even in death. The potential for medication error must be recognized and steps taken to minimize the risk. As a minimum, this will include the use of a worksheet listing the formulation ingredients and the identity of the ingredients; quantities, calculations and measurements should be double-checked by trained personnel and signatures provided. The pharmacist responsible should check the final product and label against the signed worksheet, ingredients and prescription.

- *Exercise caution in extrapolating from other formulations*

  Caution is required when extrapolating the formulation from a published study or formulary. Formulations made from APIs may be more stable than formulations made from solid dose forms and vice versa. Tablet and capsule excipients can increase or decrease the stability of the API in an oral liquid preparation. The salt form of the API used in a published study could be different to the form locally available and this may affect its solubility, bioavailability and stability. Consult publications and pharmacopoeias, and seek specialist advice, if possible.

  Similarly, the results of a published study using an API mixed with a commercial suspending base cannot generally be extrapolated to a situation where the same API is mixed with a simple base of syrup or glycerol.

  Formulations for compounded medicines based on APIs and crushed tablets are not interchangeable.

- *Dose uniformity may be a problem – explain the importance of shaking prior to use*

  If the API is poorly soluble in water, uniformity of dosing may be a problem and a suspending agent will be required. Always check that the finished preparation resuspends under in-use conditions and explain the importance of resuspension by shaking to patients or their carers.

As excipients and other formulation components can affect solubility, all compounded liquid formulations should be shaken prior to administration. Some of the API may not be in solution even if it is highly soluble in water. The only exception would be if the preparation is made from pure API and it can be assured that the entire API is in solution.

Suppositories have sometimes been melted and recast into smaller moulds. This option is associated with a risk of recrystallization and of affecting the distribution and solubility of the API, resulting in over- or underdosing. Further, re-melting may affect degradant levels. Re-melting is therefore generally discouraged.

- *Exceptionally, when no published formulation is available*

  When no published formulation is available the pharmacist must assess the risks associated with the different options and use his or her knowledge and experience to formulate a product taking into account the need to:

  – obtain information on the physicochemical properties of the API if available.

    If possible, obtain basic physicochemical information about the API, especially its aqueous solubility at the expected pH of the final preparation. This allows a judgement to be made as to whether an API solution or suspension is formed at a particular dose-relevant concentration.

  – test the physical characteristics before using the preparation to treat a patient.

    FPPs of the same medicine may vary worldwide, especially with respect to the content of excipients. Such differences can influence the safety, efficacy and acceptability of the preparation. Basic performance tests should be done before the preparation is used in a patient, particularly on formulations prepared for the first time. Tests include ease of resuspension and pouring, degree of caking on storage, and observation of physical behaviour and characteristics.

  – consider risk of microbial growth.

    All compounded liquid formulations are highly susceptible to microbial growth. Oral liquids that are not adequately preserved will support rapid growth of bacteria and fungi especially at warm to hot temperatures and can pose hazards to patients especially those who are immunosuppressed. An antimicrobial preservative should be included if the final product is likely to be used beyond 2–3 days, even when it is stored under refrigeration.

The effects of the addition of the preservative on interactions between pH, stability and effectiveness of the preservative should be carefully taken into account.

Compounded liquids should be prepared under conditions that minimize the introduction of microbial contaminants.

- *Use appropriate final containers*

  Final containers and closures should be clean and free from dust and other residues. Use of new containers is recommended. Containers that are reused should be thoroughly washed, rinsed with sterile or freshly boiled water and dried. Light-protective (e.g. dark plastic or amber glass) containers should generally be used.

  Consider the use of a light-protective wrapping such as foil if a light-protective container is not available. When selecting the final container, consider the interactions between the container and the product, for example, the possibility of adsorption to plastic containers.

- *Dosing device*

  For liquid preparations, the feasibility of appropriate dosing should be confirmed bearing in mind that not all dosing devices may allow delivery of the required volume. Most compounded liquids should be shaken prior to administration and this may introduce entrapped air in the liquid, which could cause problems with accurate measurement of small volumes.

- *Consider in-use storage*

  In-use storage conditions may vary considerably from those in a published study or formulary recommendation. Always consider whether it will be possible to store and use the preparation under the optimal conditions described in the study; usually refrigeration, protection from light and minimal possibility of in-use contamination. If these conditions are not possible locally it can be assumed that the preparation will be less stable and more susceptible to microbial growth. Reduce the shelf life according to professional judgement. If possible, obtain expert advice.

- *Expiry date*

  It is recommended that each compounded preparation be given an expiry date assigned in a conservative way and taking into account

API-specific and general stability documentation and relevant literature when available.

When an authorized medicine is used as the source of the API, stability information can be obtained from the manufacturer. Otherwise, applicable information on stability, compatibility and degradation of ingredients, and use has to be sought in the literature.

Stability may be formulation-dependent and is likely to change with any manipulation of the product. Most studies base their expiry date recommendation on chemical stability but do not address possible physical or microbiological spoilage which may be significant during actual use of the product. Whereas compounded preparations will normally be freshly prepared, the storage and shelf life during use need to be considered, in particular if it becomes impractical to prepare the product immediately prior to dispensing each time it is needed.

The assignment of an expiry date serves to ensure suitability for use and will encourage regular fresh preparations. It also allows the practitioner to regularly review the patient's use of the preparation.

The following aspects should be considered when determining an expiry date:

- nature of the API and its degradation mechanisms;
- dosage form and its components;
- potential for microbial proliferation in the preparation;
- container in which the preparation is packaged;
- expected storage conditions; and
- the intended duration of therapy.

The in-use conditions, for example, access to a refrigerator for storage, should be taken into account when establishing the expiry date.

- *Give clear instructions to caregivers and patients*

The instructions given to caregivers and patients may include instructions on storage, resuspension, changes in taste, smell, appearance, adverse effects and other pharmaceutical advice.

Compounded dosage forms are sometimes added to a small amount of liquid (e.g. water or juice) or sprinkled onto small amounts of food. Consideration should be given to the effect of food on bioavailability and to the risk that only part of the dose will be swallowed. Provide parents and carers with appropriate information.

If an oral syringe or other measuring device is used it is important to check the technique to ensure that the correct dose is administered. Advise the use of clean measuring devices and explain how to avoid contaminating the preparation when preparing the dose.

- *Label information*

  In addition to dosage instructions, include at least the following information, subject to national regulations for the labelling of medicines:

  - if applicable, the name of the pharmaceutical preparation;
  - the route of administration;
  - the name(s) of the API(s) and excipients of known pharmacological action, and adverse effects, e.g. antimicrobial agents, antioxidants;
  - if the preparation is a liquid, give the concentration(s) of the API(s), e.g. in mg/mL, and the amount or volume of the preparation in the container;
  - if the preparation is a solid, give amount(s) of the API(s) in each dose and the number of doses in the container;
  - reference or batch number (or date of preparation);
  - expiry date ("do not use after ...");
  - any special storage conditions and handling precautions that may be necessary, e.g. "to be shaken before use", "shelf life during use";
  - the pharmacy name and contact information;
  - name of the patient.

  Consider adding pictograms to supplement the label information, e.g. for "to be shaken well" and "store in the refrigerator".

- *Document concerns and share information*

  Practitioners are encouraged to maintain a dialogue with regulatory bodies and international agencies and networks about problems and concerns associated with the preparation and availability of age-appropriate medicines for children. The sharing of solutions to problems is also important.

5. Information, availability and access

A number of networks, websites and other resources are available which provide information on standards of practice, formulas for compounded preparations, manufacturers, suppliers of oral liquid formulations and responsive information services. These should be consulted by practitioners and regulators to enable them to provide the safest and most effective treatment options for children who require an age-appropriate formulation.

5.1 Standards of practice and guidelines

Some national, regional and international guidelines for extemporaneous formulations and medicines administration to children have been published. Consulting these documents may assist in forming local policies on practice and educational activities for practitioners.

5.2 Formularies and compendia

Formularies and compendia may be helpful in providing formulation advice and general advice on dosage manipulations. The information in these formularies may be difficult to transfer to a local situation where the base ingredients (e.g. commercial suspending bases, antimicrobial preservatives, pure API powder) are not readily available.

In addition to formularies and compendia, information can be sought in:

- the eMixt database (www.pharminfotech.co.nz), which provides comprehensive information for all settings and environments;
- *Handbook of extemporaneous preparations* (*11*), which contains formulations and associated stability summaries for oral liquid preparations;
- *Improving medicines for children*, by the Council of Canadian Academies, which contains a comprehensive review of paediatric medicines (*14*);
- The International Journal of Pharmaceutical Compounding, which is a general source of information. It is a subscription-only journal, but the contents can be searched on the journal's website (http://www.ijpc.com).

5.3 Source and supply

A database of sources and prices of medicines for children has been compiled by the United Nations Children's Fund (UNICEF) (*15*) and the UNICEF catalogue (https://supply.unicef.org) provides examples without being exhaustive.

Countries may also have their own database to use to find suppliers of age-appropriate formulations for paediatric use.

5.4 Networks and information services

- Local, national and international medicines information centres may respond to questions about formulation. One example is the WHO Paediatric medicines Regulatory Network (PmRN) (http://www.who.int/childmedicines/paediatric_regulators/en/). Partnerships and twinning arrangements between hospitals in poorly-resourced countries and developed countries can be explored and are often beneficial.
- Questions can be posted via the eMixt website (www.pharminfotech.co.nz).
- Sharing of information and advice on paediatric formulations should be explored whenever possible.
- International discussion lists can be useful for posting questions on formulations and their archives can be searched for previous questions and answers. Examples include eDrug and INDICES (accessed via www.asksource.info/resources/essentialdrugsorg).

References

1. Ernest TB, Craig J, Nunn A, Salunke S, Tuleu C, Breitkreutz J, et al. Preparation of medicines for children – a hierarchy of classification. Int Journal Pharm. 2012;435(2): 124–30. doi: 10.1016/j.ijpharm.2012.05.070.
2. Nunn T, Hill S, Secretary, WHO Expert Committee on the Selection and Use of Essential Medicines. Report for WHO on findings of a review of existing guidance/advisory documents on how medicines should be administered to children, including general instructions on extemporaneous preparations and manipulation of adult dosage forms. Geneva: World Health Organization; 2011 (working document QAS/11.400 – available on request) (http://www.who.int/medicines/areas/quality_safety/quality_assurance/Review-findings-PaediatricMedicnesAdmin_QAS11-400Rev1_22082011.pdf, accessed 20 November 2015).
3. MODRIC. Manipulation of drugs for children – a guideline for health professionals. Liverpool: Alder Hey Children's NHS Trust (http://www.alderhey.nhs.uk/wp-content/uploads/MODRIC_Guideline_FULL-DOCUMENT.pdf, accessed 20 November 2015).
4. Freeman MK, White W, Iranikhah M. Tablet splitting: a review of weight and content uniformity. Consult Pharm. 2012;27(5):341–52. doi: 10.4140/TCP.n.2012.341.
5. Development of paediatric medicines: points to consider in formulation. In: WHO Expert Committee on Specifications for Pharmaceutical Preparations: forty-sixth report. Geneva: World Health Organization; 2012: Annex 5 (WHO Technical Report Series, No. 970).
6. Anon. Crushing tablets or opening capsules: many uncertainties, some established dangers. Prescrire Int. 2014; 23(152): 209–11, 213–14.

7. Smith S, Sharkey I, Campbell D. Guidelines for rectal administration of anticonvulsant medication in children. Paediatr Perinatal Drug Ther. 2001;4(4):140–7.
8. WHO good manufacturing practices: main principles for pharmaceutical products. In: WHO Expert Committee on Specifications for Pharmaceutical Preparations: forty-eighth report. Geneva: World Health Organization; 2014: Annex 2 (WHO Technical Report Series, No. 986).
9. Good manufacturing practices for pharmaceutical products. In: Quality assurance of pharmaceuticals. WHO guidelines, related guidance and GXP training materials. Geneva: World Health Organization; 2015 CD-ROM.
10. Pharmaceutical Inspection Co-operation Scheme. PE 010-3 Guide to good practices for the preparation of medicinal products in healthcare establishments. PICS; 2014 (http://www.picscheme.org/bo/commun/upload/document/pe-010-4-guide-to-good-practices-for-the-preparation-of-medicinal-products-in-healthcare-establishments-1.pdf, accessed 20 November 2015).
11. Jackson M, Lowey A. Handbook of extemporaneous preparation: A guide to pharmaceutical compounding. London: Pharmaceutical Press; 2010.
12. Patel VP, Desai TR, Chavda BG, Katira RM. Extemporaneous dosage form for oral liquids. Pharmacophore. 2011;2(2):86–103.
13. Glass BD, Haywood A. Liquid dosage forms extemporaneously prepared from commercially available products – Considering new evidence on stability. J Pharm Sci. 2006;9(3):398–426.
14. Council of Canadian Academies. Improving medicines for children in Canada. Ottawa: The Expert Panel on Therapeutic Products for Infants, Children, and Youth; 2014 (http://www.scienceadvice.ca/uploads/eng/assessments%20and%20publications%20and%20news%20releases/therapeutics/therapeutics_fullreporten.pdf, accessed 20 November 2015).
15. Sources and prices of selected medicines for children, including therapeutic food, dietary vitamin and mineral supplementation – 2nd edition. Geneva: UNICEF/WHO; 2010 (http://www.who.int/medicines/publications/sources_prices/en/, accessed 20 November 2015).

Further reading

The International Pharmacopoeia, fifth edition; 2015. Available online and CD-ROM version) (http://who.int/medicines/publications/pharmacopoeia/en/index.html).

Kastango ES, Trissel LA, Bradshaw BD. An ounce of prevention: Controlling hazards in extemporaneous compounding practices. Int. J Pharm. Compounding. 2003;7(5):401–16.

Pharmaceutical development for multisource (generic) pharmaceutical products. In: WHO Expert Committee on Specifications for Pharmaceutical Preparations: forty-sixth report. Geneva: World Health Organization; 2012: Annex 3 (WHO Technical Report Series, No. 970) (http://www.who.int/medicines/areas/quality_safety/quality_assurance/en/).

Pharmaceutical Inspection Co-operation Scheme (http://www.picscheme.org/). In particular the following documents can be downloaded free of charge: PE 009-9 (Part I); PIC/S GMP guide (Part I: Basic requirements for medicinal products); PE 010-3 Guide to good practices for the preparation of medicinal products in healthcare establishments.

Report of the Informal Expert Meeting on Dosage Forms of Medicines for Children. Geneva: World Health Organization; 2008 (http://www.who.int/selection_medicines/committees/expert/17/application/paediatric/Dosage_form_report DEC2008.pdf).

The WHO Model formulary for children. Geneva: World Health Organization; 2010 (http://www.who.int/selection_medicines/list/WMFc_2010.pdf).

Appendix 1

Examples of therapeutic alternatives to extemporaneous formulations

Required (available)	Possible alternative	Notes
diclofenac oral liquid (tablet)	naproxen oral suspension; ibuprofen oral liquid	The alternatives are available in some countries.
enalapril oral liquid (tablet)	captopril oral liquid (losartan oral suspension)	Captopril oral liquid is not available in all countries. Captopril has a shorter duration of action than enalapril. Enalapril tablets can be crushed and suspended in water immediately before use. Captopril tablets can be easily dispersed in water. Losartan may be appropriate for hypertension.
ibuprofen oral liquid (tablet)	paracetamol oral liquid	For pain and fever but not as an anti-inflammatory.
levamisole oral liquid (tablet)	albendazole chewable tablet; mebendazole oral liquid; pyrantel oral liquid	
lisinopril oral liquid (tablet)	ramipril oral liquid	
omeprazole oral liquid (capsule)	esomeprazole granules; lansoprazole orodispersible tablet	
praziquantel oral liquid (tablet)	niclosamide chewable tablet	Niclosamide can also be crushed and mixed with water to form a vanilla paste.
sertraline oral liquid (tablet)	fluoxetine oral liquid	

Table *continued*

Required (available)	Possible alternative	Notes
tinidazole oral liquid (tablet)	metronidazole oral liquid	Very few reasons why tinidazole should be preferred over metronidazole.
ciprofloxacin/ dexamethasone ear drops	ciprofloxacin/hydrocortisone ear drops	

Annex 3

WHO good manufacturing practices for biological products

Replacement[1] of Annex 1 of WHO Technical Report Series, No. 822

[1] It also replaces Annex 3 of the report of the Expert Committee on Specifications for Pharmaceutical Preparations, Technical Report Series, No. 834, and forms Annex 2 of the report of the Expert Committee on Biological Standardization, Technical Report Series, No. 993.

Guidelines published by WHO are intended to be scientific and advisory in nature. Each of the following sections constitutes guidance for national regulatory authorities (NRAs) and for manufacturers of biological products. If an NRA so desires, these WHO Guidelines may be adopted as definitive national requirements, or modifications may be justified and made by the NRA.

Abbreviations

AEFI	adverse event following immunization
ATMP	advanced therapy medicinal product
BCG	bacille Calmette–Guérin
GMP	good manufacturing practice(s)
HEPA	high-efficiency particulate air
HVAC	heating, ventilation and air conditioning
IgE	immunoglobulin E
mAb	monoclonal antibody
MCB	master cell bank
MSL	master seed lot
MVS	master virus seed
NRA	national regulatory authority
PDL	population doubling level
PQR	product quality review
PQS	pharmaceutical quality system
QRM	quality risk management
rDNA	recombinant DNA
SPF	specific pathogen free
TSE	transmissible spongiform encephalopathy
WCB	working cell bank
WSL	working seed lot
WVS	working virus seed

1. Introduction

Biological products can be defined according to their source material and method of manufacture. The source materials and methods employed in the manufacture of biological products for human use therefore represent critical factors in shaping their appropriate regulatory control. Biological products are derived from cells, tissues or microorganisms and reflect the inherent variability characteristic of living materials. The active substances in biological products are often too complex to be fully characterized by utilizing physicochemical testing methods alone and may show a marked heterogeneity from one preparation and/or batch to the next. Consequently, special considerations are needed when manufacturing biological products in order to maintain consistency in product quality.

Good manufacturing practices (GMP) for biological products were first published by WHO in 1992 (*1*). This current revision reflects subsequent developments that have taken place in science and technology, and in the application of risk-based approaches to GMP (*2–14*). The content of this document should be considered complementary to the general recommendations set out in the current WHO good manufacturing practices for pharmaceutical products: main principles (*2*) and in other WHO documents related specifically to the production and control of biological products.

This document is intended to serve as a basis for establishing national guidelines for GMP for biological products. If a national regulatory authority (NRA) so desires, the guidance provided may be adopted as definitive national requirements, or modifications may be justified and made by the NRA in light of the risk–benefit balance and legal considerations in each authority. In such cases, it is recommended that any modification to the principles and technical specifications set out below should be made only on the condition that the modifications ensure product quality, safety and efficacy that are at least equivalent to that recommended in this document.

2. Scope

The guidance provided in this document applies to the manufacture, control and testing of biological products for human use – from starting materials and preparations (including seed lots, cell banks and intermediates) to the finished product.

Manufacturing procedures within the scope of this document include:

- growth of strains of microorganisms and eukaryotic cells;
- extraction of substances from biological tissues, including human, animal and plant tissues, and fungi;

- recombinant DNA (rDNA) techniques;
- hybridoma techniques;
- propagation of microorganisms in embryos or animals.

Medicinal products of biological origin manufactured by these procedures include allergens, antigens, vaccines, certain hormones, cytokines, monoclonal antibodies (mAbs), enzymes, animal immune sera, products of fermentation (including products derived from rDNA), biological diagnostic reagents for in vivo use and advanced therapy medicinal products (ATMPs) used for example in gene therapy and cell therapy.

For human whole blood, blood components and plasma-derived products for therapeutic use separate comprehensive WHO guidance is available and should be followed (*12*, *15*).

In some countries certain small-molecule medicinal products (for example, antibiotics) are not defined as biological products. Nevertheless, where the manufacturing procedures described in this document are used then the guidance provided may be followed.

The preparation of investigational medicinal products for use in clinical trials should follow the basic principles of GMP set out in these and other WHO GMP guidelines (*2*, *16*) as appropriate. However, certain other requirements (such as process and analytical method validations) could be completed before marketing authorization (*17–19*).

The current document does not provide detailed recommendations for specific classes of biological products (for example, vaccines). Attention is therefore directed to other relevant WHO documents, and in particular to WHO recommendations to assure the quality, safety and efficacy of specific products.[2]

Table 1 illustrates the typical risk-based application of the current document (*4*, *7*). It should be noted that this table is illustrative only and is not intended to describe the precise scope.

[2] See: http://www.who.int/biologicals/en/ (accessed 4 November 2015).

Table A3.1
Scope of the current document (illustrative)

Type and source of material	Example products	Application of this document to steps in manufacture			
1. Animal or plant sources: non-transgenic	Heparins, insulin, enzymes, proteins, allergen extract, ATMPs, animal immune sera	Collection of plant, organ, tissue or fluid	Cutting, mixing and/or initial processing	Isolation and purification	Formulation and filling
2. Virus or bacteria/ fermentation/cell culture	Viral or bacterial vaccines, enzymes, proteins	Establishment and maintenance of MCB, WCB, MSL/ MVS, WSL/WVS	Cell culture and/or fermentation	Inactivation when applicable, isolation and purification	Formulation and filling
3. Biotechnology fermentation/cell culture	Recombinant products, mAbs, allergens, vaccines, gene therapy (viral and non-viral vectors, plasmids)	Establishment and maintenance of MCB, WCB, MSL, WSL	Cell culture and/or fermentation	Isolation, purification and modification	Formulation and filling
4. Animal sources: transgenic	Recombinant proteins, ATMPs	Master and working transgenic bank	Collection, cutting, mixing and/or initial processing	Isolation, purification and modification	Formulation and filling
5. Plant sources: transgenic	Recombinant proteins, vaccines, allergens	Master and working transgenic bank	Growing and/or harvesting	Initial extraction, isolation, purification and modification	Formulation and filling

Table A3.1 *continued*

Type and source of material	Example products	Application of this document to steps in manufacture			
6. Human sources	Urine-derived enzymes, hormones	Collection of fluid	Mixing and/or initial processing	Isolation and purification	Formulation and filling
7. Human and/or animal sources	Gene therapy: genetically modified cells	Donation, procurement and testing of starting tissue/cellsa	Vector manufacture and cell purification and processing	Ex vivo genetic modification of cells, establish MCB, WCB or cell stock	Formulation and filling
	Somatic cell therapy	Donation, procurement and testing of starting tissue/cellsa	Establishing and maintaining MCB, WCB or cell stock	Cell isolation, culture purification and combination with non-cellular components	Formulation, combination and filling
	Tissue-engineered products	Donation, procurement and testing of starting tissue/cells[a]	Initial processing, isolation and purification, establishing and maintaining MCB, WCB, primary cell stock	Cell isolation, culture, purification and combination with non-cellular components	Formulation, combination and filling

[a] GMP guidelines, as described in this document, are not applied to this step. Other national regulations, requirements, recommendations and/or guidelines may apply as deemed necessary by the NRA.

MCB = master cell bank; MSL = master seed lot; MVS = master virus seed; WCB = working cell bank; WSL = working seed lot; WVS = working virus seed.

3. Terminology

In addition to the terms defined in WHO good manufacturing practices for pharmaceutical products: main principles (*2*) and WHO good manufacturing practices for sterile pharmaceutical products (*3*), the definitions given below apply to the terms as used in the current document. These terms may have different meanings in other contexts.

Active substance: a defined process intermediate containing the active ingredient, which is subsequently formulated with excipients to produce the drug product. This may also be referred to as "drug substance" or "active ingredient" in other documents.

Adventitious agents: contaminating microorganisms of the cell culture or source materials, including bacteria, fungi, mycoplasmas/spiroplasmas, mycobacteria, rickettsia, protozoa, parasites, transmissible spongiform encephalopathy (TSE) agents and viruses that have been unintentionally introduced into the manufacturing process of a biological product. The source of these contaminants may be the legacy of the cell line, or the raw materials used in the culture medium to propagate the cells (in banking, in production or in their legacy), the environment, personnel, equipment or elsewhere.

Allergen: a molecule capable of inducing an immunoglobulin E (IgE) response and/or a Type I allergic reaction.

Antibodies: proteins produced naturally by the B-lymphocytes that bind to specific antigens. Using rDNA technology antibodies are also produced in other (continuous) cell lines. Antibodies may be divided into two main types – monoclonal and polyclonal antibodies – based on key differences in their methods of manufacture. Also called immunoglobulins.

Antigens: substances (for example, toxins, foreign proteins, bacteria, tissue cells and venoms) capable of inducing specific immune responses.

Axenic: a single organism in culture which is not contaminated with any other organism.

Bioburden: the level and type (objectionable or not) of microorganisms present in raw materials, media, biological substances, intermediates or finished products. Regarded as contamination when the level and/or type exceed specifications.

Biohazard: any biological material considered to be hazardous to people and/or the environment.

Biological starting materials: starting materials derived from a biological source that mark the beginning of the manufacturing process of a drug, as described in a marketing authorization or licence application, and from which the active ingredient is derived either directly (for example, plasma derivatives, ascitic fluid and bovine lung) or indirectly (for example, cell substrates, host/vector production cells, eggs and viral strains).

Biosafety risk group: denotes the containment conditions required for safe handling of organisms associated with different hazards, ranging from Risk Group 1 (lowest risk, no or low individual and community risk, and unlikely to cause disease) to Risk Group 4 (highest risk, high individual and community risk, usually causes severe disease, and which is likely to spread with no prophylaxis or treatment available) (*20*).

Campaign manufacture: the manufacture of an uninterrupted sequence of batches of the same product or intermediate in a given time period, followed by strict adherence to accepted control measures before switching to another product or different serotype. The different products are not run at the same time but may be run on the same equipment.

Cell bank: a collection of appropriate containers whose contents are of uniform composition and stored under defined conditions. Each container represents an aliquot of a single pool of cells.

Cell culture: the process by which cells that are no longer organized into tissues are grown in vitro under defined and controlled conditions. Cell cultures are operated and processed under axenic conditions to ensure a pure culture absent of microbial contamination.

Cell stock: primary cells expanded to a given number of cells to be aliquoted and used as starting material for production of a limited number of lots of a cell-based medicinal product.

Containment: the concept of using a process, equipment, personnel, utilities, system and/or facility to contain product, dust or contaminants in one zone, preventing them from entering into another zone and/or escaping.

Continuous culture: a process by which the growth of cells is maintained by periodically replacing a portion of the cells and the medium so that there is no lag or saturation phase.

Control strategy: a planned set of controls derived from current product and process understanding that assures process performance and product quality. The controls can include parameters and attributes related to active substance and finished product materials and components; facility and equipment operating conditions; in-process controls; finished product specifications; and the associated methods and frequency of monitoring and control.

Cross-contamination: contamination of a starting material, intermediate product or finished product with another starting material or product during production. In multi-product facilities, cross-contamination can occur throughout the manufacturing process, from generation of the master cell bank (MCB) and working cell bank (WCB) to finished product.

Dedicated: facility, personnel, equipment or piece of equipment used only in the manufacture of a particular product or group of specified products of similar risk.

Dedicated area: an area that may be in the same building as another area but which is separated by a physical barrier and which has, for example, separate entrances, staff facilities and air-handling systems. Also referred to as "self-contained facility" in other GMP documents.

Feeder cells: cells used in co-culture to maintain pluripotent stem cells. For human embryonic stem cell culture, typical feeder layers include mouse embryonic fibroblasts or human embryonic fibroblasts that have been treated to prevent them from dividing.

Finished product: a finished dosage form that has undergone all stages of manufacture, including packaging in its final container and labelling. Also referred to as "finished dosage form", "drug product" or "final product" in other documents.

Fermentation: maintenance or propagation of microbial cells in vitro (fermenter). Fermentation is operated and progressed under axenic conditions to ensure a pure culture absent of contaminating microorganisms.

Harvesting: the procedure by which the cells, inclusion bodies or crude supernatants containing the unpurified active ingredient are recovered.

Hybridoma: an immortalized cell line that secretes desired (monoclonal) antibodies and which is typically derived by fusing B-lymphocytes with tumour cells.

Inactivation: removal or reduction to an acceptable limit of infectivity of microorganisms or detoxification of toxins by chemical or physical modification.

Master cell bank (MCB): a quantity of well-characterized cells of animal or other origin, derived from a cell seed at a specific population doubling level (PDL) or passage level, dispensed into multiple containers and stored under defined conditions. The MCB is prepared from a single homogeneously mixed pool of cells. In some cases, such as genetically engineered cells, the MCB may be prepared from a selected cell clone established under defined conditions. However, the MCB may not be clonal. The MCB is used to derive a working cell bank (WCB).

Monoclonal antibodies (mAbs): homogenous antibody population obtained from a single clone of lymphocytes or by recombinant technology and which bind to a single epitope.

Pharmaceutical quality system (PQS): management system used by a pharmaceutical company to direct and control its activities with regard to quality.

Polyclonal antibodies: antibodies derived from a range of lymphocyte clones and produced in humans and animals in response to the epitopes on most "non-self" molecules.

Primary containment: a system of containment that prevents the escape of a biological agent into the immediate working environment. It involves the use of closed containers or biological safety cabinets along with secure operating procedures.

Quality risk management (QRM): a systematic process for the assessment, control, communication and review of risks to the quality of pharmaceutical products across the product life-cycle.

Reference sample: a sample of a batch of starting material, packaging material, intermediate or finished product which is stored for the purpose of being analysed should the need arise during the shelf-life of the batch concerned.

Retention sample: a sample of a fully packaged unit from a batch of finished product. It is stored for identification purposes (for example, of presentation, packaging, labelling, patient information leaflet, batch number and expiry date) should the need arise during the shelf-life of the batch concerned.

Seed lot: a quantity of live cells or viruses which has been derived from a single culture (though not necessarily clonal), has a uniform composition and is aliquoted into appropriate storage containers from which all future products will be derived, either directly or via a seed lot system. The following derived terms are used in this document – **master seed lot (MSL):** a lot or bank of cells or viruses from which all future vaccine production will be derived. The MSL represents a well-characterized collection of cells or viruses or bacteria of uniform composition. Also referred to as "master virus seed" (MVS) for virus seeds, "master seed bank", "master seed antigen" or "master transgenic bank" in other documents; and **working seed lot (WSL):** a cell or viral or bacterial seed lot derived by propagation from the MSL under defined conditions and used to initiate production of vaccines on a lot-by-lot basis. Also referred to as "working virus seed" (WVS) for virus seeds, "working seed bank", "working seed antigen" or "working transgenic bank" in other documents.

Specific pathogen free (SPF): denoting animals or animal materials (such as chickens, embryos, eggs or cell cultures) derived from groups of animals (for example, flocks or herds) free from specified pathogens, and used for the production or quality control of biological products. Such flocks or herds are defined as animals sharing a common environment and having their own caretakers who have no contact with non-SPF groups.

Starting materials: any substances of a defined quality used in the production of a pharmaceutical product, but excluding packaging materials. In the context of biological products manufacturing, examples of starting materials may include cryo-protectants, feeder cells, reagents, growth media, buffers, serum, enzymes, cytokines, growth factors and amino acids.

Transgenic: denoting an organism that contains a foreign gene in its normal genetic component for the expression of biological pharmaceutical materials.

Vaccine: a preparation containing antigens capable of inducing an active immune response for the prevention, amelioration or treatment of infectious diseases.

Working cell bank (WCB): a quantity of well-characterized cells of animal or other origin, derived from an MCB at a specific PDL or passage level, dispensed into multiple containers and stored under defined conditions. The WCB is prepared from a single homogeneously mixed pool of cells (often, this is the MCB). One or more of the WCB containers is used for each production culture.

4. Principles and general considerations

The manufacture of biological products should be undertaken in accordance with the basic principles of GMP. The points covered by the current document should, therefore, be considered as complementary to the general recommendations set out in the current WHO good manufacturing practices for pharmaceutical products: main principles (*2*) and associated specialized guidelines and recommendations (*3*, *4*, *10*, *13*, *14*) as well as other WHO documents related specifically to the production and control of biological products established by the WHO Expert Committee on Biological Standardization.[3]

The manufacture, control and administration of biological active substances and finished products require certain specific considerations and precautions arising from the nature of these products and their processes. Unlike conventional pharmaceutical products which are manufactured using chemical and physical techniques capable of a high degree of consistency, the manufacture of biological active substances and finished products involves biological processes and materials, such as cultivation of cells or extraction from living organisms. As these biological processes may display inherent variability, the range and nature of by-products may also be variable. As a result, quality risk management (QRM) principles are particularly important for this class of materials and should be used to develop the control strategy across all stages of manufacture so as to minimize variability and reduce the opportunity for contamination and cross-contamination.

Materials and processing conditions used in cultivation processes are designed to provide conditions for the growth of target cells and microorganisms – therefore, extraneous microbial contaminants have the opportunity to grow. Furthermore, many biological products have limited ability to withstand certain purification techniques, particularly those designed to inactivate or remove adventitious viral contaminants. The design of the processes, equipment, facilities, utilities, the conditions of preparation and addition of buffers and reagents, sampling, and training of the operators are key considerations in minimizing

[3] See: http://www.who.int/biologicals/en/ (accessed 4 November 2015).

such contamination events. Specifications outlined in WHO guidelines and recommendations will determine whether and to what stage of production substances and materials can have a defined level of bioburden or need to be sterile. Similarly, manufacturing should be consistent with other specifications set out in the product summary files, marketing authorization or clinical trial approvals (for example, number of generations (expressed as doublings or passages) between the seed lot or cell bank and the finished product).

Many biological materials (such as live-attenuated bacteria and viruses) cannot be terminally sterilized by heat, gas or radiation. In addition, some products, such as certain live and adjuvanted vaccines (for example, bacille Calmette–Guérin (BCG) or cholera), may not be sterilized by filtration processes. For these axenic products, processing should be conducted aseptically to minimize the introduction of contaminants from the point where a potential contamination cannot be removed from the manufacturing process. Relevant WHO documents should be consulted on the validation of specific manufacturing steps such as virus removal or inactivation (*21*). Robust environmental controls and monitoring and, wherever feasible, in situ cleaning and sterilization systems, together with the use of closed systems can significantly reduce the risk of accidental contamination and cross-contamination.

Control usually involves biological analytical techniques, which typically have a greater variability than physicochemical determinations. The combination of variability in starting materials and the potential for subtle changes during the manufacturing process of biological products also requires an emphasis on production consistency. This is of particular concern because of the need to link consistency to original clinical trials documenting the product's safety and efficacy. A robust manufacturing process is therefore crucial and in-process controls take on a particular importance in the manufacture of biological active substances and medicinal products.

Because of the risks inherent in producing and manipulating pathogenic and transmissible microorganisms during the production and testing of biological materials, GMP should prioritize the safety of the recipient to whom the biological product is administered, the safety of personnel during operation and the protection of the environment.

Biosafety considerations should follow national guidelines and (if applicable and available) international guidelines. In most countries, the regulation of GMP and biosafety are governed by different institutions. In the context of manufacturing pathogenic biological products of Biosafety Risk Group 3 and 4, close collaboration between such institutions is especially required to assure that both product contamination and environmental contamination levels are controlled within acceptable limits. Specific recommendations regarding containment are outlined below in section 10.

5. Pharmaceutical quality system and quality risk management

Biological products, like any pharmaceutical product, should be manufactured in accordance with the requirements of a pharmaceutical quality system (PQS) based on a life-cycle approach as defined in WHO good manufacturing practices for pharmaceutical products: main principles (*2*). This approach facilitates innovation and continual improvement, and also strengthens the link between pharmaceutical development and manufacturing activities.

QRM principles should be used to develop the control strategy across all manufacturing and control stages – including materials sourcing and storage, personnel and materials flow, manufacture and packaging, quality control, quality assurance, storage and distribution activities, as described in relevant WHO guidelines (*14*) and other documents (*22*). Due to the inherent variability of biological processes and starting materials, ongoing trend analysis and periodic review are particularly important elements of PQS. Thus, special attention should be paid to starting material controls, change control, trend analysis and deviation management in order to ensure production consistency. Monitoring systems should be designed so as to provide early detection of any unwanted or unanticipated factors that may affect the quality, safety and efficacy of the product. The effectiveness of the control strategy in monitoring, reducing and managing such risks should be regularly reviewed and the systems updated as required taking into account scientific and technical progress.

6. Personnel

6.1 Personnel responsible for production and control should have an adequate background in relevant scientific disciplines such as microbiology, biology, biometry, chemistry, medicine, pharmacy, pharmacology, virology, immunology, biotechnology and veterinary medicine, together with sufficient practical experience to enable them to perform their duties.

6.2 The health status of personnel should be taken into consideration as part of ensuring product safety. Where necessary, personnel engaged in production, maintenance, testing and animal care (and inspections) should be vaccinated with appropriate specific vaccines and have regular health checks. Any changes in the health status of personnel which could adversely affect the quality of the product should preclude their working in the production area, and appropriate records kept. The scope and frequency of health monitoring should be commensurate with the risk to the product and personnel.

6.3 Training in cleaning and disinfection procedures, hygiene and microbiology should emphasize the risk of microbial and adventitious contamination and the nature of the target microorganisms and growth media routinely used.

6.4 Where required to minimize the opportunity for cross-contamination, restrictions on the movement of all personnel (including quality control, maintenance and cleaning staff) should be defined on the basis of QRM principles. In general, all personnel including those not routinely involved in the production operation (such as management, engineering staff and validation staff or auditors) should not pass from areas with exposure to live microorganisms, genetically modified microorganisms, animal tissue, toxins, venoms or animals to areas where other products (inactivated or sterile) or different organisms are handled. If such passage is unavoidable during a working day, then contamination control measures (for example, clearly defined decontamination measures such as a complete change of appropriate clothing and shoes, and showering if applicable) should be followed by all personnel visiting any such production area unless otherwise justified on the basis of QRM.

6.5 Because the risks are difficult to manage, personnel working in an animal facility should be restricted from entering production areas where potential risks of cross-contamination exist.

6.6 Staff assigned to the production of BCG products should not work with other infectious agents. In particular, they should not work with virulent strains of *Mycobacterium tuberculosis*, nor should they be exposed to a known risk of tuberculosis infection (*23*). Additionally, they should be carefully monitored, with regular health checks that screen for tuberculosis infection.

6.7 If personnel working in BCG manufacturing and in animal quarters need to be reassigned to other manufacturing units they should not be allowed into such units until they pass their health check.

7. Starting materials

7.1 The source, origin and suitability of active substances, starting materials (for example, cryo-protectants and feeder cells), buffers and media (for example, reagents, growth media, serum, enzymes, cytokines, growth factors and amino acids) and other components of the finished product should be clearly defined and controlled according to the principles set out in WHO guidance on GMP for pharmaceutical products (*2*).

7.2 Manufacturers should retain information describing the source and quality of the biological materials used for at least 1 year after the expiry date of the finished products and according to local regulations concerning biological products. It has been found that documents retained for longer periods may provide useful information related to adverse events following immunization (AEFIs) and other investigations.

7.3 All starting material suppliers (that is, manufacturers) should be initially qualified on the basis of documented criteria and a risk-based approach. Regular assessments of their status should also be carried out. Particular attention should be given to the identification and monitoring of any variability that may affect biological processes. When starting materials are sourced from brokers who could increase the risk of contamination by performing repackaging operations under GMP (*2*, *4*) they should be carefully qualified; an audit may form part of such qualification, as needed.

7.4 An identity test, or equivalent, should be performed on each batch of received starting materials prior to release. The number of containers sampled should be justified on the basis of QRM principles and in agreement with all applicable guidelines (*2*). The identification of all starting materials should be in compliance with the requirements appropriate to the stage of manufacture. The level of testing should be commensurate with the qualification level of the supplier and the nature of the materials used. In the case of starting material used to manufacture active substances the number of samples taken should be based on statistically recognized criteria and QRM principles (*2*). However, for starting materials and intermediates used in the formulation of finished product each container should be sampled for identity testing in accordance with the main principles of GMP for pharmaceutical products unless reduced testing has been validated.

7.5 The sampling process should not adversely affect the quality of the product. Incoming starting materials should be sampled under appropriate conditions in order to prevent contamination and cross-contamination.

7.6 Where justified (such as the special case of sterile starting materials) it may be acceptable to reduce the risk of contamination by not performing sampling at the time of receipt but to perform the testing later on samples taken at the time of use. In such cases, release of the finished product is conditional upon satisfactory results of these tests.

7.7 Where the necessary tests for approving starting materials take a significantly long time, it may be permissible by exception to process starting materials before the test results are available. The use of these materials should be clearly justified in a documented manner, and the risks should be understood and assessed under the principles of QRM. In such cases, release of the finished product is conditional upon satisfactory results from the tests. It must be ensured that this is not standard practice and occurs only with justification of the risk taken.

7.8 The risk of contamination of starting materials during their passage along the supply chain should be assessed, with particular emphasis on adventitious agents such as those causing TSEs (*24*). Other materials that come into direct contact with manufacturing equipment and/or with potential product contact surfaces (such as filter media, growth media during aseptic process simulations and lubricants) should also be controlled. A quality risk assessment should be performed to evaluate the potential for adventitious agents in biological starting materials.

7.9 Where required, the sterilization of starting materials should be carried out by heat whenever possible. Where necessary, other appropriate validated methods may also be used for this purpose (such as irradiation and filtration).

7.10 The controls required for ensuring the quality of sterile starting materials and of the aseptic manufacturing process should be based on the principles and guidance contained in the current WHO good manufacturing practices for sterile pharmaceutical products (*3*).

7.11 The transport of critical materials, reference materials, active substances, human tissues and cells to the manufacturing site should be controlled as part of a written quality agreement between the responsible parties if they are different commercial entities. Manufacturing sites should have documentary evidence of adherence to the specified storage and transport conditions, including cold chain requirements, if required. The required traceability – starting at tissue establishments through to the recipient(s), and including the traceability of materials in contact with the cells or tissues – should be ensured, maintained and documented.

8. Seed lots and cell banks

8.1 The recommendations set out in WHO good manufacturing practices for active pharmaceutical ingredients (*4*) should be followed – specifically section 18 on specific guidance for active pharmaceutical ingredients manufactured by cell culture/fermentation.

8.2 Where human or animal cells are used as feeder cells in the manufacturing process, appropriate controls over their sourcing, testing, transport and storage should be in place.

8.3 In order to prevent the unwanted drift of genetic properties which might result from repeated subcultures or multiple generations, the production of biological products obtained by microbial culture, cell culture or propagation in embryos and animals should be based on a system of master and working seed lots and/or cell banks; which is the beginning of the manufacturing process of certain biological products (for example, vaccines).

8.4 The number of generations (expressed as passages or doublings) between the seed lot or cell bank and the finished product, defined as maximum, should be consistent with the marketing authorization dossier and should not be exceeded.

8.5 Cell-based medicinal products are often generated from a cell stock obtained from a limited number of passages. In contrast with the two-tier system of MCBs and WCBs, the number of production runs from a cell stock is limited by the number of aliquots obtained after expansion and does not cover the entire life-cycle of the product. Cell stock changes should be covered by a validation protocol and communicated to the NRA, as applicable.

8.6 Establishment and handling of the MCBs and WCBs should be performed under conditions which are demonstrably appropriate. These should include an appropriately controlled environment to protect the seed lot and the cell bank, and the personnel handling them. To establish the minimum requirements for clean room grade and environmental monitoring in the case of vaccines see the WHO *Environmental monitoring of clean rooms in vaccine manufacturing facilities: points to consider for manufacturers of human vaccines* (*25*). During the establishment of the seed lot and cell bank, no other living or infectious material (such as viruses, cell lines or microbial strains) should be handled simultaneously in the same area or by the same persons, as set out in current WHO Recommendations (*26*).

8.7 Quarantine and release procedures for master and working cell banks/seed lots should be followed, including adequate characterization and testing for contaminants. Initially, full characterization testing of the MCB should be done, including genetic identification. A new MCB (from a previous initial clone, MCB or WCB) should be subjected to the same established testing as the original MCB, unless otherwise justified. Thereafter, the viability, purity and other stability-indicating attributes of seed lots and cell banks should be checked regularly according to justified criteria. Evidence of the stability and recovery of the seed lots and banks should be documented and records should be kept in a manner that permits trend evaluation.

8.8 Each storage container should be adequately sealed, clearly labelled and kept at an appropriate temperature. A stock inventory should be kept. The storage temperature should be recorded continuously and, where applicable, the liquid nitrogen level should be monitored. Any deviation from the set limits, and any corrective and preventive action taken, should be recorded. Temperature deviations should be detected as early as possible (for example, through the use of an alarm system for temperature and nitrogen levels).

8.9 Seed lots and cell banks should be stored and used in such a way as to minimize the risks of contamination or alteration (for example, stored in qualified ultra-low temperature freezers or liquid nitrogen storage containers). Control measures for the storage of different seeds and/or cells in the same area or equipment should prevent mix-up and should take into account the infectious nature of the materials in order to prevent cross-contamination.

8.10 MSLs, MCBs, and preferably also WSLs and WCBs, should be stored in two or more controlled separate sites in order to minimize the risk of total loss due to natural disaster, equipment malfunction or human error. A contingency plan should be in place.

8.11 The storage and handling conditions for the cell or seed banks should be defined. Access should be controlled and restricted to authorized personnel, and appropriate access records maintained. Records of location, identity and inventory of individual containers should also be kept. Once containers are removed from the seed lot/cell bank management system they should not be returned to stock.

9. Premises and equipment

9.1 In general, preparations containing live microorganisms or live viruses should not be manufactured and containers should not be filled in areas used for the processing of other pharmaceutical products. However, if the manufacturer can demonstrate and validate effective containment and decontamination of the live microorganisms and viruses then the use of multi-product facilities may be justifiable. In such cases, measures such as campaign production, closed systems and/or disposable systems should be considered and should be based on QRM principles (see sections 10 and 13 below on containment and campaign production respectively).

9.2 Documented QRM should be carried out for every additional product in a biological manufacturing multi-product facility, which may include a potency and toxicological evaluation based on cross-contamination risks. Other factors to be taken into account include facility/equipment design and use, personnel and material flows, microbiological controls, physicochemical characteristics of the active substance, process characteristics, cleaning processes and analytical capabilities relative to the relevant limits established from product evaluation. The outcome of the QRM process should be the basis for determining the necessity for premises and equipment to be dedicated to a particular product or product family, and the extent to which this should be the case. This may include dedicating specific product-contact parts. The NRA should approve the use of a manufacturing facility for the production of multiple products on case-to-case basis.

9.3 Killed vaccines, antisera and other biological products – including those made by rDNA techniques, toxoids and bacterial extracts – may, following inactivation, be manufactured on the same premises provided that adequate decontamination and cleaning measures are implemented on the basis of QRM.

9.4 Cleaning and sanitization should take into account the fact that processes often include the handling of growth media and other growth-promoting agents. Validation studies should be carried out to ensure the effectiveness of cleaning, sanitization and disinfection, including elimination of residues of used agents. Environmental and personnel safety precautions should be taken during the cleaning and sanitization processes. The use of cleaning and sanitizing agents should not pose any major risk to the performance of equipment.

The use of closed systems to improve asepsis and containment should be considered where practicable. Where open systems are utilized during processing (for example, during addition of growth supplements, media, buffers and gases, and during sampling and aseptic manipulations during the handling of live cells such as in cell-therapy products) control measures should be put in place to prevent contamination, mix-up and cross-contamination. Logical and unidirectional flows of personnel, materials and processes, and the use of clean-in-place and sterilize-in-place systems, should be considered wherever possible. Where sterile single-use systems such as bags and connectors are utilized, they should be qualified with respect to suitability, extractables, leachables and integrity.

9.5 Because of the variability of biological products, and of the corresponding manufacturing processes, approved starting materials that have to be measured or weighed for the production process (such as growth media, solutions and buffers) may be kept in small stocks in the production area for a specified period of time according to defined criteria – such as for the duration of manufacture of the batch or of the campaign. Appropriate storage conditions and controls should be maintained during such temporary storage. These materials should not be returned to the general stock. Materials used to formulate buffers, growth media and so on should be weighed and made into a solution in a contained area using local protection (such as a classified weighing booth) and outside the aseptic processing areas in order to minimize particulate contamination of the latter.

9.6 In manufacturing facilities, the mix-up of entry and exit of personnel should be avoided through the use of separate changing rooms or through procedural controls where Biosafety Risk Group 3 or 4 organisms are handled (*20*).

10. Containment

10.1 Airborne dissemination of live microorganisms and viruses used for the production process, including those from personnel, should be avoided.

10.2 Adequate precautions should be taken to avoid contamination of the drainage system with dangerous effluents. Drainage systems should be designed in such a way that effluents can be effectively neutralized or decontaminated to minimize the risk of cross-contamination. Specific and validated decontamination systems should be considered for effluents when infectious and/or potentially infectious materials are used for production. Local regulations should be complied with in order to minimize the risk of contamination of the external environment according to the risk associated with the biohazardous nature of waste materials.

10.3 Dedicated production areas should be used for the handling of live cells capable of persistence in the manufacturing environment, for pathogenic organisms of Biosafety Risk Group 3 or 4 and/or for spore-forming organisms until the inactivation process is accomplished and verified. For *Bacillus anthracis*, *Clostridium tetani* and *Clostridium botulinum* strictly dedicated facilities should be utilized for each individual product. Up-to-date information on these and other high-risk or "special" agents should be sought from major information resources (*27*). Where campaign manufacture of spore-forming organisms occurs in a facility or suite of facilities only one product should be processed at any one time.

Use of any pathogenic organism above Biosafety Risk Group 3 may be permitted by the NRA according to the biohazard classification of the organism, the risk assessment of the biological product and its emergency demand.

10.4 Production of BCG-related product should take place in a dedicated area and by means of dedicated equipment and utilities (such as heating, ventilation and air conditioning (HVAC) systems) in order to minimize the hazard of cross-contamination.

10.5 Specific containment requirements apply to poliomyelitis vaccine in accordance with the WHO global action plan to minimize poliovirus facility-associated risk (*28*) and with WHO Guidelines for the safe production and quality control of inactivated poliomyelitis vaccine manufactured from wild polioviruses (*29*). The measures and procedures necessary for containment (that is, for protecting the environment and ensuring the safety of the operator) should not conflict with those for ensuring product quality.

10.6 Air-handling systems should be designed, constructed and maintained to minimize the risk of cross-contamination between different manufacturing areas as required. The need for dedicated air-handling units or single-pass systems should be based on QRM principles, taking into account the biohazard classification and containment requirements of the relevant organism, and process and equipment risks. In the case of Biosafety Risk Group 3 organisms, air should not be recirculated to any other area in the facility and should be exhausted through high-efficiency particulate air (HEPA) filters that are regularly checked for performance. A dedicated non-recirculating ventilation system and HEPA-filtering of exhaust air are required when handling Biosafety Risk Group 4 organisms (*27*).

10.7 Primary containment equipment should be designed and initially qualified for integrity in order to ensure that the escape of biological agents and/or material into the immediate working area and outside environment is prevented. Thereafter, in line with relevant guidelines and QRM principles, periodical tests should be performed to ensure that the equipment is in proper working condition.

10.8 Activities associated with the handling of live biological agents (such as centrifugation and blending of products which can lead to aerosol formation) should be contained in such a way as to prevent contamination of other products or the egress of live agents into the working and/or outside environment. The viability of such organisms and their biohazard classification should be taken into consideration as part of the management of such risks.

Accidental spillages, especially of live organisms, must be dealt with quickly and safely. Validated decontamination measures should be available for each organism or groups of related organisms. Where different strains of a single bacteria species or very similar viruses are involved, the decontamination process may be validated with one representative strain, unless the strains vary significantly in their resistance to the decontaminating agent(s) used.

10.9 Areas where Biosafety Risk Group 3 or 4 organisms are handled should always have a negative air pressure relative to the environment. This will ensure the containment of the organism in unlikely events such as failure of the door interlock. Air-lock doors should be interlocked to prevent them being opened simultaneously. Differential pressure alarms should be present wherever required, and should be validated and monitored.

10.10 Air-vent filters should be hydrophobic and subject to integrity testing at intervals determined by a QRM approach.

10.11 Where the filtration of exhaust air is necessary, the safe changing of filters should be ensured or bag-in-bag-out housings should be employed. Once removed, filters should be decontaminated and properly destroyed. In addition to HEPA filtration other inactivation technologies such as heat inactivation and steam scavenging may be considered for exhaust air to ensure effective inactivation of pathogenic organisms of Biosafety Risk Group 3 and/or 4.

11. Clean rooms

11.1 The WHO good manufacturing practices for sterile pharmaceutical products (3) defines and establishes the required class/grade of clean areas for the manufacture of sterile products according to the operations performed, including final aseptic fill. Additionally, in order to address the specific manufacturing processes involved in the production of biological products, and particularly vaccines, the WHO *Environmental monitoring of clean rooms in vaccine manufacturing facilities: points to consider for manufacturers of human vaccines* (25) guidance document may be used to develop the environmental classification requirements for biological manufacturing processes.

As part of the control strategy, the degree of environmental control of particulate and microbial contamination of the production premises should be adapted to the intermediate or finished product, and also to the production step, taking into account the potential level of contamination of the starting materials and the risks to the finished product.

11.2 The environmental monitoring programme should be supplemented with methods to detect the presence of the specific microorganisms used for production (for example, recombinant yeast and toxin- or polysaccharide-producing bacteria). The environmental monitoring programme may also include detection of the produced organisms and adventitious agents of production organisms, especially when campaign manufacture is applied on the basis of QRM principles.

12. Production

12.1 Since cultivation conditions, media and reagents are designed to promote the growth of cells or microbial organisms, typically in an axenic state, particular attention should be paid to the control strategy for ensuring that effective steps are in place for preventing or minimizing the occurrence of unwanted bioburden, endotoxins, viruses of animal and human origin, and associated metabolites.

12.2 The QRM process should be the basis for implementing the technical and organizational measures required to control the risks of contamination and cross-contamination. These could include, though are not limited to:

- carrying out processing and filling in segregated areas;
- containing material transfer by means of an airlock and appropriate type of pass box with validated transfer procedures, clothing change and effective washing and decontamination of equipment;
- recirculation of only treated (HEPA-filtered) air;
- acquiring knowledge of the key characteristics (for example, pathogenicity, detectability, persistence and susceptibility to inactivation) of all cells, organisms and any adventitious agents within the same facility;
- when considering the acceptability of concurrent work in cases where production is characterized by multiple small batches from different starting materials (for example, cell-based products) taking into account factors such as the health status of donors and the risk of total loss of a product from or for specific patients during development of the cross-contamination control strategy;
- preventing the risk of live organisms and spores entering non-related areas or equipment by addressing all potential routes of cross-contamination (for example, through the HVAC system) through the use of single-use components and closed systems;

- conducting environmental monitoring specific to the microorganism being manufactured in adjacent areas while paying attention to cross-contamination risks arising from the use of certain monitoring equipment (such as that used for airborne particle monitoring) in areas handling live and/or spore-forming organisms;
- using campaign-based production (see section 13 below).

12.3 When applicable, the inoculum preparation area should be designed so as to effectively control the risk of contamination, and should be equipped with a biosafety hood for primary containment.

12.4 If possible, growth media should be sterilized in situ by heat or in-line microbial-retentive filters. Additionally, in-line microbial-retentive filters should be used for the routine addition of gases, media, acids, alkalis and so on to fermenters or bioreactors.

12.5 Data from continuous monitoring of certain production processes (such as fermentation) should form part of the batch record. Where continuous culture is used, special consideration should be given to parameters such as temperature, pH, pO_2, CO_2 and the rate of feed or carbon source with respect to growth of cells.

12.6 In cases where a viral inactivation or removal process is performed, measures should be taken (for example, in relation to facility layout, unidirectional flow and equipment) to avoid the risk of recontamination of treated products by non-treated products.

12.7 A wide variety of equipment and components (for example, resins, matrices and cassettes) are used for purification purposes. QRM principles should be applied to devise the control strategy regarding such equipment and associated components when used in campaign manufacture and in multi-product facilities. The reuse of components at different stages of processing of one product is discouraged but, if performed, should be validated. Acceptance criteria, operating conditions, regeneration methods, lifespan and sanitization or sterilization methods, cleaning process, and hold time between the use of reused components should be defined and validated. The reuse of components for different products is not acceptable.

12.8 Where adverse donor (human or animal) health information becomes available after procurement and/or processing, and this information relates to product quality, then appropriate measures should be taken – including product recall, if applicable.

12.9 Antibiotics may be used during the early stages of production to help prevent inadvertent microbial contamination or to reduce the bioburden of living tissues and cells. In this case, the use of antibiotics should be well justified, and they should be cleared from the manufacturing process at the stage specified in the marketing authorization. Acceptable residual levels should be defined and validated. Penicillin and other beta-lactam antibiotics should not be used at any stage of the process.

12.10 A procedure should be in place to address equipment and/or accessories failure (such as air vent filter failure) which should include a product impact review. If such failures are discovered following batch release the NRA should be notified and the need for a batch recall should be considered.

13. Campaign production

13.1 The decision to use a facility or filling line for campaign manufacture should be justified in a documented manner and should be based on a systematic risk approach for each product (or strain) taking into account the containment requirements and the risk of cross-contamination to the next product. Campaign changeover procedures, including sensitive techniques used for the determination of residues, should be validated and proper cleaning acceptance criteria should be defined on a toxicology basis of product residues from the last campaign, as applicable. Equipment assigned to continued production or to campaign production of successive batches of the same intermediate product should be cleaned at appropriate validated intervals to prevent build-up and carry-over of contaminants (such as product degradants or objectionable levels of microorganisms).

13.2 For downstream operations of certain products (for example, pertussis or diphtheria vaccines) campaign production may be acceptable if well justified. For finishing operations (formulation and filling) the need for dedicated facilities or the use of campaigns in the same facility will depend on the specific characteristics of the biological product, on the characteristics of the other products (including any non-biological products), on the filling technologies used (such as single-use closed systems) and on local NRA regulations. Labelling and packaging operations can be carried out in a multi-product facility.

13.3 Campaign changeover involves intensive decontamination/sterilization (if required) and cleaning of the equipment and manufacturing area. Decontamination/sterilization (if required) and cleaning should include all equipment and accessories used during production, as well as the facility itself. The following recommendations should be considered:

- waste should be removed from the manufacturing area or sent to the bio-waste system in a safe manner;
- materials should be transferred by a validated procedure;
- the Quality Unit should confirm area clearance by inspection, and review the campaign changeover data (including monitoring results) prior to releasing the area for the next product.

13.4 When required, the corresponding diluent for the product can be filled in the same facility in line with the defined campaign production strategy for finished product.

13.5 When campaign-based manufacturing is considered, the facility layout and the design of the premises and equipment should permit effective cleaning and decontamination/sterilization (if required) based on QRM principles and validated procedures following the production campaign. In addition, consideration may need to be given at the design stage of facility layout to the possible need for fumigation.

14. Labelling

14.1 The information provided on the inner label (also called the container label) and on the outer label (on the packaging) should be readable and legible, and the content approved by the NRA.

14.2 Minimal key information should be printed on the inner label, and additional information should be provided on the outer label (for example, carton) and/or product leaflet.

14.3 The suitability of labels for low and ultra-low storage temperatures should be verified, if applicable. The label should remain properly attached to the container under different storage conditions during the shelf-life of the product. The label and its adhesive should have no adverse effect on the quality of the product caused by leaching, migration and/or other means.

15. Validation

15.1 Biological processes, handling of live materials and using campaign-based production, if applicable, are the major aspects of biological product manufacturing which require process and cleaning validation. The validation of such processes – given the typical variability of biological products, the possible use of harmful and toxic materials and the need for inactivation processes – plays an important role in demonstrating production consistency and in proving that the critical process parameters and product attributes are controlled. Where available, WHO guidance documents should be consulted on the validation of specific manufacturing methods (for example, virus removal or inactivation (*21*)).

15.2 A QRM approach should be used to determine the scope and extent of validation.

15.3 All critical biological processes (including inoculation, multiplication, fermentation, cell disruption, inactivation, purification, virus removal, removal of toxic and harmful additives, filtration, formulation and aseptic filling) are subject, as applicable, to process validation. Manufacturing control parameters to be validated may include specific addition sequences, mixing speeds, time and temperature controls, limits of light exposure and containment.

15.4 After initial process validation studies have been finalized and routine production has begun, critical processes should be subject to monitoring and trending with the objective of assuring consistency and detecting any unexpected variability. The monitoring strategy should be defined, taking into consideration factors such as the inherent variability, complexity of quality attributes and heterogeneity of biological products. A system or systems for detecting unplanned departures from the process as designed should be in place to ensure that the process remains in a state of control. Collection and evaluation of information and data on the performance of the process will allow for detection of undesired process variability and will determine whether action should be taken to prevent, anticipate and/or correct problems so that the process remains under control.

15.5 Cleaning validation should be performed in order to confirm the effectiveness of cleaning procedures designed to remove biological substances, growth media, process reagents, cleaning agents, inactivation agents and so on. Careful consideration should be given to cleaning validation when campaign-based production is practised.

15.6 Critical processes for inactivation or elimination of potentially harmful microorganisms of Biosafety Risk Group 2 or above, including genetically modified ones, are subject to validation.

15.7 Process revalidation may be triggered by a process change as part of the change-control system. In addition, because of the variability of processes, products and methods, process revalidation may be conducted at predetermined regular intervals according to risk considerations. A detailed review of all changes, trends and deviations occurring within a defined time period – for example, 1 year, based on the regular product quality review (PQR) – may indicate a need for process revalidation.

15.8 The integrity and specified hold times of containers used to store intermediate products should be validated unless such intermediate products are freshly prepared and used immediately.

16. Quality control

16.1 As part of quality control sampling and testing procedures for biological materials and products, special consideration should be given to the nature of the materials being sampled (for example, the need to avoid contamination, ensure biocontainment and/or cold chain requirements) in order to ensure that the testing carried out is representative.

16.2 Samples for post-release use typically fall into one of two categories – reference samples or retention samples – for the purposes of analytical testing and identification respectively. For finished products the reference and retention samples will in many instances be presented identically as fully packaged units. In such circumstances, reference and retention samples may be regarded as interchangeable.

Reference samples of biological starting materials should be retained under the recommended storage conditions for at least 1 year beyond the expiry date of the corresponding finished product. Reference samples of other starting materials (other than solvents, gases and water) as well as intermediates for which critical parameters cannot be tested in the final product should be retained for at least 2 years after the release of the product if their stability allows for this storage period. Certain starting materials such as components of growth media need not necessarily be retained.

Retention samples of a finished product should be stored in their final packaging at the recommended storage conditions for at least 1 year after the expiry date.

16.3 For cell-based products, microbiological tests (for example, sterility tests or purity checks) should be conducted on cultures of cells or cell banks free of antibiotics and other inhibitory substances in order to provide evidence of the absence of bacterial and fungal contamination, and to be able to detect fastidious organisms where appropriate. Where antibiotics are used, they should be removed by filtration at the time of testing.

16.4 The traceability, proper use and storage of reference standards should be ensured, defined and recorded. The stability of reference standards should be monitored, and their performance trended. The WHO Recommendations for the preparation, characterization and establishment of international and other biological reference standards (*30*) should be followed.

16.5 All stability studies – including real-time/real-condition stability, accelerated stability and stress testing – should be carried out according to relevant WHO and other guidelines (*31*) or other recognized documents. Trend analysis of the test results from the stability monitoring programme should assure the early detection of any process or assay drift, and this information should be part of the PQR of biological products.

16.6 For products where ongoing stability monitoring would normally require testing using animals, and no appropriate alternative or validated techniques are available, the frequency of testing may take into account a risk-based approach. The principle of bracketing and matrix designs may be applied if scientifically justified in the stability protocol.

16.7 All analytical methods used in the quality control and in-process control of biological products should be well characterized, validated and documented to a satisfactory standard in order to yield reliable results. The fundamental parameters of this validation include linearity, accuracy, precision, selectivity/specificity, sensitivity and reproducibility (*32–35*).

16.8 For test methods described in relevant pharmacopoeial monographs, qualification of the laboratory test equipment and personnel should be performed. In addition, repeat precision and comparability precision should be shown in the case of animal tests. Repeatability and reproducibility should also be demonstrated by reviewing retrospective test data.

In addition to the common parameters typically used for validating assays (such as accuracy and precision) additional measurements (for example, of the performance of references, critical reagents and/or cell lines) should be considered during the validation of bioassays based on the biological nature of the assay and reagents used.

17. Documentation (batch processing records)

17.1 In general, the processing records of regular production batches should provide a complete account of the manufacturing activities of each batch of biological product showing that it has been produced, tested and dispensed into containers in accordance with the approved procedures.

In the case of vaccines, a batch processing record and a summary protocol should be prepared for each batch for the purpose of lot release by the NRA. The information included in the summary protocol should follow the WHO Guidelines for independent lot release of vaccines by regulatory authorities (*36*). The summary protocol and all associated records should be of a type approved by the NRA.

17.2 Manufacturing batch records should be retained for at least 1 year after the expiry date of the batch of the biological product and should be readily retrievable for inspection by the NRA. It has been found that documents retained for longer periods may provide useful information related to AEFI and other investigations.

17.3 Starting materials may require additional documentation on source, origin, supply chain, method of manufacture and controls applied in order to ensure an appropriate level of control, including of microbiological quality if applicable.

17.4 Some product types may require a specific definition of what materials constitute a batch – particularly somatic cells in the context of ATMPs. For autologous and donor-matched situations, the manufactured product should be viewed as a batch.

18. Use of animals

18.1 A wide range of animals is used for the manufacture or quality control of biological products. Special considerations are required when animal facilities are present at a manufacturing site.

18.2 The presence of live animals in the production area should be avoided unless otherwise justified. Embryonated eggs are allowed in the production area, if applicable. If the extraction of tissues or organs from animals is required then particular care should be taken to prevent contamination of the production area (for example, appropriate disinfection procedures should be undertaken).

18.3 Areas used for performing tests involving animals or microorganisms should be well separated from premises used for the manufacturing of products and should have completely separate ventilation systems and separate staff. The separation of different animal species before and during testing should be considered, as should the necessary animal acclimatization process, as part of the test requirements.

18.4 In addition to monitoring compliance with TSE regulations (*24*) other adventitious agents that are of concern (including those causing zoonotic diseases and diseases in source animals) should also be monitored and recorded in line with specialist advice on establishing such programmes. Instances of ill health occurring in the source/donor animals should be investigated with respect to their suitability, and the suitability of in-contact animals, for continued use (for example, in manufacture, as sources of starting materials, and for quality control and safety testing). Decisions should be documented.

18.5 A look-back procedure should be in place in relation to the decision-making process used to evaluate the continued suitability of the biological active substance or finished product in which animal-sourced starting materials have been used or incorporated. This decision-making process may include the retesting of reference samples from previous collections from the same donor animal (where applicable) to establish the last negative donation. The withdrawal period of therapeutic agents used to treat source/donor animals should be documented and should be taken into account when considering the removal of those animals from the programme for defined periods.

18.6 Particular care should be taken to prevent and monitor infections in source/donor animals. Measures taken should cover aspects such as sourcing, facilities, husbandry, biosafety procedures, testing regimes, control of bedding and feed materials, 100% fresh air supply, appropriate design of the HVAC system, water supply and appropriate temperature and humidity conditions for the species being handled. This is of special relevance to SPF animals where pharmacopoeial monograph requirements should be met. Housing and health monitoring should also be defined for other categories of animals (for example, healthy flocks or herds).

18.7 For products manufactured from transgenic animals, traceability should be maintained in the creation of such animals from the source animals. Note should be taken of national requirements for animal quarters, care and quarantine.

18.8 For different animal species and lines, key criteria should be defined, monitored and recorded. These may include the age, sex, weight and health status of the animals.

18.9 Animals, biological agents and tests carried out should be appropriately identified to prevent any risk of mix-up and to control all identified hazards.

18.10 The facility layout should ensure a unidirectional and segregated flow of healthy animals, inoculated animals and waste-decontamination areas. Personnel and visitors should also follow a defined flow in order to avoid cross-contamination.

19. Authors and acknowledgements

The scientific basis for the revision of these WHO Guidelines was discussed at a working group meeting held in Bangkok, Thailand, 10–13 September 2007 and attended by: Dr M.M.F. Ahmed, Center for Control of Biologicals and Vaccines, Egypt; Dr H. Alitamsar, PT Bio Farma, Indonesia; Mr P. Angtrakool, Ministry of Public Health, Thailand; Dr D. Buckley, Consultant, Monash, Australia; Dr M. Dennehy, The Biovac Institute, South Africa; Ms X. Dong, Beijing Tiantan Biological Products Co. Ltd, China; Dr H.J.M. van de Donk, Consultant, Den Haag, Netherlands; Dr M. Gheisarzardeh, Ministry of Health and Medical Education, the Islamic Republic of Iran; Dr H.T. Hong, National Institute for Control of Vaccine and Biologicals, Viet Nam; Mrs W. Jariyapan, WHO Regional Office for South-East Asia, India; Mr M. Javadekar, Serum Institute of India Ltd, India; Dr D. Jiang, State Food and Drug Administration, China; Mrs T. Jivapaisarnpong, Ministry of Public Health, Thailand; Dr A. Khadem, Pasteur Institute of Iran, the Islamic Republic of Iran; Professor S. Khomvilai, Thai Red Cross Society, Thailand; Dr K-H. Kim, Korean Food and Drug Administration, Republic of Korea; Dr Kustantinah, National Agency of Drug and Food Control, Indonesia; Professor C.K. Lee, Advisor to the Korean Food and Drug Administration, Republic of Korea; Mrs J. Li, Sinovac Biotech Co. Ltd, China; V.G. Maqueda, Biologist, Buenos Aires, Argentina; Dr K-I. Min, Korean Food and Drug Administration, Republic of Korea; Mr I. Rees, Medicines and Healthcare Products Regulatory Agency, the United Kingdom; Dr C.H. Sia, Health Sciences Authority, Singapore; Dr M. Suhardono, PT Bio Farma, Indonesia; Ms J. Teo, Centre for Drug Administration, Singapore; Ms P.S. Thanaphollert, Ministry of Public Health, Thailand; Mr S. Thirapakpoomanunt, Ministry of Public Health, Thailand; Ms A.R.T. Utami, National Agency of Drug and Food Control, Indonesia; Dr D.T.H. Van, Institute for Vaccine and Biologicals, Viet Nam; Mr B. Wibisono, National Agency of Drug and Food Control, Indonesia; Mr J. Yang, Kunming Institute of Medical Biology, China; Mr Y. Yu, Kunming Institute of Medical Biology, China; and Dr I. Knezevic and Dr S. Lambert, World Health Organization, Switzerland – and a WHO drafting group meeting held in Geneva, Switzerland, 30–31 October 2013 and attended by: Mr R. Acs, Central Drugs Standard Control Organisation, India; Mr M. Eisenhawer, WHO Regional Office for South-East Asia, India; Dr S. Fakhrzadeh, Ministry of Health and Medical Education, the Islamic Republic of Iran; V.G. Maqueda, Biologist, Buenos Aires, Argentina; Mrs K. Porkaew, Ministry of Public Health, Thailand; Dr S.O. Rumiano, Consultant, Buenos Aires, Argentina; Dr Y. Wang, National Institutes for Food and Drug Control, China; Mr B. Wibisono, National Agency of Drug and Food Control, Indonesia; and Dr A. Chawla, Dr A.R. Khadem, Dr I. Knezevic, Dr S. Kopp and Dr D. Lei, World Health Organization, Switzerland.

Based upon the principles defined in the above working group and drafting group meetings the first draft of these Guidelines was prepared by Mr R. Acs, Central Drugs Standard Control Organisation, India; Dr B. Yáñez Chamizo, Centro para el Control Estatal de Medicamentos, Equipos y Dispositivos Médicos, Cuba; Dr S. Fakhrzadeh, Ministry of Health and Medical Education, the Islamic Republic of Iran; Mrs K. Porkaew, Ministry of Public Health, Thailand; Dr S.O. Rumiano, Consultant, Buenos Aires, Argentina; Dr Y. Wang, National Institutes for Food and Drug Control, China; Mr B. Wibisono, National Agency of Drug and Food Control, Indonesia; Mr M. Eisenhawer, WHO Regional Office for South-East Asia, India; Dr A. Chawla, Consultant, Greater Noida, India; Dr A.R. Khadem, World Health Organization, Switzerland; V.G. Maqueda, Biologist, Buenos Aires, Argentina; and Dr D. Lei, World Health Organization, Switzerland.

A second draft was then prepared by V.G. Maqueda, Biologist, Buenos Aires, Argentina; Dr B. Yáñez Chamizo, Centro para el Control Estatal de Medicamentos, Equipos y Dispositivos Médicos, Cuba; Dr S. Fakhrzadeh, Ministry of Health and Medical Education, the Islamic Republic of Iran; Dr S.O. Rumiano, Consultant, Buenos Aires, Argentina; Dr Y. Wang, National Institutes for Food and Drug Control, China; Mr B. Wibisono, National Agency of Drug and Food Control, Indonesia; Mr M. Eisenhawer, WHO Regional Office for South-East Asia, India; Dr A. Chawla, Consultant, Greater Noida, India; and Dr A.R. Khadem and Dr D. Lei, World Health Organization, Switzerland following a consultation held in Tunis, Tunisia, 22–24 July 2014 and attended by: Dr H. Baiao, National Authority for Medicines and Health Products, Portugal; Mrs R. Bose, Ministry of Health and Family Welfare, India; Mr C. Cabral, Butantan Institute, Brazil; Dr R. Chaplinsky, GSK Vaccines, Belgium; Dr A. Chawla, Consultant, Greater Noida, India; Mr M. Diagne, Direction de la Pharmacie et des Laboratoires, Senegal; Mr M. Eisenhawer, WHO Regional Office for South-East Asia, India; Dr S. Fakhrzadeh, Ministry of Health and Medical Education, the Islamic Republic of Iran; Mrs R. Frikha, Directorate of Pharmacy Inspection, Tunisia; Dr M. Gershman, Pfizer, the USA; Ms A.R. Cornelio Geyer, Agência Nacional de Vigilância Sanitária, Brazil; Dr E. Griffiths, Consultant, Kingston-upon-Thames, the United Kingdom; Dr N. Harjee, Consultant, Ontario, Canada; Ms D.T.M. Hang, Ministry of Health, Viet Nam; Dr H. Langar, WHO Regional Office for the Eastern Mediterranean, Egypt; Dr P. Lauer, Sanofi Pasteur, France; Dr C.K. Lee, Korea Food and Drug Administration, Republic of Korea; Dr H. Leng, Medicines Regulatory Authority, South Africa; Dr M.G. Lopez Santos, Comisión Federal para la Protección contra Riesgos Sanitarios, Mexico; V.G. Maqueda, Biologist, Buenos Aires, Argentina; Dr A. Mihaylova, Bulgarian Drug Agency, Bulgaria; Dr J. Miteva, Bulgarian Drug Agency, Bulgaria; Dr S. Pagliusi, DCVMN International, Switzerland; Dr V.A. Pessanha, Oswaldo Cruz Foundation, Brazil; Mrs K. Porkaew, Ministry of Public Health, Thailand; Dr S. Ramanan, Amgen, the USA; Dr P. Rampignon,

GSK Vaccines, Belgium; Dr D. Rebeski, The Biovac Institute, South Africa; Dr M. Refaat, Central Administration for Pharmaceutical Affairs, Egypt; Dr S.O. Rumiano, Consultant, Buenos Aires, Argentina; Dr A.L. Salvati, Agenzia Italiana del Farmaco, Italy; Dr J. Shin, WHO Regional Office for the Western Pacific, Philippines; Dr W. Stevens, Health Canada, Canada; Dr I. Susanti, PT Bio Farma, Indonesia; Ms C.S. Takata, Butantan Institute, Brazil; Dr S. Uddin, Directorate General of Drug Administration, Bangladesh; Dr Y. Wang, National Institutes for Food and Drug Control, China; Mr B. Wibisono, National Agency of Drug and Food Control, Indonesia; and Dr A.K. Broojerdi, Dr D. Lei, Dr I. Streipa-Nauman and Dr D.J. Wood, World Health Organization, Switzerland.

The document WHO/BS/2015.2253, incorporating comments received from regulators and industry following public consultation on the WHO Biologicals website, was prepared by V.G. Maqueda, Biologist, Buenos Aires, Argentina; Dr B. Yáñez Chamizo, Centro para el Control Estatal de Medicamentos, Equipos y Dispositivos Médicos, Cuba; Dr S. Fakhrzadeh, Ministry of Health and Medical Education, the Islamic Republic of Iran; Dr S.O. Rumiano, Consultant, Buenos Aires, Argentina; Dr Y. Wang, National Institutes for Food and Drug Control, China; Dr A. Chawla, Consultant, Greater Noida, India; Dr M. Refaat, Central Administration for Pharmaceutical Affairs, Egypt; Dr A. Khadem, Pasteur Institute of Iran, the Islamic Republic of Iran; and Dr M. Chafai, Dr D. Lei, Dr D. Mubangizi and Dr I.R. Thrussell, World Health Organization, Switzerland.

Further changes were subsequently made to document WHO/BS/2015.2253 by the WHO Expert Committee on Biological Standardization.

20. References[4]

1. Good manufacturing practices for biological products. In: WHO Expert Committee on Biological Standardization: forty-second report. Geneva: World Health Organization; 1992: Annex 1 (WHO Technical Report Series, No. 822; http://www.who.int/biologicals/publications/trs/areas/vaccines/gmp/WHO_TRS_822_A1.pdf?ua=1, accessed 8 November 2015).
2. WHO good manufacturing practices for pharmaceutical products: main principles. In: WHO Expert Committee on Specifications for Pharmaceutical Preparations: forty-eighth report. Geneva: World Health Organization; 2013: Annex 2 (WHO Technical Report Series, No. 986; http://www.who.int/medicines/areas/quality_safety/quality_assurance/TRS986annex2.pdf?ua=1, accessed 8 November 2015).
3. WHO good manufacturing practices for sterile pharmaceutical products. In: WHO Expert Committee on Specifications for Pharmaceutical Preparations: forty-fifth report. Geneva: World Health Organization; 2011: Annex 6 (WHO Technical Report Series, No. 961; http://www.who.int/medicines/areas/quality_safety/quality_assurance/GMPSterilePharmaceuticalProductsTRS961Annex6.pdf?ua=1, accessed 8 November 2015).

[4] All WHO GXPs and guidelines for medicines can also be found on the WHO CD-ROM on *Quality assurance of pharmaceuticals. WHO guidelines, good practices, related regulatory guidance and GXP training materials.*

4. WHO good manufacturing practices for active pharmaceutical ingredients. In: WHO Expert Committee on Specifications for Pharmaceutical Preparations: forty-fourth report. Geneva: World Health Organization; 2010: Annex 2 (WHO Technical Report Series, No. 957; http://www.who.int/medicines/areas/quality_safety/quality_assurance/GMPActivePharmaceutical IngredientsTRS957Annex2.pdf?ua=1, accessed 8 November 2015).
5. Guide to good manufacturing practice for medicinal products. Part I, Annex 2. Manufacture of biological medicinal substances and products for human use. Pharmaceutical Inspection Convention and Pharmaceutical Inspection Co-operation Scheme (PIC/S); 1 March 2014 (http://www.fda.gov.ph/attachments/article/224762/pe-009-11-gmp-guide-xannexes.pdf, accessed 8 November 2015).
6. Guide to good manufacturing practice for medicinal products, Part II. Pharmaceutical Inspection Convention and Pharmaceutical Inspection Co-operation Scheme (PIC/S); 1 March 2014 (http://www.medsafe.govt.nz/regulatory/Guideline/PE_009-8_GMP_Guide%20_Part_II_Basic_Requirements_for_API.pdf, accessed 8 November 2015).
7. EU Guidelines for good manufacturing practice for medicinal products for human and veterinary use. Annex 2: Manufacture of biological active substances and medicinal products for human use. Brussels: European Commission; 2013.
8. EU Guidelines for good manufacturing practice for medicinal products for human and veterinary use. Part I. Chapter 6: Quality control. Brussels: European Commission; 2005.
9. Current good manufacturing practice for finished pharmaceuticals. Code of Federal Regulations Title 21, Vol. 4, revised 1 April 2014. Silver Spring, MD: United States Food and Drug Administration; 2014 (http://www.accessdata.fda.gov/scripts/cdrh/cfdocs/cfcfr/CFRSearch.cfm?CFRPart=211&showFR=1, accessed 4 July 2015).
10. WHO good practices for pharmaceutical quality control laboratories. In: WHO Expert Committee on Specifications for Pharmaceutical Preparations: forty-fourth report. Geneva: World Health Organization; 2010: Annex 1 (WHO Technical Report Series, No. 957; http://www.who.int/medicines/areas/quality_safety/quality_assurance/Goodpractices PharmaceuticalQualityControlLaboratoriesTRS957Annex1.pdf?ua=1, accessed 2 February 2016).
11. Good manufacturing practice for drugs (2010 revision). Beijing: China Food and Drug Administration; 2011 (http://eng.sfda.gov.cn/WS03/CL0768/65113.html, accessed 8 November 2015).
12. WHO guidelines on good manufacturing practices for blood establishments. In: WHO Expert Committee on Specifications for Pharmaceutical Preparations: forty-fifth report. Geneva: World Health Organization; 2011: Annex 4 (WHO Technical Report Series, No. 961; http://www.who.int/bloodproducts/publications/GMP_Bloodestablishments.pdf?ua=1, accessed 2 February 2016).
13. WHO good distribution practices for pharmaceutical products. In: WHO Expert Committee on Specifications for Pharmaceutical Preparations: forty-fourth report. Geneva: World Health Organization; 2010: Annex 5 (WHO Technical Report Series, No. 957; http://www.who.int/medicines/areas/quality_safety/quality_assurance/GoodDistributionPracticesTRS957Annex5.pdf?ua=1, accessed 2 February 2016).
14. WHO guidelines on quality risk management. In: WHO Expert Committee on Specifications for Pharmaceutical Preparations: forty-seventh report. Geneva: World Health Organization; 2013: Annex 2 (WHO Technical Report Series, No. 981; http://www.who.int/medicines/areas/quality_safety/quality_assurance/Annex2TRS-981.pdf?ua=1, accessed 2 February 2016).
15. Recommendations for the production, control and regulation of human plasma for fractionation. In: WHO Expert Committee on Biological Standardization: fifty-sixth report. Geneva: World Health Organization; 2007: Annex 4 (WHO Technical Report Series, No. 941; http://www.who.int/bloodproducts/publications/TRS941Annex4blood.pdf?ua=1, accessed 2 February 2016).

16. Good manufacturing practices: supplementary guidelines for the manufacture of investigational pharmaceutical products for clinical trials in humans. In WHO Expert Committee on Specifications for Pharmaceutical Preparations: thirty-fourth report. Geneva: World Health Organization; 1996: Annex 7 (WHO Technical Report Series, No. 863; http://www.who.int/medicines/areas/quality_safety/quality_assurance/Investigational PharmaceuticalProductsClinicalTrialsHumansTRS863Annex7.pdf?ua=1, accessed 2 February 2016).
17. WHO guidelines on nonclinical evaluation of vaccines. In: WHO Expert Committee on Biological Standardization: fifty-fourth report. Geneva: World Health Organization; 2005: Annex 1 (WHO Technical Report Series, No. 927; http://www.who.int/biologicals/publications/trs/areas/vaccines/nonclinical_evaluation/ANNEX%201Nonclinical.P31-63.pdf?ua=1, accessed 8 November 2015).
18. Guidelines on clinical evaluation of vaccines: regulatory expectations. In: WHO Expert Committee on Biological Standardization: fifty-second report. Geneva: World Health Organization; 2004: Annex 1 (WHO Technical Report Series, No. 924; http://www.who.int/biologicals/publications/trs/areas/vaccines/clinical_evaluation/035-101.pdf?ua=1, accessed 2 February 2016).
19. Guidelines on the nonclinical evaluation of vaccine adjuvants and adjuvanted vaccines. In: WHO Expert Committee on Biological Standardization: sixty-fourth report. Geneva: World Health Organization; 2014: Annex 2 (WHO Technical Report Series, No. 987; http://www.who.int/biologicals/areas/vaccines/TRS_987_Annex2.pdf?ua=1, accessed 2 February 2016).
20. Laboratory biosafety manual, third edition. Geneva: World Health Organization; 2004 (http://www.who.int/csr/resources/publications/biosafety/Biosafety7.pdf, accessed 8 November 2015).
21. Guidelines on viral inactivation and removal procedures intended to assure the viral safety of human blood plasma products. In: WHO Expert Committee on Biological Standardization: fifty-second report. Geneva: World Health Organization; 2004: Annex 4 (WHO Technical Report Series, No. 924; http://www.who.int/bloodproducts/publications/WHO_TRS_924_A4.pdf?ua=1, accessed 21 January 2016).
22. ICH Harmonised Tripartite Guideline Q10. Pharmaceutical quality system. Geneva: International Conference on Harmonisation of Technical Requirements for Registration of Pharmaceuticals for Human Use; June 2008 (http://www.ich.org/fileadmin/Public_Web_Site/ICH_Products/Guidelines/Quality/Q10/Step4/Q10_Guideline.pdf, accessed 8 November 2015).
23. Recommendations to assure the quality, safety and efficacy of BCG vaccines. In: WHO Expert Committee on Biological Standardization: sixty-second report. Geneva: World Health Organization; 2013: Annex 3 (WHO Technical Report Series, No. 979; http://www.who.int/biologicals/areas/vaccines/TRS_979_Annex_3.pdf?ua=1, accessed 21 January 2016).
24. WHO Guidelines on transmissible spongiform encephalopathies in relation to biological and pharmaceutical products. Geneva: World Health Organization; 2003 (http://www.who.int/biologicals/publications/en/whotse2003.pdf?ua=1, accessed 2 February 2016).
25. Environmental monitoring of clean rooms in vaccine manufacturing facilities: points to consider for manufacturers of human vaccines. Geneva: World Health Organization; 2012 (http://www.who.int/immunization_standards/vaccine_quality/env_monitoring_cleanrooms_final.pdf?ua=1, accessed 2 February 2016).
26. Recommendations for the evaluation of animal cell cultures as substrates for the manufacturer of biological medicinal products and for the characterization of cell banks. In: WHO Expert Committee on Biological Standardization: sixty-first report. Geneva: World Health Organization; 2013: Annex 3 (WHO Technical Report Series, No. 978; http://www.who.int/biologicals/vaccines/TRS_978_Annex_3.pdf?ua=1, accessed 2 February 2016).
27. Biosafety [website]. Atlanta, GA: Centers for Disease Control and Prevention (http://www.cdc.gov/biosafety/, accessed 8 November 2015).

28. WHO Global Action Plan to minimize poliovirus facility-associated risk after type-specific eradication of wild polioviruses and sequential cessation of OPV use. Geneva: World Health Organization; 2015 (http://www.polioeradication.org/Portals/0/Document/Resources/PostEradication/GAPIII_2014.pdf, accessed 8 November 2015).
29. Guidelines for the safe production and quality control of inactivated poliomyelitis vaccine manufactured from wild polioviruses (Addendum, 2003, to the Recommendations for the production and quality control of poliomyelitis vaccine (inactivated)). In: WHO Expert Committee on Biological Standardization: fifty-third report. Geneva: World Health Organization; 2004: Annex 2 (WHO Technical Report Series, No. 926; http://www.who.int/biologicals/publications/trs/areas/vaccines/polio/Annex%202%20(65-89)TRS926Polio2003.pdf?ua=1, accessed 2 February 2016).
30. Recommendations for the preparation, characterization and establishment of international and other biological reference standards (revised 2004). In: WHO Expert Committee on Biological Standardization: fifty-fifth report. Geneva: World Health Organization; 2006: Annex 2 (WHO Technical Report Series, No. 932; http://www.who.int/immunization_standards/vaccine_reference_preparations/TRS932Annex%202_Inter%20_biol%20ef%20standards%20rev2004.pdf?ua=1, accessed 2 February 2016).
31. Guidelines on stability evaluation of vaccines. In: WHO Expert Committee on Biological Standardization: fifty-seventh report. Geneva: World Health Organization; 2011: Annex 3 (WHO Technical Report Series, No. 962; http://www.who.int/biologicals/vaccines/Annex_3_WHO_TRS_962-3.pdf?ua=1, accessed 21 January 2016).
32. Supplementary guidelines on good manufacturing practices: validation. In: WHO Expert Committee on Specifications for Pharmaceutical Preparations: fortieth report. Geneva: World Health Organization; 2006: Annex 4 (WHO Technical Report Series, No. 937; http://www.who.int/medicines/areas/quality_safety/quality_assurance/SupplementaryGMPValidationTRS937Annex4.pdf?ua=1, accessed 2 February 2016).
33. A WHO guide to good manufacturing practice (GMP) requirements. Part 2: Validation. Geneva: World Health Organization; 1997 (WHO/VSQ/97.02; http://apps.who.int/iris/bitstream/10665/64465/2/WHO_VSQ_97.02.pdf?ua=1, accessed 2 February 2016).
34. Guideline on bioanalytical method validation. Committee for Medicinal Products for Human Use. London: European Medicines Agency; 2009 (EMEA/CHMP/EWP/192217/2009 Rev.1; http://www.ema.europa.eu/docs/en_GB/document_library/Scientific_guideline/2011/08/WC500109686.pdf, accessed 8 November 2015).
35. Guidance for industry. Bioanalytical method validation. Rockville, MD: Center for Veterinary Medicine; 2013 (http://www.fda.gov/downloads/drugs/guidancecomplianceregulatoryinformation/guidances/ucm368107.pdf, accessed 8 November 2015).
36. Guidelines for independent lot release of vaccines by regulatory authorities. In: WHO Expert Committee on Biological Standardization: sixty-first report. Geneva: World Health Organization; 2013: Annex 2 (WHO Technical Report Series, No. 978; http://www.who.int/biologicals/TRS_978_Annex_2.pdf?ua=1, accessed 2 February 2016).

Annex 4

Guidance on good manufacturing practices: inspection report

Background

The need for revision of the *Guidance on good manufacturing practices: inspection report* (World Health Organization (WHO) Technical Report Series, No. 908, Annex 6, 2003) was brought to the attention of the WHO Expert Committee on Specifications for Pharmaceutical Preparations. The intent of this update is to bring it in line with the current format used by the Prequalification Team (PQT) for its inspections and the formats currently used internationally in national and regional inspectorates. In addition, the concepts of risk management, as, for example, included in the *WHO guidelines on quality risk management* (WHO Technical Report Series, No. 986, Annex 6, 2014), have been taken into consideration.

1. Introduction

1.1 This guidance describes general principles and a recommended format for inspection reports for use by organizations performing pharmaceutical inspections. It aims to support convergence of practices in drawing up inspection reports so as to facilitate cooperation and information sharing.

2. Scope

2.1 These guidelines apply to reports on inspections of active pharmaceutical ingredients (APIs) and finished pharmaceutical products (FPPs). A separate template may be used for inspections of contract research organizations and quality control laboratories.

3. Glossary

The definitions given below apply to the terms used in these guidelines. They may have different meanings in other contexts.

correction. A correction is any action that is taken to eliminate a nonconformity. However, corrections do not address causes. When applied to products, corrections can include reworking products, reprocessing them, regrading them, assigning them to a different use, or simply destroying them.

corrective action. Corrective actions are steps that are taken to eliminate the causes of existing nonconformities in order to prevent recurrence. The corrective action process tries to make sure that existing nonconformities and potentially undesirable situations do not happen again. While corrective actions prevent recurrence, *preventive actions* prevent occurrence. Both types of actions are intended to prevent nonconformities.

corrective and preventive action. A system for implementing corrective actions and preventive actions resulting from an investigation of complaints, product rejections, non-conformances, recalls, deviations, audits, regulatory inspections and findings, and trends from process performance and product quality monitoring.

deficiency. Non-fulfilment of a requirement. In this sense this term can be used interchangeably with “nonconformity”.

inspection observation. An inspection observation is a finding or a statement of fact made during an inspection and substantiated by objective evidence. Such findings may be positive or negative. Positive observations should take the form of a description of the processes that the firm is carrying out particularly well and that may be considered examples of particularly good practice. Negative observations are findings of non-compliance with requirements.

nonconformity. Nonconformity refers to a failure to comply with requirements. A requirement is a need, expectation or obligation. It can be stated or implied by an organization, its customers or other interested parties. There are many types of requirements. These include quality requirements, customer requirements, management requirements, product requirements, process requirements and legal requirements. Whenever an organization fails to meet one of these requirements, a nonconformity occurs.

preventive action. Preventive actions are steps that are taken to remove the causes of potential nonconformities or potential situations that are undesirable.

4. General principles

4.1 When a site at which pharmaceutical products are manufactured is inspected, the inspector(s) responsible should draw up a report. The inspection report should include the items shown in the proposed model inspection report (Appendix 1), adapted as appropriate, according to the national or regional settings and to the scope and purpose of the inspection. Where relevant the appropriate system of good manufacturing practices (GMP) or the nationally appropriate legal basis for GMP, should be indicated.

4.2 The purpose of an inspection report is to provide a factual and objective record of the inspection that includes what was done, the inspection observations or findings (positive and negative) for each activity inspected, as communicated to the company before the end of the inspection, and a conclusion that is applicable at the time that the report is written. Positive findings may include praise for noteworthy efforts in areas that are seen as excellent examples of implementation of the requirements of the guidelines. They could also be conveyed when the company has shown significant improvement in certain areas compared to the findings from previous inspections. Noteworthy efforts do not require any action. Their inclusion in the inspection report is done to highlight areas of strength for future tracking of improvements or areas of decline and to show the organization what areas it can feel proud of.

4.3 The report should be prepared in a timely manner after an inspection, with the participation of all members of the inspection team under the coordination of the lead inspector. The report should be reviewed in accordance with the quality system of the inspectorate.

4.4 The inspection report should, as appropriate, be written in the third person, passive voice and the past tense.

Example: "Cleaning logs for rooms and equipment *were maintained* in all areas of the factory."

4.5 All the observations that are considered as deficiencies/noncompliances should be listed under Part 3 of the report. Each observation included in an inspection report should be referenced to the relevant GMP text, WHO guidelines or conditions or commitments under the marketing authorization. An observation that cannot be reasonably referenced should not be listed as a deficiency.

4.6 The non-compliance statement should include the requirement (R), evidence (E) and deficiency (D).

Example: (R) The relevant cleaning records and source data should be kept in cleaning validation reports; (E) the source of three samples taken for recovery testing during the process equipment validation was not traceable; (D) cleaning validation reports did not include sufficient data.

4.7 Deficiencies/noncompliance statements should distinguish whether the defect lies in the system itself or in a failure to comply with the system. For instance, when cleaning is found to be suboptimal, it is important to know whether the standard operating procedures (SOPs) are inadequate or lacking, or whether adequate written procedures exist but are not being followed by personnel.

4.8 Where more than one deficiency relates to the same basic quality system failure, the deficiencies should be grouped and listed as a single observation, under a heading that reflects the basic system failure.

4.9 Deficiencies should be reported with a focus on risk to patient health and/ or need for corrective and preventive action (CAPA).

4.10 The report should not include comments that could be construed as proposed specific solutions to issues raised. Recommendations should relate to recommended regulatory action as appropriate.

4.11 Each deficiency should be classified as critical, major or other, according to the following definitions, which may be adapted according to the national or regional legal context.

4.11.1 A *critical* deficiency may be defined as an observation that has produced, or may result in a significant risk of producing, a product that is harmful to the user.

4.11.2 A *major* deficiency may be defined as a non-critical observation that:

a) has produced or may produce a product that does not comply with its marketing authorization and/or prequalification application (including variations);
b) indicates a major deviation from the GMP guide;
c) indicates a failure to carry out satisfactory procedures for release of batches;
d) indicates a failure of the person responsible for quality assurance/ quality control to fulfil his or her duties;
e) consists of several other deficiencies, none of which on its own may be major, but which together may represent a major deficiency and should be explained and reported as such.

4.11.3 A deficiency may be classified as *other* if it cannot be classified as either *critical* or *major*, but indicates a departure from GMP. A deficiency may be *other* either because it is judged as minor or because there is insufficient information to classify it as *major* or *critical*.

4.11.4 Classification of a deficiency is based on the assessed risk level and may vary depending on the nature of the products manufactured, e.g. in some circumstances an example of an *other* deficiency may be categorized as *major*.

4.11.5 A deficiency that was reported at a previous inspection and was not corrected may be reported with a higher classification.

4.11.6 One-off minor lapses or less significant issues are usually not formally reported, but are brought to the attention of the manufacturer during the inspection.

4.11.7 The status of compliance with WHO GMP guidelines should be determined by the nature and number of deficiencies:

a) When there are *other* deficiencies only:

i. the site is considered to be operating at an acceptable level of GMP compliance,
ii. the manufacturer is expected to provide CAPAs,
iii. CAPAs are evaluated and followed up during the next routine inspection.

b) When there are *other* and a few *major* deficiencies (e.g. < 6[1]):

   i. the site is compliant with GMP after assessing the CAPAs,
   ii. CAPAs for *all* deficiencies to include actions implemented and/or planned, timelines and documented evidence of completion, as appropriate,
   iii. CAPAs are evaluated on paper and may or may not include an on-site, follow-up inspection.

c) When there are *critical* or several *major* deficiencies (e.g. ≥ 6):

   i. the site is considered to be operating at an unacceptable level of compliance with GMP guidelines,
   ii. another inspection will normally be required,
   iii. administrative and/or legal enforcement actions are applied as necessary.

4.12 The next date for inspection of the site should be determined depending on the level of compliance and risk category as defined under national or regional procedures. Appendix 2 provides an example of how the next inspection date may be determined. Other approaches may be used.

4.13 The report shall be signed by all inspection team members, but may be signed by the lead inspector after consultation with and on behalf of the inspection team, and reviewed in accordance with the quality system of the inspectorate.

[1] The number six is related to the six systems to be inspected, as listed in Appendix 1.

Appendix 1

Guidance on good manufacturing practices: inspection report

Model inspection report

Part 1	General information
Manufacturer details	
Company information	Name of manufacturer Corporate address of manufacturer (including telephone, fax, email and 24-hour telephone numbers) Contact person, telephone number and email address
Inspected site	Address of inspected manufacturing site if different from that given above (including global positioning system (GPS) coordinates in World Geodetic System (WGS) 84: latitude and longitude expressed in decimal degrees, taken at the main entrance of the site; data universal numbering system (D-U-N-S) number: NNNNNNNNN, where each N represents a number from 0–9, if available) and specific production blocks or workshops inspected if the whole site was not inspected Site number (e.g. unit number, site master file number or number allocated by the responsible authority) Manufacturing licence number (if applicable) Key personnel
Summary of activities performed at the site	For example, manufacture of active pharmaceutical ingredient(s) (APIs), manufacture of finished pharmaceutical products (FPPs), intermediates or bulk packaging, laboratory testing, batch release, distribution and importer activities
Inspection details	
Date(s) of inspection(s)	...
Type of inspection	For example, initial, routine, follow-up, special
Inspector(s)	Name(s) and agency affiliations of lead inspector, inspector(s), accompanying experts and observers

Table *continued*

Part 1	General information
Competent regulatory authority	For foreign inspections, state whether the national regulatory authority (NRA) of the country where the inspection took place was informed and whether it took part in the inspection
GMP guidelines used for assessing compliance	List the relevant guidelines stating the title of the guidelines, the title of the publication and web address where the guidelines can be accessed, for example: 1. WHO good manufacturing practices for pharmaceutical products: main principles. In: WHO Expert Committee on Specifications for Pharmaceutical Preparations: forty-eighth report. Geneva: World Health Organization; 2014: Annex 2 (WHO Technical Report Series, No. 986; http://www.who.int/entity/medicines/areas/quality_safety/quality_assurance/TRS986annex2.pdf?ua=1)
Introduction	
Brief summary of the manufacturing activities	Description of main activities (including, e.g. FPP(s) or API(s) manufactured and their reference/registration/active pharmaceutical ingredient master file (APIMF)/drug master file (DMF)/certificate of suitability to the monographs of the European Pharmacopoeia (CEP) numbers, as appropriate); other manufacturing activities carried out on the site (e.g. manufacture of cosmetics, research and development); use of outside scientific, analytical or other technical assistance in manufacture and quality control Brief description of the quality management system of the firm responsible for manufacture. Reference can be made to a site master file if one is available
History	Previous inspection date and history of regulatory agency inspections Summary of past inspections; observations on CAPA from previous inspection Major change since previous inspection and planned future changes GMP-related recalls from the market of any product in the past two years

Table *continued*

Part 1	General information
Brief report of inspection activities undertaken	
Scope and limitations	For example, blocks inspected, areas of interest, focus of inspection Out-of-scope: areas, activities or product lines not inspected Restrictions: constraints noted in inspecting specific areas
Areas inspected	For example, dosage form(s) included in the inspection
Key persons met	Names and job titles

Part 2	Brief summary of the findings and recommendations (where applicable)
	This part of the report is arranged based on the WHO Guidance for good manufacturing practices: main principles. It may also be arranged according to six inspection systems, namely: 1. pharmaceutical quality system, 2. production system, 3. facilities and equipment system, 4. laboratory control system, 5. materials system, 6. packaging and labelling system.The observations made during the inspection that are considered to be non-compliant with GMP should be listed. Where positive observations are included in the report, a clear distinction should be made between positive and non-compliant. Non-compliant observations can be classified, e.g. as *critical*, *major* and *other* if the Member State concerned has defined these terms The date by which corrective action and completion are requested in accordance with the policy of the NRA should be given.
1. Pharmaceutical quality system	Describe the pharmaceutical quality system (PQS) in place and how well the elements are institutionalized and implemented, including the quality risk management (QRM) and product quality review (PQR)

Table *continued*

Part 2	Brief summary of the findings and recommendations (where applicable)
2. Good manufacturing practices for pharmaceutical products	Briefly describe how the elements of GMP are implemented
3. Sanitation and hygiene	Describe procedures and records relating to sanitation and hygiene for personnel, premises, equipment, production materials, cleaning materials and others that could become a source of contamination
4. Qualification and validation	Describe policies, procedures, records and any other evidence for qualification and validation and how the validation status is monitored and maintained
5. Complaints	Describe procedures, responsibilities and records for handling complaints, including extension of investigation to other batches, possibility of counterfeits, trending and consideration for recall and notification of competent authorities
6. Product recalls	Describe the existence of a recall procedure and evidence of its effectiveness; provisions for notification of customers and competent authorities and segregation of recalled products
7. Contract production, analysis and other activities	Describe how contractors are evaluated, how compliance with marketing authorization is ensured, existence of comprehensive contracts and clarity of responsibilities and limits
8. Self-inspection, quality audits and suppliers' audits and approval	a) Self-inspection: describe the procedures and items for self-inspection and quality audits; constitution of self-inspection team(s); frequency of self-inspection; existence of self-inspection schedules and report; system for monitoring follow-up actions. b) Suppliers' audits and approval: describe procedures for evaluation and approval of suppliers including applications of risk management principles, especially determining the need and frequency for on-site audits.

Table *continued*

Part 2	Brief summary of the findings and recommendations (where applicable)
9. Personnel	Describe availability of adequate numbers of sufficiently qualified and experienced personnel, clarity of their responsibilities, limits and reporting hierarchy. Qualifications, experience and responsibilities of key personnel (head of production, head(s) of the quality unit(s), authorized person) and procedures for delegation of their responsibilities
10. Training	Describe comprehensiveness of procedures and records for induction, specialized and continuing training and evaluation of its effectiveness; coverage of GMP and concepts of quality assurance during training; training of visitors and evaluation consultants and contract staff
11. Personal hygiene	Describe system in place for initial and regular health examination of staff appropriate to their responsibilities. Measures and facilities to impart, maintain and monitor knowledge of a high level of personal hygiene. Measures to ensure personnel do not become a source of contamination to the product, including hand-washing and gowning. Appropriate restriction of smoking, eating, drinking, chewing and related materials from production, laboratory and storage areas
12. Premises	Description of the appropriateness of the location, design, construction and maintenance of premises to minimize errors, avoid cross-contamination, permit effective cleaning and maintenance; measures for dust control; specific measures for ancillary areas, storage areas, weighing areas, production areas and quality control areas; measures for appropriate segregation and restricted access; provisions for appropriate lighting, effective ventilation and air-control to prevent contamination and cross-contamination, as well as control of temperature and, where necessary, humidity
13. Equipment	Describe the adequacy of the numbers, type, location, design and construction, and maintenance of equipment to minimize errors, avoid cross-contamination, permit effective cleaning and maintenance; use, cleaning and maintenance procedures, records and logs; calibration of balances and other measuring instruments; status labelling

Table *continued*

Part 2	Brief summary of the findings and recommendations (where applicable)
14. Materials	Describe measures in place to select, store, approve and use materials (including water) of appropriate quality and how these measures cover starting materials, packaging materials, intermediate and bulk products, finished products, reagents, culture media and reference standards. Describe also the measures for the handling and control of rejected, recovered, reprocessed and reworked materials; recalled products; returned goods; and waste materials
15. Documentation	Describe the comprehensiveness and adequacy of the documentation system in place (labels; specifications and testing procedures, starting, packaging materials, intermediate, bulk products and finished products; master formulas; packaging instructions; batch processing and packaging records; standard operating procedures (SOPs) and records) and how principles of good documentation and data management (attributable, legible, contemporaneous, original, accurate (ALCOA)) are institutionalized, implemented and maintained
16. Good practices in production	Describe procedures, facilities and controls in place for production (processing and packaging); prevention of risk of mix-up, cross-contamination and bacterial contamination during production
17. Good practices in quality control	Describe the extent of the organizational and functional independence of the quality control function and the adequacy of its resourcing. Describe the procedures, facilities, organization and documentation in place which ensure that the necessary and relevant tests are actually carried out and that materials are not released for use, nor products released for sale or supply, until their quality has been judged to be compliant with the requirements. Describe the procedures for the control of starting materials and intermediate, bulk and finished products; test requirements; procedures and responsibilities for batch record review; procedures, records and facilities for initial and ongoing stability studies; policy, procedures, facilities and records for retention samples.

Table *continued*

Part 2	**Brief summary of the findings and recommendations (where applicable)**	
Samples taken	(if applicable)	
Assessment of the site master file	(if applicable)	
Annexes attached	...	

Part 3	**List of deficiencies**	
List of deficiencies	Deficiencies should be listed by category with reference to the relevant section(s) of GMP guidelines. This may be presented in a tabular format, giving references to the relevant GMP requirement:	
	Deficiencies	References
1. Critical	1.1 ... 1.2 ...	... ...
2. Major	2.1 ... 2.2 ...	... ...
3. Other	3.1 ... 3.2 ...	... ...

Part 4	**Outcome**
Initial conclusion	Statement regarding the GMP status, including information on any restrictions in scope. The following guidance may be used to determine the outcome of the inspection based on the nature and number of deficiencies observed: • *other* deficiencies only: operating at an acceptable level of compliance with GMP guidelines; • *other* and a few (e.g. < 6) *major* deficiencies: decision on level of compliance to be made after receipt and evaluation of CAPAs; • *any critical* or several (e.g. ≥ 6) *major* deficiencies: operating at an unacceptable level of compliance with GMP guidelines.

Part 5	List of GMP guidelines referenced in the inspection
References	List of GMP guidelines referred to in the inspection, for example: 1. WHO good manufacturing practices for pharmaceutical products: main principles. In: WHO Expert Committee on Specifications for Pharmaceutical Preparations: forty-eighth report. Geneva: World Health Organization; 2014: Annex 2 (WHO Technical Report Series, No. 986; http://www.who.int/medicines/publications/pharmprep/en/index.html) 2. WHO good manufacturing practices for sterile pharmaceutical products. In: WHO Expert Committee on Specifications for Pharmaceutical Preparations: forty-fifth report. Geneva: World Health Organization; 2011: Annex 6 (WHO Technical Report Series, No. 961; http://www.who.int/medicines/publications/pharmprep/en/index.html) 3. WHO good manufacturing practices for active pharmaceutical ingredients. In: WHO Expert Committee on Specifications for Pharmaceutical Preparations: forty-fourth report. Geneva: World Health Organization; 2010: Annex 3 (WHO Technical Report Series, No. 957; http://www.who.int/medicines/publications/pharmprep/en/index.html) 4. WHO good manufacturing practices: water for pharmaceutical use. In: WHO Expert Committee on Specifications for Pharmaceutical Preparations: forty-sixth report. Geneva: World Health Organization; 2012: Annex 2 (WHO Technical Report Series, No. 970; http://www.who.int/medicines/publications/pharmprep/en/index.html) 5. WHO guidelines on good manufacturing practices for heating, ventilation and air-conditioning systems for non-sterile pharmaceutical dosage forms. In: WHO Expert Committee on Specifications for Pharmaceutical Preparations: forty-fifth report. Geneva: World Health Organization; 2011: Annex 5 (WHO Technical Report Series, No. 961; http://www.who.int/medicines/publications/pharmprep/en/index.html) 6. General guidelines for the establishment maintenance and distribution of chemical reference substances. In: WHO Expert Committee on Specifications for Pharmaceutical Preparations: forty-first report. Geneva: World Health Organization; 2011: Annex 3 (WHO Technical Report Series, No. 937; http://www.who.int/medicines/publications/pharmprep/en/index.html)

Part 6	Assessment of company response, final conclusion, risk rating and next due date
Brief narrative on the adequacy of the company's response to issues to be addressed	...
Final conclusion	Final statement of GMP compliance, including information on any restrictions in scope
Risk rating following the inspection	For example, low (L), medium (M), high (H), critical (C)
Date next inspection due (for planning purposes)	The inspectorate may decide to include this information for internal use only
Name(s) (all inspectors or lead inspector)	
Signature(s) (all inspectors or lead inspector)	
Date	

Appendix 2

Example of a risk category assessment of the site depending on level of compliance and inspection frequency

Risk category of the site	GMP compliance rating and related inspection frequency (in months)			
	Acceptable			Unacceptable
	Good	Satisfactory	Basic	
Critical (C)	24	18	12	Determine on a case-by-case basis
High (H)	30	20	15	Determine on a case-by-case basis
Medium (M)	36	24	18	Determine on a case-by-case basis
Low (L)	48	36	24	Determine on a case-by-case basis

Annex 5

Guidance on good data and record management practices

Background

During an informal consultation on inspection, good manufacturing practices and risk management guidance in medicines' manufacturing held by the World Health Organization (WHO) in Geneva in April 2014, a proposal for new guidance on good data management was discussed and its development recommended. The participants included national inspectors and specialists in the various agenda topics, as well as staff of the Prequalification Team (PQT)–Inspections.

The WHO Expert Committee on Specifications for Pharmaceutical Preparations received feedback from this informal consultation during its forty-ninth meeting in October 2014. A concept paper was received from PQT–Inspections describing the proposed structure of a new guidance document, which was discussed in detail. The concept paper consolidated existing normative principles and gave some illustrative examples of their implementation. In the Appendix to the concept paper, extracts from existing good practices and guidance documents were combined to illustrate the current relevant guidance on assuring the reliability of data and related GXP (good (anything) practice) matters. In view of the increasing number of observations made during inspections that relate to data management practices, the Committee endorsed the proposal.

Following this endorsement, a draft document was prepared by members of PQT–Inspection and a drafting group, including national inspectors. This draft was discussed at a consultation on data management, bioequivalence, good manufacturing practices and medicines' inspection held from 29 June to 1 July 2015.

A revised draft document was subsequently prepared by the authors in collaboration with the drafting group, based on the feedback received during this consultation, and the subsequent WHO workshop on data management.

Collaboration is being sought with other organizations towards future convergence in this area.

1. Introduction

1.1 Medicines regulatory systems worldwide have always depended upon the knowledge of organizations that develop, manufacture and package, test, distribute and monitor pharmaceutical products. Implicit in the assessment and review process is trust between the regulator and the regulated that the information submitted in dossiers and used in day-to-day decision-making is comprehensive, complete and reliable. The data on which these decisions are based should therefore be complete as well as being attributable, legible, contemporaneous, original and accurate, commonly referred to as "ALCOA".

1.2 These basic ALCOA principles and the related good practice expectations that assure data reliability are not new and much high- and mid-level normative guidance already exists. However, in recent years, the number of observations made regarding good data and record management practices (GDRP) during inspections of good manufacturing practice (GMP) (*1*), good clinical practice (GCP) and good laboratory practice (GLP) has been increasing. The reasons for the increasing concern of health authorities regarding data reliability are undoubtedly multifactorial and include increased regulatory awareness and concern regarding gaps between industry choices and appropriate and modern control strategies.

1.3 Contributing factors include failures by organizations to apply robust systems that inhibit data risks, to improve the detection of situations where data reliability may be compromised, and/or to investigate and address root causes when failures do arise. For example, organizations subject to medical product good practice requirements have been using validated computerized systems for many decades but many fail to adequately review and manage original electronic records and instead often only review and manage incomplete and/or inappropriate printouts. These observations highlight the need for industry to modernize control strategies and apply modern quality risk management (QRM) and sound scientific principles to current business models (such as outsourcing and globalization) as well as technologies currently in use (such as computerized systems).

1.4 Examples of controls that may require development and strengthening to ensure good data management strategies include, but are not limited to:

- a QRM approach that effectively assures patient safety and product quality and validity of data by ensuring that management aligns expectations with actual process capabilities. Management should take responsibility for good data management by first setting realistic and achievable expectations for the true and current capabilities of a process, a method, an environment, personnel, or technologies, among others;

- monitoring of processes and allocation of the necessary resources by management to ensure and enhance infrastructure, as required (for example, to continuously improve processes and methods, to ensure adequate design and maintenance of buildings, facilities, equipment and systems; to ensure adequate reliable power and water supplies; to provide necessary training for personnel; and to allocate the necessary resources to the oversight of contract sites and suppliers to ensure adequate quality standards are met). Active engagement of management in this manner remediates and reduces pressures and possible sources of error that may increase data integrity risks;
- adoption of a quality culture within the company that encourages personnel to be transparent about failures so that management has an accurate understanding of risks and can then provide the necessary resources to achieve expectations and meet data quality standards: a reporting mechanism independent of management hierarchy should be provided for;
- mapping of data processes and application of modern QRM and sound scientific principles throughout the data life cycle;
- ensuring that all site personnel are kept up to date about the application of good documentation practices (GDocP) to ensure that the GXP principles of ALCOA are understood and applied to electronic data in the same manner that has historically been applied to paper records;
- implementation and confirmation during validation of computerized systems and subsequent change control, that all necessary controls for GDocP for electronic data are in place and that the probability of the occurrence of errors in the data is minimized;
- training of personnel who use computerized systems and review electronic data in basic understanding of how computerized systems work and how to efficiently review the electronic data, which includes metadata and audit trails;
- definition and management of appropriate roles and responsibilities for quality agreements and contracts entered into by contract givers and contract acceptors, including the need for risk-based monitoring of data generated and managed by the contract acceptor on behalf of the contract giver;
- modernization of quality assurance inspection techniques and gathering of quality metrics to efficiently and effectively identify risks and opportunities to improve data processes.

2. Aims and objectives of this guidance

2.1 This guidance consolidates existing normative principles and gives detailed illustrative implementation guidance to bridge the gaps in current guidance. Additionally, it gives explanations as to what these high-level requirements mean in practice and what should be demonstrably implemented to achieve compliance.

2.2 These guidelines highlight, and in some instances clarify, the application of data management procedures. The focus is on those principles that are implicit in existing WHO guidelines and that if not robustly implemented can impact on data reliability and completeness and undermine the robustness of decision-making based upon those data. Illustrative examples are provided as to how these principles may be applied to current technologies and business models. These guidelines do not define all expected controls for assuring data reliability and this guidance should be considered in conjunction with existing WHO guidelines and other related international references.

2.3 This guidance is of an evolutionary, illustrative nature and will therefore be subject to periodic review based upon experience with its implementation and usefulness, as well as the feedback provided by the stakeholders, including national regulatory authorities (NRAs).

3. Glossary

The definitions given below apply to the terms used in these guidelines. They may have different meanings in other contexts.

ALCOA. A commonly used acronym for "attributable, legible, contemporaneous, original and accurate".

ALCOA-plus. A commonly used acronym for "attributable, legible, contemporaneous, original and accurate", which puts additional emphasis on the attributes of being complete, consistent, enduring and available – implicit basic ALCOA principles.

archival. Archiving is the process of protecting records from the possibility of being further altered or deleted, and storing these records under the control of independent data management personnel throughout the required retention period. Archived records should include, for example, associated metadata and electronic signatures.

archivist. An independent individual designated in good laboratory practice (GLP) who has been authorized by management to be responsible for the management of the archive, i.e. for the operations and procedures for archiving. GLP requires a designated archivist (i.e. an individual); however, in other GXPs the roles and responsibilities of the archivist are normally fulfilled by several designated personnel or groups of personnel (e.g. both quality assurance document control personnel and information technology (IT) system administrators) without there being one single person assigned responsibility for control as is required in GLP.

It is recognized that in certain circumstances it may be necessary for the archivist to delegate specific archiving tasks, for example, the management of electronic data, to specific IT personnel. Tasks, duties and responsibilities should be specified and detailed in standard operating procedures. The responsibilities of the archivist and the staff to whom archival tasks are delegated include – for both paper and electronic data – ensuring that access to the archive is controlled, ensuring that the orderly storage and retrieval of records and materials is facilitated by a system of indexing, and ensuring that movement of records and materials into and out of the archives is properly controlled and documented. These procedures and records should be periodically reviewed by an independent auditor.

audit trail. The audit trail is a form of metadata that contains information associated with actions that relate to the creation, modification or deletion of GXP records. An audit trail provides for secure recording of life-cycle details such as creation, additions, deletions or alterations of information in a record, either paper or electronic, without obscuring or overwriting the original record. An audit trail facilitates the reconstruction of the history of such events relating to the record regardless of its medium, including the "who, what, when and why" of the action.

For example, in a paper record, an audit trail of a change would be documented via a single-line cross-out that allows the original entry to remain legible and documents the initials of the person making the change, the date of the change and the reason for the change, as required to substantiate and justify the change. In electronic records, secure, computer-generated, time-stamped audit trails should allow for reconstruction of the course of events relating to the creation, modification and deletion of electronic data. Computer-generated audit trails should retain the original entry and document the user identification, the time/date stamp of the action, as well as the reason for the change, as required to substantiate and justify the action. Computer-generated audit trails may include discrete event logs, history files, database queries or reports or other mechanisms that display events related to the computerized system, specific electronic records or specific data contained within the record.

backup. A backup means a copy of one or more electronic files created as an alternative in case the original data or system are lost or become unusable (for example, in the event of a system crash or corruption of a disk). It is important to note that backup differs from archival in that back-up copies of electronic records are typically only temporarily stored for the purposes of disaster recovery and may be periodically overwritten. Such temporary back-up copies should not be relied upon as an archival mechanism.

computerized system. A computerized system collectively controls the performance of one or more automated processes and/or functions. It includes computer hardware, software, peripheral devices, networks and documentation, e.g. manuals and standard operating procedures, as well as the personnel interfacing with the hardware and software, e.g. users and information technology support personnel.

control strategy. A planned set of controls, derived from current protocol, test article or product and process understanding, which assures protocol compliance, process performance, product quality and data reliability, as applicable. The controls should include appropriate parameters and quality attributes related to study subjects, test systems, product materials and components, technologies and equipment, facilities, operating conditions, specifications and the associated methods and frequency of monitoring and control.

corrective and preventive action (**CAPA**, also sometimes called **corrective action/preventive action**) refers to the actions taken to improve an organization's processes and to eliminate causes of non-conformities or other undesirable situations. CAPA is a concept common across the GXPs (good laboratory practices, good clinical practices and good manufacturing practices), and numerous International Organization for Standardization business standards. The process focuses on the systematic investigation of the root causes of identified problems or identified risks in an attempt to prevent their recurrence (for corrective action) or to prevent occurrence (for preventive action).

data. Data means all original records and true copies of original records, including source data and metadata and all subsequent transformations and reports of these data, which are generated or recorded at the time of the GXP activity and allow full and complete reconstruction and evaluation of the GXP activity. Data should be accurately recorded by permanent means at the time of the activity. Data may be contained in paper records (such as worksheets and logbooks), electronic records and audit trails, photographs, microfilm or microfiche, audio- or video-files or any other media whereby information related to GXP activities is recorded.

data governance. The totality of arrangements to ensure that data, irrespective of the format in which they are generated, are recorded, processed, retained and used to ensure a complete, consistent and accurate record throughout the data life cycle.

data integrity. Data integrity is the degree to which data are complete, consistent, accurate, trustworthy and reliable and that these characteristics of the data are maintained throughout the data life cycle. The data should be collected and maintained in a secure manner, such that they are attributable, legible, contemporaneously recorded, original or a true copy and accurate. Assuring data integrity requires appropriate quality and risk management systems, including adherence to sound scientific principles and good documentation practices.

data life cycle. All phases of the process by which data are created, recorded, processed, reviewed, analysed and reported, transferred, stored and retrieved and monitored until retirement and disposal. There should be a planned approach to assessing, monitoring and managing the data and the risks to those data in a manner commensurate with potential impact on patient safety, product quality and/or the reliability of the decisions made throughout all phases of the data life cycle.

dynamic record format. Records in dynamic format, such as electronic records, that allow for an interactive relationship between the user and the record content. For example, electronic records in database formats allow the user to track, trend and query data; chromatography records maintained as electronic records allow the user (with proper access permissions) to reprocess the data and expand the baseline to view the integration more clearly.

fully-electronic approach. This term refers to use of a computerized system in which the original electronic records are electronically signed.

good data and record management practices. The totality of organized measures that should be in place to collectively and individually ensure that data and records are secure, attributable, legible, traceable, permanent, contemporaneously recorded, original and accurate and that if not robustly implemented can impact on data reliability and completeness and undermine the robustness of decision-making based upon those data records.

good documentation practices. In the context of these guidelines, good documentation practices are those measures that collectively and individually ensure documentation, whether paper or electronic, is secure, attributable, legible, traceable, permanent, contemporaneously recorded, original and accurate.

GXP. Acronym for the group of good practice guides governing the preclinical, clinical, manufacturing, testing, storage, distribution and post-market activities for regulated pharmaceuticals, biologicals and medical devices, such as good laboratory practices, good clinical practices, good manufacturing practices, good pharmacovigilance practices and good distribution practices.

hybrid approach. This refers to the use of a computerized system in which there is a combination of original electronic records and paper records that comprise the total record set that should be reviewed and retained. An example of a hybrid approach is where laboratory analysts use computerized instrument systems that create original electronic records and then print a summary of the results. The hybrid approach requires a secure link between all record types, including paper and electronic, throughout the records retention period. Where hybrid approaches are used, appropriate controls for electronic documents, such as templates, forms and master documents, that may be printed, should be available.

metadata. Metadata are data about data that provide the contextual information required to understand those data. These include structural and descriptive metadata. Such data describe the structure, data elements, interrelationships and other characteristics of data. They also permit data to be attributable to an individual. Metadata necessary to evaluate the meaning of data should be securely linked to the data and subject to adequate review. For example, in weighing, the number 8 is meaningless without metadata, i.e. the unit, mg. Other examples of metadata include the time/date stamp of an activity, the operator identification (ID) of the person who performed an activity, the instrument ID used, processing parameters, sequence files, audit trails and other data required to understand data and reconstruct activities.

quality metrics. Quality metrics are objective measures used by management and other interested parties to monitor the overall state of quality of a GXP organization, activity or process or study conduct, as applicable. They include measures to assess the effective functioning of quality system controls and of the performance, quality and safety of medicinal products and reliability of data.

quality risk management. A systematic process for the assessment, control, communication and review of risks to the quality of the pharmaceutical product throughout the product life cycle.

senior management. Person(s) who direct and control a company or site at the highest levels with the authority and responsibility to mobilize resources within the company or site.

static record format. A static record format, such as a paper or pdf record, is one that is fixed and allows little or no interaction between the user and the record content. For example, once printed or converted to static pdfs, chromatography records lose the capability of being reprocessed or enabling more detailed viewing of baselines.

true copy. A true copy is a copy of an original recording of data that has been verified and certified to confirm it is an exact and complete copy that preserves the entire content and meaning of the original record, including, in the case of electronic data, all essential metadata and the original record format as appropriate.

4. Principles

4.1 GDRP are critical elements of the pharmaceutical quality system and a systematic approach should be implemented to provide a high level of assurance that throughout the product life cycle, all GXP records and data are complete and reliable.

4.2 The data governance programme should include policies and governance procedures that address the general principles listed below for a good data management programme. These principles are clarified with additional detail in the sections below.

4.3 **Applicability to both paper and electronic data.** The requirements for GDRP that assure robust control of data validity apply equally to paper and electronic data. Organizations subject to GXP should be fully aware that reverting from automated or computerized to manual or paper-based systems does not in itself remove the need for robust management controls.

4.4 **Applicability to contract givers and contract acceptors.** The principles of these guidelines apply to contract givers and contract acceptors. Contract givers are ultimately responsible for the robustness of all decisions made on the basis of GXP data, including those made on the basis of data provided to them by contract acceptors. Contract givers should therefore perform risk-based, due diligence to assure themselves that contract acceptors have in place appropriate programmes to ensure the veracity, completeness and reliability of the data provided.

4.5 **Good documentation practices.** To achieve robust decisions, the supporting data set needs to be reliable and complete. GDocP should be followed in order to ensure all records, both paper and electronic, allow the full reconstruction and traceability of GXP activities.

4.6 **Management governance.** To establish a robust and sustainable good data management system it is important that senior management ensure that appropriate data management governance programmes are in place (for details see Section 6).

Elements of effective management governance should include:

- application of modern QRM principles and good data management principles that assure the validity, completeness and reliability of data;
- application of appropriate quality metrics;
- assurance that personnel are not subject to commercial, political, financial and other organizational pressures or incentives that may adversely affect the quality and integrity of their work;
- allocation of adequate human and technical resources such that the workload, work hours and pressures on those responsible for data generation and record keeping do not increase errors;
- ensure staff are aware of the importance of their role in ensuring data integrity and the relationship of these activities to assuring product quality and protecting patient safety.

4.7 **Quality culture.** Management, with the support of the quality unit, should establish and maintain a working environment that minimizes the risk of non-compliant records and erroneous records and data. An essential element of the quality culture is the transparent and open reporting of deviations, errors, omissions and aberrant results at all levels of the organization, irrespective of hierarchy. Steps should be taken to prevent, and to detect and correct weaknesses in systems and procedures that may lead to data errors so as to continually improve the robustness of scientific decision-making within the organization. Senior management should actively discourage any management practices that might reasonably be expected to inhibit the active and complete reporting of such issues, for example, hierarchical constraints and blame cultures.

4.8 **Quality risk management and sound scientific principles.** Robust decision-making requires appropriate quality and risk management systems, and adherence to sound scientific and statistical principles, which must be based upon reliable data. For example, the scientific principle of being an objective, unbiased observer regarding the outcome of a sample analysis requires that suspect results be investigated and rejected from the reported results only if they are clearly attributable to an identified cause. Adhering to good data and record-keeping principles requires that any rejected results be recorded, together with a documented justification for their rejection, and that this documentation is subject to review and retention.

4.9 **Data life cycle management.** Continual improvement of products to ensure and enhance their safety, efficacy and quality requires a data governance approach to ensure management of data integrity risks throughout all phases of the process by which data are created, recorded, processed, transmitted, reviewed, reported, archived and retrieved and this management process is subject to regular review. To ensure that the organization, assimilation and analysis of data into information facilitates evidence-based and reliable decision-making, data governance should address data ownership and accountability for data process(es) and risk management of the data life cycle.

4.10 To ensure that the organization, assimilation and analysis of data into a format or structure that facilitates evidence-based and reliable decision-making, data governance should address data ownership and accountability for data process(es) and risk management of the data life cycle.

4.11 **Design of record-keeping methodologies and systems.** Record-keeping methodologies and systems, whether paper or electronic, should be designed in a way that encourages compliance with the principles of data integrity.

4.12 Examples include, but are not restricted to:

- restricting the ability to change any clock used for recording timed events, for example, system clocks in electronic systems and process instrumentation;
- ensuring controlled forms used for recording GXP data (e.g. paper batch records, paper case report forms and laboratory worksheets) are accessible at the locations where an activity is taking place, at the time that the activity is taking place, so that ad hoc data recording and later transcription is not necessary;
- controlling the issuance of blank paper templates for data recording of GXP activities so that all printed forms can be reconciled and accounted for;
- restricting user access rights to automated systems to prevent (or audit trail) data amendments;
- ensuring automated data capture or printers are attached and connected to equipment, such as balances, to ensure independent and timely recording of the data;
- ensuring proximity of printers to sites of relevant activities;
- ensuring ease of access to locations of sampling points (e.g. sampling points for water systems) to allow easy and efficient performance of sampling by the operators and therefore minimizing the temptation to take shortcuts or falsify samples;
- ensuring access to original electronic data for staff performing data checking activities.

4.13 Data and record media should be durable. For paper records, the ink should be indelible. Temperature-sensitive or photosensitive inks and other erasable inks should not be used. Paper should also not be temperature-sensitive, photosensitive or easily oxidizable. If this is not feasible or limited (as may be the case in printouts from legacy printers of balance and other instruments in quality control laboratories), then true or certified copies should be available until this equipment is retired or replaced.

4.14 **Maintenance of record-keeping systems.** The systems implemented and maintained for both paper and electronic record-keeping should take account of scientific and technical progress. Systems, procedures and methodology used to record and store data should be periodically reviewed for effectiveness and updated as necessary.

5. Quality risk management to ensure good data management

5.1 All organizations performing work subject to GXP are required by applicable existing WHO guidance to establish, implement and maintain an appropriate quality management system, the elements of which should be documented in their prescribed format, such as a quality manual or other appropriate documentation. The quality manual, or equivalent documentation, should include a quality policy statement of management's commitment to an effective quality management system and to good professional practice. These policies should include a code of ethics and code of proper conduct to assure the reliability and completeness of data, including mechanisms for staff to report any quality and compliance questions or concerns to management.

5.2 Within the quality management system, the organization should establish the appropriate infrastructure, organizational structure, written policies and procedures, processes and systems to both prevent and detect situations that may impact on data integrity and, in turn, the risk-based and scientific robustness of decisions based upon those data.

5.3 QRM is an essential component of an effective data and record validity programme. The effort and resources assigned to data and record management should be commensurate with the risk to product quality. The risk-based approach to record and data management should ensure that adequate resources are allocated and that control strategies for the assurance of the integrity of GXP data are commensurate with their potential impact on product quality and patient safety and related decision-making.

5.4 Strategies that promote good practices and prevent record and data integrity issues from occurring are preferred and are likely to be the most effective and cost-effective. For example, access controls that allow only people with the appropriate authorization to alter a master processing formula will reduce the probability of invalid and aberrant data being generated. Such preventive measures, when effectively implemented, also reduce the amount of monitoring required to detect uncontrolled change.

5.5 Record and data integrity risks should be assessed, mitigated, communicated and reviewed throughout the data life cycle in accordance with the principles of QRM. Examples of approaches that may enhance data reliability are given in these guidelines but should be viewed as recommendations. Other approaches may be justified and shown to be equally effective in achieving satisfactory control of risk. Organizations should therefore design appropriate tools and strategies for the management of data integrity risks based upon their own GXP activities, technologies and processes.

5.6 A data management programme developed and implemented upon the basis of sound QRM principles is expected to leverage existing technologies to their full potential. This in turn will streamline data processes in a manner that not only improves data management but also the business process efficiency and effectiveness, thereby reducing costs and facilitating continual improvement.

6. Management governance and quality audits

6.1 Assuring robust data integrity begins with management, which has the overall responsibility for the technical operations and provision of resources to ensure the required quality of GXP operations. Senior management has the ultimate responsibility for ensuring that an effective quality system is in place to achieve the quality objectives, and that staff roles, responsibilities and authorities, including those required for effective data governance programmes, are defined, communicated and implemented throughout the organization. Leadership is essential to establish and maintain a company-wide commitment to data reliability as an essential element of the quality system.

6.2 The building blocks of behaviours, procedural/policy considerations and basic technical controls together form the foundation of good data governance, upon which future revisions can be built. For example, a good data governance programme requires the necessary management arrangements to ensure personnel are not subject to commercial, political, financial and other pressures or conflicts of interest that may adversely affect the quality of their work and integrity of their data. Management should also make staff aware of the relevance of data integrity and the importance of their role in protecting the safety of patients and the reputation of their organization for quality products and services.

6.3 Management should create a work environment in which staff are encouraged to communicate failures and mistakes, including data reliability issues, so that corrective and preventive actions can be taken and the quality of an organization's products and services enhanced. This includes ensuring adequate information flow between staff at all levels. Senior management should actively discourage any management practices that might reasonably be expected to inhibit the active and complete reporting of such issues, for example, hierarchical constraints and blame cultures.

6.4 Management reviews and regular reporting of quality metrics facilitate meeting these objectives. This requires designation of a quality manager who has direct access to the highest level of management and can directly communicate risks, so that senior management is made aware of any issues and can allocate resources to address them. To fulfil this role the quality unit should conduct and report to management formal, documented risk reviews of the key performance indicators of the quality management system. These should include metrics related to data integrity that will help identify opportunities for improvement. For example:

- tracking and trending of invalid and aberrant data may reveal unforeseen variability in processes and procedures previously believed to be robust, opportunities to enhance analytical procedures and their validation, validation of processes, training of personnel or sourcing of raw materials and components;
- adequate review of audit trails, including those reviewed as part of key decision-making steps (e.g. GMP batch release, issuance of a GLP study report or approval of case report forms), may reveal incorrect processing of data, help prevent incorrect results from being reported and identify the need for additional training of personnel;
- routine audits and/or self-inspections of computerized systems may reveal gaps in security controls that inadvertently allow personnel to access and potentially alter time/date stamps. Such findings help raise awareness among management of the need to allocate resources to improve validation controls for computerized systems;
- monitoring of contract acceptors and tracking and trending of associated quality metrics for these sites help to identify risks that may indicate the need for more active engagement and allocation of additional resources by the contract giver to ensure quality standards are met.

6.5 Quality audits of suppliers, self-inspections and risk reviews should identify and inform management of opportunities to improve foundational systems and processes that have an impact on data reliability. Allocation of resources by management to these improvements of systems and processes may efficiently reduce data integrity risks. For example, identifying and addressing technical difficulties with the equipment used to perform multiple GXP operations may greatly improve the reliability of data for all of these operations. Another example relates to identifying conflicts of interests affecting security. Allocating independent technical support personnel to perform system administration for computerized systems, including managing security, backup and archival, reduces potential conflicts of interest and may greatly streamline and improve data management efficiency.

6.6 All GXP records held by the GXP organization are subject to inspection by the responsible health authorities. This includes original electronic data and metadata, such as audit trails maintained in computerized systems. Management of both contract givers and contract acceptors should ensure that adequate resources are available and that procedures for computerized systems are available for inspection. System administrator personnel should be available to readily retrieve requested records and facilitate inspections.

7. Contracted organizations, suppliers and service providers

7.1 The increasing outsourcing of GXP work to contracted organizations, e.g. contract research organizations, suppliers and other service providers, emphasizes the need to establish and robustly maintain defined roles and responsibilities to assure complete and accurate data and records throughout these relationships. The responsibilities of the contract giver and acceptor, should comprehensively address the processes of both parties that should be followed to ensure data integrity. These details should be included in the contract described in the WHO GXPs relevant to the outsourced work performed or the services provided.

7.2 The organization that outsources work has the responsibility for the integrity of all results reported, including those furnished by any subcontracting organization or service provider. These responsibilities extend to any providers of relevant computing services. When outsourcing databases and software provision, the contract giver should ensure that any subcontractors have been agreed upon and are included in the quality agreement with the contract accepter, and are appropriately qualified and trained in GRDP. Their activities should be monitored on a regular basis at intervals determined through risk assessment. This also applies to cloud-based service providers.

7.3 To fulfil this responsibility, in addition to having their own governance systems, outsourcing organizations should verify the adequacy of the governance systems of the contract acceptor, through an audit or other suitable means. This should include the adequacy of the contract acceptor's controls over suppliers and a list of significant authorized third parties working for the contract acceptor.

7.4 The personnel who evaluate and periodically assess the competence of a contracted organization or service provider should have the appropriate background, qualifications, experience and training to assess data integrity governance systems and to detect validity issues. The nature and frequency of the evaluation of the contract acceptor and the approach to ongoing monitoring of their work should be based upon documented assessment of risk. This assessment should include an assessment of relevant data processes and their risks.

7.5 The expected data integrity control strategies should be included in quality agreements and in written contract and technical arrangements, as appropriate and applicable, between the contract giver and the contract acceptor. These should include provisions for the contract giver to have access to all data held by the contracted organization that are relevant to the contract giver's product or service as well as all relevant quality systems records. This should include ensuring access by the contract giver to electronic records, including audit trails, held in the contracted organization's computerized systems as well as any printed reports and other relevant paper or electronic records.

7.6 Where data and document retention is contracted to a third party, particular attention should be paid to understanding the ownership and retrieval of data held under this arrangement. The physical location where the data are held, and the impact of any laws applicable to that geographical location, should also be considered. Agreements and contracts should establish mutually agreed consequences if the contract acceptor denies, refuses or limits the contract giver's access to their records held by the contract acceptor. The agreements and contracts should also contain provisions for actions to be taken in the event of business closure or bankruptcy of the third party to ensure that access is maintained and the data can be transferred before the cessation of all business activities.

7.7 When outsourcing databases, the contract giver should ensure that if subcontractors are used, in particular cloud-based service providers, they are included in the quality agreement and are appropriately qualified and trained in GRDP. Their activities should be monitored on a regular basis at intervals determined through risk assessment.

8. Training in good data and record management

8.1 Personnel should be trained in data integrity policies and agree to abide by them. Management should ensure that personnel are trained to understand and distinguish between proper and improper conduct, including deliberate falsification, and should be made aware of the potential consequences.

8.2 In addition, key personnel, including managers, supervisors and quality unit personnel, should be trained in measures to prevent and detect data issues. This may require specific training in evaluating the configuration settings and reviewing electronic data and metadata, such as audit trails, for individual computerized systems used in the generation, processing and reporting of data. For example, the quality unit should learn how to evaluate configuration settings that may intentionally or unintentionally allow data to be overwritten or obscured through the use of hidden fields or data annotation tools. Supervisors responsible for reviewing electronic data should learn which audit trails in the system track significant data changes and how these might be most efficiently accessed as part of their review.

8.3 Management should also ensure that, at the time of hire and periodically afterwards, as needed, all personnel are trained in procedures to ensure GDocP for both paper and electronic records. The quality unit should include checks for adherence to GDocP for both paper records and electronic records in their day-to-day work, system and facility audits and self-inspections and report any opportunities for improvement to management.

9. Good documentation practices

9.1 The basic building blocks of good GXP data are to follow GDocP and then to manage risks to the accuracy, completeness, consistency and reliability of the data throughout their entire period of usefulness – that is, throughout the data life cycle.

Personnel should follow GDocP for both paper records and electronic records in order to assure data integrity. These principles require that documentation has the characteristics of being attributable, legible, contemporaneously recorded, original and accurate (sometimes referred to as ALCOA). These essential characteristics apply equally for both paper and electronic records.

9.2 **Attributable.** Attributable means information is captured in the record so that it is uniquely identified as executed by the originator of the data (e.g. a person or a computer system).

9.3 **Legible, traceable and permanent.** The terms legible and traceable and permanent refer to the requirements that data are readable, understandable, and allow a clear picture of the sequencing of steps or events in the record so that all GXP activities conducted can be fully reconstructed by the people reviewing these records at any point during the records retention period set by the applicable GXP.

9.4 **Contemporaneous.** Contemporaneous data are data recorded at the time they are generated or observed.

9.5 **Original.** Original data include the first or source capture of data or information and all subsequent data required to fully reconstruct the conduct of the GXP activity. The GXP requirements for original data include the following:

- original data should be reviewed;
- original data and/or true and verified copies that preserve the content and meaning of the original data should be retained;
- as such, original records should be complete, enduring and readily retrievable and readable throughout the records retention period.

9.6 **Accurate.** The term "accurate" means data are correct, truthful, complete, valid and reliable.

9.7 Implicit in the above-listed requirements for ALCOA are that the records should be **complete, consistent, enduring and available** (to emphasize these requirements, this is sometimes referred to as ALCOA-plus).

9.8 Further guidance to aid understanding as to how these requirements apply in each case and the special risk considerations that may need to be taken into account during implementation are provided in Appendix 1.

10. Designing and validating systems to assure data quality and reliability

10.1 Record-keeping methodologies and systems, whether paper or electronic, should be designed in a way that encourages compliance and assures data quality and reliability. All requirements and controls necessary to ensure GDRP should be adhered to for both paper and electronic records.

Validation to assure good documentation practices for electronic data

10.2 To assure the integrity of electronic data, computerized systems should be validated at a level appropriate for their use and application. Validation should address the necessary controls to ensure the integrity of data, including original electronic data and any printouts or PDF reports from the system. In particular, the approach should ensure that GDocP will be implemented and that data integrity risks will be properly managed throughout the data life cycle.

10.3 The "Supplementary guidelines on good manufacturing practices: validation" (WHO Technical Report Series, No. 937, 2006, Annex 4 (*2–4*)[1] provide a more comprehensive presentation of validation considerations. The key aspects of validation that help assure GDocP for electronic data include, but are not limited to, the following.

10.4 **User involvement.** Users should be adequately involved in validation activities to define critical data and data life cycle controls that assure data integrity.

- Examples of activities to engage users may include: prototyping, user specification of critical data so that risk-based controls can be applied, user involvement in testing to facilitate user acceptance and knowledge of system features, and others.

10.5 **Configuration and design controls.** The validation activities should ensure configuration settings and design controls for GDocP are enabled and managed across the computing environment (including both the software application and operating systems environments).

Activities include, but are not limited to:

- documenting configuration specifications for commercial off-the-shelf systems as well as user-developed systems, as applicable;
- restricting security configuration settings for system administrators to independent personnel, where technically feasible;
- disabling configuration settings that allow overwriting and reprocessing of data without traceability;
- restricting access to time/date stamps.

[1] Currently under review.

For systems to be used in clinical trials, configuration and design controls should be in place to protect the blinding of the trial, for example, by restricting access to randomization data that may be stored electronically.

10.6 **Data life cycle.** Validation should include assessing risk and developing quality risk mitigation strategies for the data life cycle, including controls to prevent and detect risks throughout the steps of:

- data generation and capture;
- data transmission;
- data processing;
- data review;
- data reporting, including handling of invalid and atypical data;
- data retention and retrieval;
- data disposal.

Activities might include, but are not limited to:

- determining the risk-based approach to reviewing electronic data and audit trails based upon process understanding and knowledge of potential impact on products and patients;
- writing SOPs defining review of original electronic records and including meaningful metadata such as audit trails and review of any associated printouts or PDF records;
- documenting the system architecture and data flow, including the flow of electronic data and all associated metadata, from the point of creation through archival and retrieval;
- ensuring that the relationships between data and metadata are maintained intact throughout the data life cycle.

10.7 **SOPs and training.** The validation activities should ensure that adequate training and procedures are developed prior to release of the system for GXP use. These should address:

- computerized systems administration;
- computerized systems use;
- review of electronic data and meaningful metadata, such as audit trails, including training that may be required in system features that enable users to efficiently and effectively process data and review electronic data and metadata.

10.8 Other validation controls to ensure good data management for both electronic data and associated paper data should be implemented as deemed appropriate for the system type and its intended use.

11. Managing data and records throughout the data life cycle

11.1 Data processes should be designed to adequately mitigate and control and continuously review the data integrity risks associated with the steps of acquiring, processing, reviewing and reporting data, as well as the physical flow of the data and associated metadata during this process through storage and retrieval.

11.2 QRM of the data life cycle requires understanding the science and technology of the data process and their inherent limitations. Good data process design, based upon process understanding and the application of sound scientific principles, including QRM, would be expected to increase the assurance of data integrity and to result in an effective and efficient business process.

11.3 Data integrity risks are likely to occur and to be highest when data processes or specific data process steps are inconsistent, subjective, open to bias, unsecured, unnecessarily complex or redundant, duplicated, undefined, not well understood, hybrid, based upon unproven assumptions and/or do not adhere to GDRP.

11.4 Good data process design should consider, for each step of the data process, ensuring and enhancing controls, whenever possible, so that each step is:

- consistent;
- objective, independent and secure;
- simple and streamlined;
- well-defined and understood;
- automated;
- scientifically and statistically sound;
- properly documented according to GDRP.

Examples of considerations for each phase of the data life cycle are provided below.

11.5 **Data collection and recording.** All data collection and recording should be performed following GDRP and should apply risk-based controls to protect and verify critical data.

11.6 *Example consideration.*

Data entries, such as the sample identification for laboratory tests or the recording of source data for inclusion of a patient in a clinical trial, should be verified by a second person or entered through technical means such as barcoding, as appropriate for the intended use of these data. Additional controls may include locking critical data entries after the data are verified and review of audit trails for critical data to detect if they have been altered.

11.7 **Data processing.** To ensure data integrity, data processing should be done in an objective manner, free from bias, using validated/qualified or verified protocols, processes, methods, systems, equipment and according to approved procedures and training programmes.

11.8 *Example considerations.*

GXP organizations should take precautions to discourage testing or processing data towards a desired outcome. For example:

- to minimize potential bias and ensure consistent data processing, test methods should have established sample acquisition and processing parameters, established in default version-controlled electronic acquisition and processing method files, as appropriate. Changes to these default parameters may be necessary during sample processing, but these changes should be documented (who, what, when?) and justified (why?);
- system suitability runs should include only established standards or reference materials of known concentration to provide an appropriate comparator for the potential variability of the instrument. If a sample (e.g. a well-characterized secondary standard) is used for system suitability or a trial run, written procedures should be established and followed and the results included in the data review process. The article under test should not be used for trial run purposes or to evaluate suitability of the system;
- clinical and safety studies should be designed to prevent and detect statistical bias that may occur through improper selection of data to be included in statistical calculations.

11.9 **Data review and reporting.** Data should be reviewed and, where appropriate, evaluated statistically after completion of the process to determine whether outcomes are consistent and compliant with established standards. The evaluation should take into consideration all data, including atypical, suspect or rejected data, together with the reported data. This includes a review of the original paper and electronic records.

11.10 For example, during self-inspection, some key questions to ask are: Am I collecting all my data? Am I considering all my data? If I have excluded some data from my decision-making process, what is the justification for doing so, and are all the data retained, including both rejected and reported data?

11.11 The approach to reviewing specific record content, such as critical data fields and metadata such as cross-outs on paper records and audit trails in electronic records, should meet all applicable regulatory requirements and be risk-based.

11.12 Whenever out-of-trend or atypical results are obtained they should be investigated. This includes investigating and determining corrective and preventive actions for invalid runs, failures, repeats and other atypical data. All data should be included in the dataset unless there is a documented scientific explanation for their exclusion.

11.13 During the data life cycle, data should be subject to continuous monitoring, as appropriate, to enhance process understanding and facilitate knowledge management and informed decision-making.

11.14 *Example considerations*

To ensure that the entire set of data is considered in the reported data, the review of original electronic data should include checks of all locations where data may have been stored, including locations where voided, deleted, invalid or rejected data may have been stored.

11.15 **Data retention and retrieval.** Retention of paper and electronic records is discussed in the section above, including measures for backup and archival of electronic data and metadata.

11.16 *Example consideration*

1) Data folders on some stand-alone systems may not include all audit trails or other metadata needed to reconstruct all activities. Other metadata may be found in other electronic folders or in operating system logs. When archiving electronic data, it is important to ensure that associated metadata are archived with the relevant data set or securely traceable to the data set through appropriate documentation. The ability to successfully retrieve from the archives the entire data set, including metadata, should be verified.

2) Only validated systems are used for storage of data; however, the media used for the storage of data do not have an indefinite lifespan. Consideration must be given to the longevity of media and the environment in which they are stored. Examples include the fading of microfilm records, the decreasing readability of the coatings of optical media such as compact disks (CDs) and digital versatile/video disks (DVDs), and the fact that these media may become brittle. Similarly, historical data stored on magnetic media will also become unreadable over time as a result of deterioration.

12. Addressing data reliability issues

12.1 When issues with data validity and reliability are discovered, it is important that their potential impact on patient safety and product quality and on the reliability of information used for decision-making and applications is examined as a top priority. Health authorities should be notified if the investigation identifies material impact on patients, products, reported information or on application dossiers.

12.2 The investigation should ensure that copies of all data are secured in a timely manner to permit a thorough review of the event and all potentially related processes.

12.3 The people involved should be interviewed to better understand the nature of the failure and how it occurred and what might have been done to prevent and detect the issue sooner. This should include discussions with the people involved in data integrity issues, as well as supervisory personnel, quality assurance and management staff.

12.4 The investigation should not be limited to the specific issue identified but should also consider potential impact on previous decisions based upon the data and systems now found to be unreliable. In addition, it is vital that the deeper, underlying root cause(s) of the issue be considered, including potential management pressures and incentives, for example, a lack of adequate resources.

12.5 Corrective and preventive actions taken should not only address the identified issue, but also previous decisions and datasets that are impacted, as well as deeper, underlying root causes, including the need for realignment of management expectations and allocation of additional resources to prevent risks from recurring in the future.

References and further reading

References

1. WHO good manufacturing practices for pharmaceutical products: main principles. In: WHO Expert Committee on Specifications for Pharmaceutical Preparations: forty-eighth report. Geneva: World Health Organization; 2014: Annex 2 (WHO Technical Report Series, No. 986), also available on CD-ROM and online.
2. Supplementary guidelines on good manufacturing practice: validation. In: WHO Expert Committee on Specifications for Pharmaceutical Preparations: fortieth report. Geneva: World Health Organization; 2006: Annex 4 (WHO Technical Report Series, No. 937).
3. Supplementary guidelines on good manufacturing practice: validation. Qualification of systems and equipment. In: WHO Expert Committee on Specifications for Pharmaceutical Preparations: fortieth report. Geneva: World Health Organization; 2006: Annex 4, Appendix 6 (WHO Technical Report Series, No. 937).
4. Supplementary guidelines on good manufacturing practices: validation. Validation of computerized systems. In: WHO Expert Committee on Specifications for Pharmaceutical Preparations: fortieth report. Geneva: World Health Organization; 2006: Annex 4, Appendix 5 (WHO Technical Report Series, No. 937).

Further reading

Computerised systems. In: The rules governing medicinal products in the European Union. Volume 4: Good manufacturing practice (GMP) guidelines: Annex 11. Brussels: European Commission (http://ec.europa.eu/enterprise/pharmaceuticals/eudralex/vol-4/pdfs-en/anx11en.pdf).

Good automated manufacturing practice (GAMP) good practice guide: electronic data archiving. Tampa (FL): International Society for Pharmaceutical Engineering (ISPE); 2007.

Good automated manufacturing practice GAMP good practice guide: A risk-based approach to GxP compliant laboratory computerized systems, 2nd edition. Tampa (FL): International Society for Pharmaceutical Engineering (ISPE); 2012.

MHRA GMP data integrity definitions and guidance for industry. London: Medicines and Healthcare Products Regulatory Agency; March 2015 (https://www.gov.uk/government/uploads/system/uploads/attachment_data/file/412735/Data_integrity_definitions_and_guidance_v2.pdf).

OECD series on principles of good laboratory practice (GLP) and compliance monitoring. Paris: Organisation for Economic Co-operation and Development (http://www.oecd.org/chemicalsafety/testing/oecdseriesonprinciplesofgoodlaboratorypracticeglpandcompliancemonitoring.htm).

Official Medicines Control Laboratories Network of the Council of Europe: Quality assurance documents: PA/PH/OMCL (08) 69 3R – Validation of computerised systems – core document (https://www.edqm.eu/sites/default/files/medias/fichiers/Validation_of_Computerised_Systems_Core_Document.pdf) and its annexes:

- PA/PH/OMCL (08) 87 2R – Annex 1: Validation of computerised calculation systems: example of validation of in-house software (https://www.edqm.eu/sites/default/files/medias/fichiers/NEW_Annex_1_Validation_of_computerised_calculation.pdf).
- PA/PH/OMCL (08) 88 R – Annex 2: Validation of databases (DB), laboratory information management systems (LIMS) and electronic laboratory notebooks (ELN) (https://www.edqm.eu/sites/default/files/medias/fichiers/NEW_Annex_2_Validation_of_Databases_DB_Laboratory_.pdf).

- PA/PH/OMCL (08) 89 R – Annex 3: Validation of computers as part of test equipment (https://www.edqm.eu/sites/default/files/medias/fichiers/NEW_Annex_3_Validation_of_computers_as_part_of_tes.pdf).

Title 21 Code of Federal Regulations (21 CFR Part 11): Electronic records; electronic signatures. US Food and Drug Administration. The current status of 21 CFR Part 11 Guidance is located under Regulations and Guidance at: http://www.fda.gov/cder/gmp/index.htm — see background: http://www.fda.gov/OHRMS/DOCKETS/98fr/03-4312.pdf.

PIC/S guide to good manufacturing practice for medicinal products annexes: Annex 11 – Computerised systems. Geneva: Pharmaceutical Inspection Co-operation Scheme.

PIC/S PI 011-3 Good practices for computerised systems in regulated GxP environments. Geneva: Pharmaceutical Inspection Co-operation Scheme.

WHO good manufacturing practices for active pharmaceutical ingredients. In: WHO Expert Committee on Specifications for Pharmaceutical Preparations: forty-fourth report. Geneva: World Health Organization; 2010: Annex 2 (WHO Technical Report Series, No. 957).

WHO good practices for pharmaceutical quality control laboratories. In: WHO Expert Committee on Specifications for Pharmaceutical Preparations: forty-fourth report. Geneva: World Health Organization; 2010: Annex 1 (WHO Technical Report Series, No. 957).

Appendix 1

Expectations and examples of special risk management considerations for the implementation of ALCOA (-plus) principles in paper-based and electronic systems

Organizations should follow good documentation practices (GDocP) in order to assure the accuracy, completeness, consistency and reliability of the records and data throughout their entire period of usefulness – that is, throughout the data life cycle. The principles require that documentation should have the characteristics of being attributable, legible, contemporaneously recorded, original and accurate (sometimes referred to as ALCOA).

The tables in this appendix provide further guidance on the implementation of the general ALCOA requirements for both paper and electronic records and systems. In addition, examples of special risk management considerations as well as several illustrative examples are provided of how these measures are typically implemented.

These illustrative examples are provided to aid understanding of the concepts and of how successful risk-based implementation might be achieved. These examples should not be taken as setting new normative requirements.

Attributable. Attributable means information is captured in the record so that it is uniquely identified as having been executed by the originator of the data (e.g. a person or computer system).

Attributable	
Expectations for paper records	**Expectations for electronic records**
Attribution of actions in paper records should occur, as appropriate, through the use of: • initials; • full handwritten signature; • personal seal; • date and, when necessary, time.	Attribution of actions in electronic records should occur, as appropriate, through the use of: • unique user logons that link the user to actions that create, modify or delete data; • unique electronic signatures (can be either biometric or non-biometric); • an audit trail that should capture user identification (ID) and date and time stamps; • signatures, which must be securely and permanently linked to the record being signed.

Special risk management considerations for controls to ensure that actions and records are attributed to a unique individual

- For legally-binding signatures, there should be a verifiable, secure link between the unique, identifiable (actual) person signing and the signature event. Signatures should be permanently linked to the record being signed. Systems which use one application for signing a document and another to store the document being signed should ensure that the two remain linked to ensure that the attribution is not broken.
- Signatures and personal seals should be executed at the time of review or performance of the event or action being recorded.
- Use of a personal seal to sign documents requires additional risk management controls, such as handwritten dates and procedures that require storage of the seal in a secure location with access limited only to the assigned individual, or equipped with other means of preventing potential misuse.
- Use of stored digital images of a person's handwritten signature to sign a document is not acceptable. This practice compromises confidence in the authenticity of these signatures when these stored images are not maintained in a secure location, access to which is limited only to the assigned individual, or equipped with other means of preventing potential misuse, and instead are placed in documents and emails where they can be easily copied and reused by others. Legally binding, handwritten signatures should be dated at the time of signing and electronic signatures should include the time/date stamp of signing to record the contemporaneous nature of the signing event.
- The use of hybrid systems is discouraged, but where legacy systems are awaiting replacement, mitigating controls should be in place. The use of shared and generic logon credentials should be avoided to ensure that actions documented in electronic records can be attributed to a unique individual. This would apply to the software application level and all applicable network environments where personnel may perform actions (e.g. workstation and server operating systems). Where such technical controls are not available or feasible, for example, in legacy electronic systems or where logon would terminate an application or stop the process running, combinations of paper and electronic records should be used to meet the requirements to attribute actions to the individuals concerned. In such cases, original records generated during the course of GXP

activities must be complete and must be maintained throughout the records retention period in a manner that allows the full reconstruction of the GXP activities.

- A hybrid approach might exceptionally be used to sign electronic records when the system lacks features for electronic signatures, provided adequate security can be maintained. The hybrid approach is likely to be more burdensome than a fully-electronic approach; therefore, utilizing electronic signatures, whenever available, is recommended. For example, the execution and attribution of an electronic record by attachment of a handwritten signature may be performed through a simple means that would create a single-page controlled form associated with the written procedures for system use and data review. The document should list the electronic dataset reviewed and any metadata subject to review, and would provide fields for the author, reviewer and/or approver of the dataset to insert a handwritten signature. This paper record with the handwritten signatures should then be securely and traceably linked to the electronic dataset, either through procedural means, such as use of detailed archives indexes, or technical means, such as embedding a true-copy scanned image of the signature page into the electronic dataset.
- Replacement of hybrid systems should be a priority.
- The use of a scribe to record an activity on behalf of another operator should be considered only on an exceptional basis and should only take place where:
  - the act of recording places the product or activity at risk, e.g. documenting line interventions by aseptic area operators;
  - to accommodate cultural differences or mitigate staff literacy/ language limitations, for instance, where an activity is performed by an operator, but witnessed and recorded by a supervisor or officer.

In both situations, the supervisory recording should be contemporaneous with the task being performed and should identify both the person performing the observed task and the person completing the record. The person performing the observed task should countersign the record wherever possible, although it is accepted that this countersigning step will be retrospective. The process for supervisory (scribe) documentation completion should be described in an approved procedure which should also specify the activities to which the process applies.

Legible, traceable and permanent

The terms legible, traceable and permanent refer to the requirements that data are readable, understandable and allow a clear picture of the sequencing of steps or events in the record so that all GXP activities conducted can be fully reconstructed by people reviewing these records at any point during the records retention period set by the applicable GXP.

Legible, traceable, permanent	
Expectations for paper records	**Expectations for electronic records**
Legible, traceable and permanent controls for paper records include, but are not limited to: • use of permanent, indelible ink; • no use of pencil or erasures; • use of single-line cross-outs to record changes with name, date and reason recorded (i.e. the paper equivalent to the audit trail); • no use of opaque correction fluid or otherwise obscuring the record; • controlled issuance of bound, paginated notebooks with sequentially numbered pages (i.e. that allow detection of missing or skipped pages); • controlled issuance of sequentially numbered copies of blank forms (i.e. that allow all issued forms to be accounted for); • archival of paper records by independent, designated personnel in secure and controlled paper archives (archivist is the term used for these personnel in quality control, good laboratory practices (GLP) and good clinical practices (GCP) settings. In good manufacturing practices (GMP) settings this role is normally designated to specific individual(s) in the quality assurance unit);	Legible, traceable and permanent controls for electronic records include, but are not limited to: • designing and configuring computer systems and writing standard operating procedures (SOPs), as required, that enforce the saving of electronic data at the time of the activity and before proceeding to the next step of the sequence of events (e.g. controls that prohibit generation and processing and deletion of data in temporary memory and that instead enforce the committing of the data at the time of the activity to durable memory before moving to the next step in the sequence); • use of secure, time-stamped audit trails that independently record operator actions and attribute actions to the logged-on individual; • configuration settings that restrict access to enhanced security permissions (such as the system administrator role that can be used to potentially turn off the audit trails or enable overwriting and deletion of data), only to persons independent of those responsible for the content of the electronic records; • configuration settings and SOPs, as required, to disable and prohibit the ability to overwrite data, including prohibiting overwriting of preliminary and intermediate processing of data;

Table *continued*

Legible, traceable, permanent	
Expectations for paper records	**Expectations for electronic records**
• preservation of paper/ink that fades over time where their use is unavoidable.	• strictly controlled configuration and use of data annotation tools in a manner that prevents data in displays and printouts from being obscured; • validated backup of electronic records to ensure disaster recovery; • validated archival of electronic records by independent, designated archivist(s) in secure and controlled electronic archives.

Special risk management considerations for legible, traceable and permanent recording of GXP data

- When computerized systems are used to generate electronic data, it should be possible to associate all changes to data with the people who make those changes, and those changes should be time-stamped and a reason for the change recorded where applicable. This traceability of user actions should be documented via computer-generated audit trails or in other metadata fields or system features that meet these requirements.
- Users should not be able to amend or switch off the audit trails or alternative means of providing traceability of user actions.
- The need for the implementation of appropriate audit trail functionality should be considered for all new computerized systems. Where an existing computerized system lacks computer-generated audit trails, personnel may use alternative means such as procedurally-controlled use of logbooks, change control, record version control or other combinations of paper and electronic records to meet GXP regulatory expectations for traceability to document the what, who, when and why of an action. Procedural controls should include written procedures, training programmes, review of records and audits and self-inspections of the governing process(es).

- When archival of electronic records is used, the archiving process should be done in a controlled manner to preserve the integrity of the records. Electronic archives should be validated, secured and maintained in a state of control throughout the data life cycle. Electronic records archived manually or automatically should be stored in secure and controlled electronic archives, accessible only by independent, designated archivists or by their approved delegates.

  Appropriate separation of duties should be established so that business process owners, or other users who may have a conflict of interest, are not granted enhanced security access permissions at any system level (e.g. operating system, application and database). Further, highly privileged system administrator accounts should be reserved for designated technical personnel, e.g. information technology (IT) personnel, who are fully independent of the personnel responsible for the content of the records, as these types of accounts may include the ability to change settings to overwrite, rename, delete, move data, change time/date settings, disable audit trails and perform other system maintenance functions that turn off the good data and record management practices (GDRP) controls for legible and traceable electronic data. Where it is not feasible to assign these independent security roles, other control strategies should be used to reduce data validity risks.

  - To avoid conflicts of interest, these enhanced system access permissions should only be granted to personnel with system maintenance roles (e.g. IT, metrology, records control, engineering), that are fully independent of the personnel responsible for the content of the records (e.g. laboratory analysts, laboratory management, clinical investigators, study directors, production operators and production management). Where these independent security role assignments are not feasible, other control strategies should be used to reduce data validity risks.

It is particularly important that individuals with enhanced access permissions understand the impact of any changes they make using these privileges. Personnel with enhanced access should therefore also be trained in data integrity principles.

Contemporaneous

Contemporaneous data are data recorded at the time they are generated or observed.

Contemporaneous	
Expectations for paper records	**Expectations for electronic records**
Contemporaneous recording of actions in paper records should occur, as appropriate, through use of: • written procedures, and training and review and audit and self-inspection controls that ensure personnel record data entries and information *at the time of the activity directly in official controlled documents* (e.g. laboratory notebooks, batch records, case report forms); • procedures requiring that activities be recorded in paper records with the date of the activity (and time as well, if it is a time-sensitive activity); • good document design, which encourages good practice: documents should be appropriately designed and the availability of blank forms/documents in which the activities are recorded should be ensured; • recording of the date and time of activities using synchronized time sources (facility and computerized system clocks) which cannot be changed by unauthorized personnel. Where possible, data and time recording of manual activities (e.g. weighing) should be done automatically.	Contemporaneous recording of actions in electronic records should occur, as appropriate, through use of: • configuration settings, SOPs and controls that ensure that data recorded in temporary memory are committed to durable media upon completion of the step or event and before proceeding to the next step or event in order to ensure the permanent recording of the step or event at the time it is conducted; • secure system time/date stamps that cannot be altered by personnel; • procedures and maintenance programmes that ensure time/date stamps are synchronized across the GXP operations; • controls that allow for the determination of the timing of one activity relative to another (e.g. time zone controls); • availability of the system to the user at the time of the activity.

Special risk management considerations for contemporaneous recording of GXP data

- Training programmes in GDocP should emphasize that it is unacceptable to record data first in unofficial documentation (e.g. on a scrap of paper) and later transfer the data to official documentation (e.g. the laboratory notebook). Instead, original data should be recorded directly in official records, such as approved analytical worksheets, immediately at the time of the GXP activity.
- Training programmes should emphasize that it is unacceptable to backdate or forward date a record. Instead the date recorded should be the actual date of the data entry. Late entries should be indicated as such with both the date of the activity and the date of the entry being recorded. If a person makes mistakes on a paper document he or she should make single-line corrections, sign and date them, provide reasons for the changes and retain this record in the record set.
- If users of stand-alone computerized systems are provided with full administrator rights to the workstation operating systems on which the original electronic records are stored, this may inappropriately grant permission to users to rename, copy or delete files stored on the local system and to change the time/date stamp. For this reason, validation of the stand-alone computerized system should ensure proper security restrictions to protect time/date settings and ensure data integrity in all computing environments, including the workstation operating system, the software application and any other applicable network environments.

Original

Original data include the first or source capture of data or information and all subsequent data required to fully reconstruct the conduct of the GXP activity. The GXP requirements for original data include the following:

- original data should be reviewed;
- original data and/or true and verified copies that preserve the content and meaning of the original data should be retained;
- as such, original records should be complete, enduring and readily retrievable and readable throughout the records retention period.

Examples of original data include original electronic data and metadata in stand-alone computerized laboratory instrument systems (e.g. ultraviolet/visible spectrophotometry (UV/Vis), Fourier transform infrared spectroscopy (FT-IR), electrocardiogram (ECG), liquid chromatography-tandem mass spectrometry (LC/MS/MS) and haematology and chemistry analysers), original electronic data and metadata in automated production systems (e.g. automated filter integrity testers, supervisory control and data acquisition (SCADA) and distributed control system (DCS)), original electronic data and metadata in network database systems (e.g. laboratory information management system (LIMS), enterprise resource planning (ERP), manufacturing execution systems (MES), electronic case report form/electronic data capture (eCRF/EDC), toxicology databases, and deviation and corrective and preventive action (CAPA) databases), handwritten sample preparation information in paper notebooks, printed recordings of balance readings, electronic health records and paper batch records.

Review of original records	
Expectations for paper records	**Expectations for electronic records**
Controls for review of original paper records include, but are not limited to: • written procedures and training and review and audit and self-inspection controls to ensure that personnel conduct an adequate review and approval of original paper records, including those used to record the contemporaneous capture of information; • data review procedures describing review of relevant metadata. For example, written procedures for review should require that personnel evaluate changes made to original information on paper records (such as changes documented in cross-out or data correction) to ensure these changes are appropriately documented, and justified with substantiating evidence and investigated when required;	Controls for review of original electronic records include, but are not limited to: • written procedures and training and review and audit and inspection controls that ensure personnel conduct an adequate review and approval of original electronic records, including human readable source records of electronic data; • data review procedures describing review of original electronic data and relevant metadata. For example, written procedures for review should require that personnel evaluate changes made to original information in electronic records (such as changes documented in audit trails or history fields or found in other meaningful metadata) to ensure these changes are appropriately documented and justified with substantiating evidence and investigated when required;

Table *continued*

Review of original records	
Expectations for paper records	**Expectations for electronic records**
• documentation of data review. For paper records this is typically signified by signing the paper records that have been reviewed. Where record approval is a separate process this should also be similarly signed. Written procedures for data review should clarify the meaning of the review and approval signatures to ensure that the people concerned understand their responsibility as reviewers and approvers to assure the integrity, accuracy, consistency and compliance with established standards of the paper records subject to review and approval;	• documentation of data review. For electronic records, this is typically signified by electronically signing the electronic data set that has been reviewed and approved. Written procedures for data review should clarify the meaning of the review and approval signatures to ensure that the personnel concerned understand their responsibility as reviewers and approvers to assure the integrity, accuracy, consistency and compliance with established standards of the electronic data and metadata subject to review and approval;
• a procedure describing the actions to be taken if data review identifies an error or omission. This procedure should enable data corrections or clarifications to be made in a GXP-compliant manner, providing visibility of the original record and audit-trailed traceability of the correction, using ALCOA principles.	• a procedure describing the actions to be taken if data review identifies an error or omission. This procedure should enable data corrections or clarifications to be made in a GXP-compliant manner, providing visibility of the original record and audit trailed traceability of the correction, using ALCOA principles.

Special risk management considerations for review of original records

- Data integrity risks may occur when people choose to rely solely upon paper printouts or PDF reports from computerized systems without meeting applicable regulatory expectations for original records. Original records should be reviewed – this includes electronic records. If the reviewer only reviews the subset of data provided as a printout or PDF, risks may go undetected and harm may occur.
- Although original records should be reviewed, and all personnel involved are fully accountable for the integrity and reliability of the subsequent decisions made based upon original records, a risk-based review of the content of original records is recommended.

- Systems typically include many metadata fields and audit trails. It is expected that during validation of the system the organization will establish – based upon a documented and justified risk assessment – the frequency, roles and responsibilities, and the approach used to review the various types of meaningful metadata, such as audit trails. For example, under some circumstances, an organization may justify periodic review of audit trails that track system maintenance activities, whereas audit trails that track changes to critical GXP data with a direct impact on patient safety or product quality would be expected to be reviewed each and every time the associated data set is being reviewed and approved – and prior to decision-making. Certain aspects of defining the audit trail review process (e.g. frequency) may be initiated during validation and then adjusted over time during the system life cycle, based upon risk reviews and to ensure continual improvement.
- A risk-based approach to reviewing data requires process understanding and knowledge of the key quality risks in the given process that may impact patients, products, compliance and the overall accuracy, consistency and reliability of GXP decision-making. When original records are electronic, a risk-based approach to reviewing original electronic data also requires an understanding of the computerized system, the data and metadata, and the data flows.
- When determining a risk-based approach to reviewing audit trails in GXP computerized systems, it is important to note that some software developers may design mechanisms for tracking user actions related to the most critical GXP data using metadata features and may not have named these "audit trails" but may instead have used the naming convention "audit trail" to track other computer system and file maintenance activities. For example, changes to scientific data may sometimes be most readily viewed by running various database queries or by viewing metadata fields labelled "history files" or by review of designed and validated system reports, and the files designated by the software developer as audit trails alone may be of limited value for an effective review. The risk-based review of electronic data and metadata, such as audit trails, requires an understanding of the system and the scientific process governing the data life cycle so that the *meaningful metadata* are subject to review, regardless of the naming conventions used by the software developer.
- Systems may be designed to facilitate audit trail review by various means; for example, the system design may permit audit trails to be reviewed as a list of relevant data or by a validated exception reporting process.

- Written procedures for data review should define the frequency, roles and responsibilities and approach to review of meaningful metadata, such as audit trails. These procedures should also describe how aberrant data are to be handled if found during the review. Personnel who conduct such reviews should have adequate and appropriate training in the review process as well as in the software systems containing the data subject to review. The organization should make the necessary provisions for personnel reviewing the data to access the system(s) containing the electronic data and metadata.
- Quality assurance should also review a sample of relevant audit trails, raw data and metadata as part of self-inspection to ensure ongoing compliance with the data governance policy and procedures.
- Any significant variation from expected outcomes should be fully recorded and investigated.
- In the hybrid approach, which is not the preferred approach, paper printouts of original electronic records from computerized systems may be useful as summary reports if the requirements for original electronic records are also met. To rely upon these printed summaries of results for future decision-making, a second person would have to review the original electronic data and any relevant metadata such as audit trails, to verify that the printed summary is representative of all results. This verification would then be documented and the printout could be used for subsequent decision-making.
- The GXP organization may choose a fully electronic approach to allow more efficient, streamlined record review and record retention. This would require authenticated and secure electronic signatures to be implemented for signing records where required. This, in turn, would require preservation of the original electronic records, or true copy, as well as the necessary software and hardware or other suitable reader equipment to view the records during the records retention period.
- System design and the manner of data capture can significantly influence the ease with which data consistency can be assured. For example, and where applicable, the use of programmed edit checks or features such as drop-down lists, check boxes or branching of questions or data fields based on entries are useful in improving data consistency.
- Data and their metadata should be maintained in such a way that they are available for review by authorized individuals, and in a format that is suitable for review for as long as the data retention requirements apply. It is desirable that the data should be maintained

and available in the original system in which they were generated for the longest possible period of time. When the original system is retired or decommissioned, migration of the data to other systems or other means of preserving the data should be used in a manner that preserves the context and meaning of the data, allowing the relevant steps to be reconstructed. Checks of accessibility to archived data, irrespective of format, and including relevant metadata, should be undertaken to confirm that the data are enduring, and continue to be available, readable and understandable by a human being.

Retention of original records or true copies	
Expectations for paper records	**Expectations for electronic records**
Controls for retention of original paper records or true copies of original paper records include, but are not limited to: • controlled and secure storage areas, including archives, for paper records; • a designated paper archivist(s) who is independent of GXP operations is required by GLP guidelines; in other GXPs the roles and responsibilities for archiving GXP records should be defined and monitored (and should normally be the responsibility of the quality assurance function or an independent documentation control unit); • indexing of records to permit ready retrieval; • periodic tests at appropriate intervals based upon risk assessment, to verify the ability to retrieve archived paper or static format records; • the provision of suitable reader equipment when required, such as microfiche or microfilm readers if original paper records are copied as true copies to microfilm or microfiche for archiving;	Controls for retention of original electronic records or true copies of original electronic records include, but are not limited to: • routine back-up copies of original electronic records stored in another location as a safeguard in case of disaster that causes loss of the original electronic records; • controlled and secure storage areas, including archives, for electronic records; • a designated electronic archivist(s) such as is required in GLP guidelines who is independent of GXP operations (the designated personnel should be suitably qualified and have relevant experience and appropriate training to perform their duties); • indexing of records to permit ready retrieval; • periodic tests to verify the ability to retrieve archived electronic data from storage locations. The ability to retrieve archived electronic data from storage locations should be tested during the validation of the electronic archive. After validation the ability to retrieve archived electronic data from the storage locations should be periodically reconfirmed, including retrieval from third-party storage;

Table *continued*

Retention of original records or true copies	
Expectations for paper records	**Expectations for electronic records**
• written procedures, training, review and audit, and self-inspection of processes defining conversion, as needed, of an original paper record to true copy should include the following steps: – a copy/copies is/are made of the original paper record(s), preserving the original record format, the *static format*, as required (e.g. photocopy, scan), – the copy/copies need to be compared with the original record(s) to determine if the copy preserves the entire content and meaning of the original record, that metadata are included, that no data are missing in the copy. The way that the record format is preserved is important for record meaning if the copy is to meet the requirements of a true copy of the original paper record(s), – the verifier documents the verification in a manner securely linked to the copy/copies indicating it is a true copy, or provides equivalent certification.	• the provision of suitable reader equipment, such as software, operating systems and virtualized environments, to view the archived electronic data when required; • written procedures, training, review and audit and self-inspection of processes defining conversion, as needed, of original electronic records to true copy to include the following steps: – a copy/copies is/are made of the original electronic data set, preserving the original record format, the *dynamic format*, as required (e.g. archival copy of the entire set of electronic data and metadata made using a validated back-up process), – a second person verifier or technical verification process (such as use of *technical hash*) to confirm successful backup) whereby a comparison is made of the electronic archival copy with the original electronic data set to confirm the copy preserves the entire content and meaning of the original record (i.e. all of the data and metadata are included, no data are missing in the copy, any dynamic record format that is important for record meaning and interpretation is preserved and the file was not corrupted during the execution of the validated back-up process), – if the copy meets the requirements as a true copy of the original, then the verifier or technical verification process should document the verification in a manner that is securely linked to the copy/copies, certifying that it is a true copy.

Special risk management considerations for retention of original records and/or true copies

- Data and document retention arrangements should ensure the protection of records from deliberate or inadvertent alteration or loss. Secure controls should be in place to ensure the data integrity of the record throughout the retention period. Archival processes should be defined in written procedures and validated where appropriate.
- Data collected or recorded (manually and/or by recording instruments or computerized systems) during a process or procedure should show that all the defined and required steps have been taken and that the quantity and quality of the output are as expected, and should enable the complete history of the process or material to be traced and be retained in a comprehensible and accessible form. That is, original records and/or true copies should be complete, consistent and enduring.
- A true copy of original records may be retained in lieu of the original records only if the copy has been compared to the original records and verified to contain the entire content and meaning of the original records, including applicable metadata and audit trails.
- If true copies of original paper records are made by scanning the original paper and conversion to an electronic image, such as PDF, then additional measures to protect the electronic image from further alteration are required (e.g. storage in a secure network location with access limited to electronic archivist personnel only, and measures taken to control potential use of annotation tools or other means of preventing further alteration of the copy).
- Consideration should be given to preservation where necessary of the full content and meaning of original hand-signed paper records, especially when the handwritten signature is an important aspect of the overall integrity and reliability of the record and in accordance with the value of the record over time. For example, in a clinical trial it may be important to preserve original hand-signed informed consent records throughout the useful life of this record as an essential aspect of the trial and related application integrity.
- True copies of electronic records should preserve the dynamic format of the original electronic data as this is essential to preserving the meaning of the original electronic data, e.g. if the old software or equipment is retired. For example, the original dynamic electronic spectral files created by instruments such as FT-IR, UV/

Vis, chromatography systems and others can be reprocessed, but a pdf or printout is fixed or static and the ability to expand baselines, view the full spectrum, reprocess and interact dynamically with the data set would be lost in the PDF or printout. As another example, preserving the dynamic format of clinical study data captured in an eCRF system allows searching and querying of data, whereas a pdf of the eCRF data, even if it includes a PDF of audit trails, would lose this aspect of the content and meaning of the original eCRF data. Clinical investigators should have access to original records throughout the study and records retention period in a manner that preserves the full content and meaning of the source information. It may be decided to maintain complete copies of electronic data as well as PDF/printed summaries of these electronic data in the archives to mitigate risks of a complete loss of ability to readily view the data should the software and hardware be retired. However, under these circumstances, especially for data that support critical decision-making, even if PDF/printed summaries are maintained, the complete copies of electronic data should continue to be maintained throughout the records retention period to allow for investigations that may be necessary under unexpected circumstances, such as application integrity investigations.

- Preserving the original electronic data in electronic form is also important because data in dynamic format facilitate usability of the data for subsequent processes. For example, having temperature logger data maintained electronically facilitates subsequent tracking and trending and monitoring of temperatures in statistical process control charts.
- In addition to the option of creating true copies of original electronic data as verified back-up copies that are then secured in electronic archives, another option for creating a true copy of original electronic data would be to migrate the original electronic data from one system to another and to verify and document that the validated data migration process preserved the entire content, including all meaningful metadata, as well as the meaning of the original electronic data.
- Electronic signature information should be retained as part of the original electronic record. This should remain linked to the record and be readable throughout the retention period, regardless of the system used for archiving the records.

Accurate

The term "accurate" means data are correct, truthful, complete, valid and reliable.

For both paper and electronic records, achieving the goal of accurate data requires adequate procedures, processes, systems and controls that comprise the quality management system. The quality management system should be appropriate to the scope of its activities and risk-based.

Controls that assure the accuracy of data in paper records and electronic records include, but are not limited to:

- qualification, calibration and maintenance of equipment, such as balances and pH meters, that generate printouts;
- validation of computerized systems that generate, process, maintain, distribute or archive electronic records;
- systems must be validated to ensure their integrity while transmitting between/among computerized systems;
- validation of analytical methods;
- validation of production processes;
- review of GXP records;
- investigation of deviations and doubtful and out-of-specifications results; and
- many other risk management controls within the quality management system.

Examples of these controls applied to the data life cycle are provided below.

Special risk management considerations for assuring accurate GXP records

- The entry of critical data into a computer by an authorized person (e.g. entry of a master processing formula) requires an additional check on the accuracy of the data entered manually. This check may be done by independent verification and release for use by a second authorized person or by validated electronic means. For example, to detect and manage risks associated with critical data, procedures would require verification by a second person, such as a member of the quality unit staff, of: calculation formulas entered into spreadsheets; master data entered into LIMS such as fields for specification ranges used to flag out-of-specification values on the certificate of analysis; and other critical master data, as appropriate.

In addition, once verified, these critical data fields would be locked to prevent further modification, when feasible and appropriate, and only modified through a formal change control process.

- The validity of the data capture process is fundamental to ensuring that high-quality data are produced.
- Where used, standard dictionaries and thesauruses, tables (e.g. units and scales) should be controlled.
- The process of data transfer between systems should be validated.
- The migration of data into and export from systems requires specific planned testing and control.
- Time may not be critical for all activities. When the activity is time-critical, printed records should display the time/date stamp.

For example: To ensure the accuracy of sample weights recorded on a paper printout from the balance, the balance would be appropriately calibrated before use and properly maintained. In addition, synchronizing and locking the metadata settings on the balance for the time/date settings would ensure accurate recordings of time/date on the balance printout.

Annex 6

Good trade and distribution practices for pharmaceutical starting materials

Introduction

Good manufacturing practices for active pharmaceutical ingredients were published in 2000 by The International Conference on Harmonisation of Technical Requirements for Registration of Pharmaceuticals for Human Use (ICH), in ICH Q7 (*1*). Section 17 of this ICH text includes guidelines for agents, brokers, traders, distributors, repackers and relabellers. This section was written based on the outcome of the World Health Organization (WHO) investigation into deaths resulting from the intentional relabelling of industrial grade ethylene glycol as pharmaceutical grade material. This material was subsequently formulated into a paediatric medicine that caused many deaths. Section 17 of this good manufacturing practice (GMP) guide for active pharmaceutical ingredients (APIs) applies to any party other than the original manufacturer which may trade and/or take possession, repack, relabel, manipulate, distribute or store an API or API intermediate. The scope of ICH Q7 does not include excipients.

Following a number of incidents involving diethylene glycol and a World Health Assembly resolution (WHA52.19), WHO published the *Good trade and distribution practices for pharmaceutical starting materials* in 2004 (*2*). At the time of publication of these guidelines, WHO had not yet adopted the text from ICH Q7 as GMP for APIs. The WHO guidance for excipients (*3*), published in 1999, did not cover trade and distribution practices for excipients.

In 2010, WHO published *Good manufacturing practices for active pharmaceutical ingredients* (*4*), which reflect the text from ICH Q7 and include Section 17 of that document, to replace the existing WHO GMP for APIs.[1]

The WHO Expert Committee on Specifications for Pharmaceutical Preparations discussed the revision of the *Good trade and distribution practices for pharmaceutical starting materials* at several meetings. The scope of this WHO guidance on *Good trade and distribution practices for pharmaceutical starting materials* is applicable to any ingredient that is used in the manufacture of a medicinal product, including APIs, excipients and any others.

Note: Material deriving from non-pharmaceutical grades, such as food, industrial or technical grades, should not be designated as pharmaceutical grade when it is not produced under the required manufacturing conditions and quality system. For finished pharmaceutical products (FPPs), details can be found in the WHO good distribution practices for pharmaceutical products (*5*).

[1] It is important to note that any party that engages in repackaging or blending of an API is considered to be a manufacturer and must submit appropriate registration documents for such manufacturing. He or she must also comply with the GMP for APIs as stated in WHO Technical Report Series, No. 957, Annex 2, 2010 (*4*).

1. Quality management

1.1 Within an organization, quality assurance serves as a management tool. In contractual situations, quality assurance also serves to generate confidence in the supplier. There should be a documented quality policy describing the overall intentions and direction of the distributor regarding quality, which should be formally expressed and authorized by management. The quality policy should clearly indicate that the distributor implements and maintains good trade and distribution practices (GTDP) as described in these guidelines, within the organization and its services.

1.2 Quality management should include:

- an appropriate infrastructure or "quality system", encompassing the organizational structure, procedures, processes and resources. The size, structure and complexity of the distributor and its activities should be taken into consideration when developing or modifying the quality system;
- an independent quality unit (or designee), which is responsible for all quality-related matters;
- an appropriate quality risk management (QRM) system to enable a systematic process for the assessment, control, communication and review of risks to the quality of the product. The extent of application of the QRM system should reflect the operations performed;
- a validation/qualification system to ensure that the resulting product is capable of meeting the requirements for the specified application;
- systematic actions necessary to ensure adequate confidence that a material (or service) and relevant documentation will satisfy given requirements for quality – the totality of these actions is termed quality assurance;
- a clear documented procedure for selecting, approving, disqualifying and re-approving suppliers of pharmaceutical starting materials and services;
- a robust deviation management and change control programme designed to ensure that quality is continually assessed and maintained: these should include a customer notification where appropriate;
- a system ensuring traceability of products and associated documentation throughout the entire supply chain.

1.3 The system should cover for example, but not be limited to, the quality assurance principles in these guidelines.

1.4 All parties involved in the manufacture and supply chain must exercise responsibility to ensure the quality and safety of the materials and products, and that they are fit for their intended use in accordance with their specifications.

1.5 The responsibilities placed on any one individual should not be so extensive as to present any risk to quality. In the event of a supplier having a limited number of staff, some duties may be delegated or contracted out to designated persons who are appropriately qualified. There should, however, be no gaps or unexplained overlaps related to the application of GTDP for pharmaceutical starting materials as described in these guidelines.

1.6 Where electronic commerce (e-commerce) is used, defined procedures and adequate systems should be in place to ensure confidence in the quality of the material and its traceability.

1.7 Authorized release procedures should be in place to ensure that when material is released for its intended purpose, it is of an appropriate quality, meets its specifications and is sourced from approved suppliers.

1.8 Implementation of QRM principles using appropriate tools such as hazard analysis and critical control point (HACCP); inspection and certification of compliance with an appropriate quality system such as applicable International Organization for Standardization (ISO) series, and recognition of compliance with national and/or regional standards by external bodies is recommended. However, this should not be seen as a substitute for the implementation of these guidelines or for conforming, for example, to pharmaceutical GMP and good storage practices (GSP) requirements, as applicable.

1.9 A system should be in place for the performance of regular internal audits with the aim of continuous improvement. The findings of the audit and any corrective and preventive actions taken, including verification of their effectiveness, should be documented and brought to the attention of the responsible management.

2. Organization and personnel

2.1 There should be an adequate organizational structure and a sufficient number of personnel should be employed to carry out all the tasks for which the supplier is responsible.

2.2 Individual responsibilities should be clearly defined, understood by the individuals concerned and recorded in writing (as job descriptions or in a contract). Certain activities, such as supervision of performance of activities in accordance with local legislation, may require special attention. Personnel should be suitably qualified, trained and authorized to undertake their duties and responsibilities.

2.3 All personnel should be aware of the principles of the appropriate guidelines, including but not limited to GTDP.

2.4 Personnel should receive initial and continuing training relevant to their tasks. Training should be provided by qualified trainers in accordance with a training programme. The effectiveness of training should be verified where appropriate. Training records should be maintained. All personnel should be motivated to support the establishment and maintenance of quality standards.

2.5 Personnel dealing with hazardous materials (such as highly active, toxic, infectious or sensitizing materials) should be given specific training and should be provided with the necessary protective equipment. Documented policies and procedures for the use of personal protective equipment should be followed to decrease exposure of workers working directly with products and those in the immediate environment.

2.6 Personnel who may be exposed to materials from open containers should maintain good hygiene, have no open wounds and should wear appropriate protective garments, gloves, masks and goggles.

3. Premises

3.1 Premises, including laboratory facilities, must be located, designed, constructed, adapted and maintained to suit the operations to be carried out. Their layout and design must aim to minimize the risk of errors and permit effective cleaning and maintenance in order to avoid contamination, cross-contamination, mix ups, build-up of dust, dirt or waste and, in general, any adverse effect on the quality of materials.

3.2 Measures should be in place to prevent unauthorized persons from entering the premises.

3.3 Premises should be designed, equipped and maintained so as to afford maximum protection against the entry of insects, rodents or other animals. A pest control programme should be implemented and maintained. Its effectiveness should be monitored.

3.4 Suitable supporting facilities and utilities (such as air control, ventilation and lighting) should be in place and appropriate to the activities performed, in order to avoid contamination, cross-contamination and degradation of the material. Utilities that could affect product quality should be identified and monitored.

3.5 If sampling of pharmaceutical starting materials is performed, the sampling area should be separate and in a controlled environment. Sampling should only be performed in a storage area if it can be conducted in such a way that there is no risk of contamination or cross-contamination. Adequate cleaning procedures should be in place for the sampling areas.

4. Procurement, warehousing and storage

Note: GSP are applicable in all circumstances in which, and in all areas where, materials are stored.

4.1 Materials should be purchased from approved suppliers in accordance with mutually agreed formal specifications.

4.2 Actions should be taken to minimize the risk of falsified or non-conforming materials entering the supply chain.

4.3 There should be authorized procedures describing the activities relating to the receipt, storage and distribution of materials. Steps should be taken to ensure and document that the arriving consignment is correct and that the products originate from approved suppliers. Deliveries should be examined to check that containers have not been damaged, altered or tampered with, and that closures and security seals are intact.

4.4 Storage areas should have sufficient capacity to allow orderly storage of the various categories of materials.

4.5 Receipt and dispatch bays should be equipped with the means to protect materials from adverse environmental conditions. Reception areas should be designed and equipped to allow containers of incoming materials to be cleaned before storage if appropriate. Upon receipt, material should be segregated until released by the quality unit.

4.6 Segregated areas should be provided for the storage of received, quarantined, rejected, recalled and returned material, including materials with damaged packaging. Any system replacing physical segregation, such as electronic segregation based on a computerized system, should provide equivalent security and should be appropriately qualified and validated.

4.7 The storage areas should be kept clean and dry.

4.8 Segregated areas and materials should be appropriately identified.

4.9 The required storage conditions, as specified for the material, should be maintained within acceptable limits at all times during storage. Appropriate checks to confirm that required shipping conditions have been met should be conducted as soon as possible after receipt.

The product should be transferred to appropriate storage facilities immediately after checks to be made in the goods receiving area have been conducted.

4.10 Where special storage conditions are required (e.g. particular temperature, humidity or protection from light) these should be provided, monitored and recorded as appropriate.

4.11 Highly active materials, narcotics, other dangerous drugs and substances presenting special risks of abuse, fire or explosion should be stored in safe, dedicated and secure areas. In addition and where applicable, international conventions and national legislation are to be adhered to.

4.12 Special attention should be given to the design, use, cleaning and maintenance of all equipment for bulk handling and storage, such as tanks and silos.

4.13 Products should be packed in such a way as to avoid breakage, contamination, tampering or theft. The packing should be adequate to maintain the quality of the product during transport. If special shipping conditions have to be met they should be defined, provided and controlled. The containers in which products are shipped should be sealed and should clearly indicate the authenticity of the product and its supplier.

4.14 Spillages should be cleaned up as soon as possible to prevent possible cross-contamination and hazard.

4.15 Provision should be made for the proper and safe storage of waste materials awaiting disposal. Toxic substances and flammable materials should be stored in suitably designed, separate, closed containers in enclosed areas, taking into account the relevant national legislation.

4.16 A default system should be in place to ensure that those materials due to expire first are sold or distributed first (earliest expiry/first out). Where no expiry dates are specified for the materials, the first in/first out principle should be applied.

4.17 A process should be in place to ensure that materials that have reached their expiry or retest date should be withdrawn immediately from saleable stock. Materials with a retest date should be retested according to the appropriate specifications. Materials with an expiry date should not be retested or used after that date.

4.18 Stock inventory should be checked regularly, at least for quantity, overall condition and retesting or expiration dates. Any discrepancies should be investigated.

4.19 Controls should be in place to ensure that the correct product is picked, packed and distributed. The material should have an appropriate remaining shelf life. All batch numbers should be recorded.

4.20 Storage areas should be clean and free from accumulated waste and from vermin. A written sanitation programme should be available, indicating the frequency of cleaning and the methods to be used to clean the premises and storage areas.

5. Equipment

5.1 Equipment must be located, designed, constructed, adapted, qualified, used, cleaned and maintained to suit the operations to be carried out. Its layout, design and use should aim to minimize the risk of errors and permit effective cleaning and maintenance so as to avoid cross-contamination, build-up of dust or dirt and any adverse effect on the quality of materials.

5.2 Defective equipment should not be used and should either be removed or labelled as defective. Equipment should be disposed of in such a way as to prevent any misuse.

5.3 The status of the equipment should be readily identifiable.

5.4 Fixed pipework should be clearly labelled to indicate the contents and, where applicable, the direction of flow.

5.5 All services, piping and devices should be adequately marked and special attention paid to the provision of non-interchangeable connections or adaptors for dangerous gases, liquids and other materials.

5.6 Balances and other measuring equipment of an appropriate range and precision should be available and should be calibrated in accordance with a suitable schedule.

5.7 Dedicated equipment should be used where appropriate when handling and/or processing pharmaceutical starting materials. Where non-dedicated equipment is used cleaning validation should be performed.

5.8 Closed equipment should be used when possible. If open equipment is used, suitable measures should be taken to prevent contamination.

5.9 Procedures should be in place for the operation and maintenance of equipment. Lubricants and other materials used on surfaces that come into direct contact with the materials should be of the appropriate grade, e.g. food-grade oil, and should not alter the quality of the materials.

5.10 Washing and cleaning equipment should be chosen and used such that it cannot be a source of contamination.

6. Documentation

6.1 Documents, in particular instructions and procedures relating to any activity that might have an impact on the quality of materials, should be designed, completed, reviewed and distributed with care. Documents should be completed, approved, signed and dated by appropriate authorized persons and should not be changed without authorization. Specifications for materials, including packaging materials, should be available, reviewed and revised on a regular basis.

6.2 Documents should have unambiguous contents: their title, nature and purpose should be clearly stated. They should be laid out in an orderly manner and be easy to check.

6.3 Certificates of analysis (COAs) issued by the original manufacturer should be provided. If additional testing is done, all COAs should be provided.

COAs should document product traceability back to the manufacturer by naming the original manufacturer and the manufacturing site. COAs should indicate which results were obtained by testing the original material and which results came from skip-lot testing or other testing and should specify the organization responsible for issuing the COA.

6.4 Before any material is sold or distributed, the supplier should ensure that the COAs and results are available and that the results meet the required specifications.

6.5 The original manufacturer and the intermediaries handling the material should always be traceable and transparent; and this information should be made available to authorities and end-users, downstream and upstream, when requested.

6.6 Depending upon risk assessment, and in accordance with the national requirements, quality agreements should form the basis of the relationship for all parties involved in the supply chain. The agreements should include mechanisms to allow transfer of information, e.g. quality or regulatory information and change control.

6.7 Labels applied to containers should be clear, unambiguous, permanently fixed and should be printed in the company's agreed format. The information on the label should be indelible.

6.8 Each container should be identified by labelling bearing at least the following information:

- the name of the pharmaceutical starting material (including grade and reference to pharmacopoeias where relevant);
- if applicable, the International Nonproprietary Name (INN);
- the amount (weight or volume);
- the batch number assigned by the original manufacturer or the batch number assigned by the repacker, if the material has been repacked and relabelled;
- the retest date or expiry date (where applicable);
- the storage conditions;
- handling precautions, where necessary;
- identification of the original manufacturing site;
- name and contact details of the supplier.

6.9 Relevant storage and handling information and safety data sheets should be available.

6.10 Records should be kept and must be readily available upon request in accordance with GMP and GSP (*6*).

7. Repackaging and relabelling

7.1 Operations, such as combining into a homogeneous batch, repackaging and/or relabelling, are manufacturing processes and are not recommended. In circumstances where they are to be conducted, their performance should be in compliance with GMP.

Note: It is important to note that any party who engages in repackaging or blending of an API is considered to be a manufacturer and must submit appropriate registration documents for such manufacturing. They must also comply with the GMP for APIs as set out in WHO Technical Report Series, No. 957, Annex 2, 2010 (*4*).

7.2 Special attention should be given to the following points:

- prevention of contamination, cross-contamination and mix ups;
- appropriate environmental conditions for dispensing, packaging and sampling;
- security of stocks of labels, line clearance checks, online inspections, destruction of excess batch-printed labels and label reconciliation;
- good sanitation and hygiene practices;
- maintaining batch integrity (mixing of different batches of the same solid material should normally not be done);
- as part of batch records, all labels that were removed from the original container during operations, and a sample of the new label, should be kept;
- if more than one batch of labels is used in one operation, samples of each batch should be kept;
- maintaining product identity, integrity and traceability.

7.3 Upon receipt, packaging materials should be placed in quarantine and should not be used prior to release. There should be procedures for the inspection, approval and release of the packaging materials.

7.4 When different batches of a material from the same original manufacturing site are received by a distributor and combined into a homogeneous batch, the conformity of each batch with its specification should be confirmed before it is added.

7.5 Only materials from the same manufacturing site, received by a distributor and conforming to the same specifications, can be mixed. If different batches of the same material are mixed to form a homogeneous batch it should be defined as a new batch, tested and supplied with a batch certificate of analysis. In such cases the customer should be informed that the material supplied is a mixture of manufacturers' batches.

7.6 In all cases, traceability back to the manufacturer should be documented by identifying the original manufacturer of the specific batch of the material and its manufacturing site.

7.7 If batches are combined or mixed, the oldest batch should determine the expiry or retest date assigned to the combined or mixed batch.

7.8 If the integrity and quality of the batch is maintained during repackaging and relabelling, then the original COA of the original manufacturer should be provided.

If retesting is done, both the original and the new COA should be provided as long as the batch integrity is maintained. The batch referred to on the new COA should be traceable to the original COA.

7.9 Repackaging of materials should be carried out using approved packaging materials for which the quality and suitability have been established as being equal to or better than those of the original container.

7.10 The reuse of containers should be discouraged unless they have been cleaned using a validated procedure. Recycled containers should not be used unless there is evidence that the quality of the material packed in them will not be adversely affected.

7.11 Materials should be repackaged only if efficient environmental control exists to ensure that there is no possibility of contamination, cross-contamination, degradation, physicochemical changes and/or mix ups. The quality of air supplied to the area should be suitable for the activities performed, e.g. there should be efficient filtration.

7.12 Suitable procedures should be followed to ensure proper label control.

7.13 Containers of repackaged material and relabelled containers should bear both the name of the original manufacturing site and the name of the distributor/repacker.

7.14 Procedures should be in place to ensure maintenance of the identity and quality of the material by appropriate means, both before and after repackaging operations.

7.15 Each batch of repackaged material should be tested to ensure that the material conforms to documented specifications.

7.16 There should be a procedure to ensure that appropriate repackaging documentation, in addition to the test results, is evaluated prior to release of the repackaged material.

7.17 Sampling, analytical testing and batch release procedures should be in accordance with GMP.

7.18 Only official pharmacopoeial methods or validated analytical test methods should be used for the analysis. Where alternatives to the test methods specified in a monograph are used to provide test results, those alternative methods should be demonstrated to be suitable and equivalent.

7.19 Out-of-specification test results should be investigated and documented.

7.20 Samples of pharmaceutical starting materials in appropriate quantities should be kept for at least one year after the expiry or retest date, or for three years after distribution is complete.

7.21 The repacker and relabeller should ensure that the stability of the material is not adversely affected by the repackaging or relabelling. Stability studies to justify assigned expiration or retest dates should be conducted if the pharmaceutical starting material is repackaged in a container different from that used by the original manufacturer. It is recognized that some excipients may not need additional stability studies.

8. Complaints

8.1 All complaints and other information concerning potentially defective materials must be carefully reviewed according to written procedures that describe the action to be taken and specify the criteria on which a decision to recall a product should be based. Records of complaints should be retained and evaluated for trends at defined intervals.

8.2 Any complaint concerning a material defect should be recorded and thoroughly investigated to identify the origin or reason for the complaint (e.g. the repackaging procedure or the original manufacturing process). Corrective and preventive actions should be taken where appropriate, and recorded.

8.3 If a defect in a pharmaceutical starting material is discovered or suspected, consideration should be given to whether other batches should be checked.

8.4 Where necessary, appropriate follow-up action, possibly including a recall, should be taken after investigation and evaluation of the complaint.

8.5 The manufacturer and customers should be informed if action is needed following possible faulty manufacturing, packaging, deterioration or any other serious quality problems with a pharmaceutical starting material.

9. Recalls

9.1 There should be a system for recalling promptly and effectively from the market, materials known or suspected to be defective.

9.2 The original manufacturer should be informed in the event of a recall.

9.3 There should be detailed written procedures for the organization of any recall activity. These procedure(s) should be regularly reviewed and updated.

9.4 All recalled materials should be stored in a secure area while their fate is decided.

9.5 In the event of serious or potentially life-threatening situations, all customers and competent authorities in all countries to which a given material may have been distributed should be promptly informed of any intention to recall the material.

9.6 All records should be readily available to the designated person(s) responsible for recalls. These records should contain sufficient information on materials supplied to customers (including exported materials).

9.7 The effectiveness of the arrangements for recalls should be evaluated at regular intervals.

10. Returned goods

10.1 Goods returned to the supplier should be appropriately identified and quarantined. The conditions under which returned goods have been stored and shipped should be evaluated to determine the quality of the returned goods.

10.2 The quality unit or designee should decide on the disposition of the returned goods following a formal and documented investigation process. Corrective and preventive actions should be taken where appropriate.

11. Handling of non-conforming materials

11.1 Non-conforming materials should be handled in accordance with a procedure that will prevent their introduction or reintroduction into the market. Records covering all activities, including destruction, disposal, return and reclassification, should be maintained.

11.2 An investigation should be performed to establish whether any other batches are also affected. Corrective and preventive measures should be taken where necessary.

11.3 The disposition of the material, including downgrading to other suitable purposes, should be documented.

11.4 Non-conforming materials should never be blended with materials that do comply with specifications.

12. Dispatch and transport

12.1 Materials should be loaded, unloaded and transported in a manner that will ensure the maintenance of controlled conditions where applicable (e.g. temperature, protection from the environment). The transport process should not adversely affect the materials. Any carrier used for transport should be approved according to a written procedure unless the carrier has been selected by the customer.

12.2 Requirements for special transport and/or storage conditions should be stated on the label and/or in the transport documentation. If the pharmaceutical starting material is intended to be transferred outside the control of the manufacturer's materials management system, the name and address of the manufacturer, quality of contents, special transport conditions and any special legal requirements should also be included on the label and/or in the transport documentation.

12.3 The supplier of the materials should ensure that the contract acceptor for transportation of the materials is aware of and provides the appropriate storage and transport conditions, e.g. through audits.

12.4 Procedures should be in place to ensure proper cleaning and prevention of cross-contamination when liquids (tanks) and bulk or packed materials are transported.

12.5 The bulk transport of pharmaceutical starting materials requires numerous precautions to avoid contamination and cross-contamination. The best practice is to use dedicated equipment, tanks or containers.

12.6 Packaging materials and transportation containers should be suitable to prevent damage to the pharmaceutical starting materials during transport.

12.7 For bulk transport, validated cleaning procedures should be used between loadings, and a list of restricted previous cargoes must be supplied to the transport companies.

12.8 Steps should be taken to prevent unauthorized access to the materials being transported.

12.9 General international requirements regarding safety aspects (e.g. prevention of explosion and of contamination of the environment) should be observed.

13. Contract activities

13.1 Any activity performed, as referenced in the GMP and GTDP guidelines, delegated to another party, should be agreed upon in a written contract.

13.2 The contract giver should evaluate the proposed contract acceptor's compliance with GTDP before entering into an agreement.

13.3 All contract acceptors should comply with the requirements in these guidelines. Special consideration should be given to the prevention of cross-contamination and to maintaining traceability.

13.4 There should be a written and approved contract or formal agreement between the contract giver and contract acceptor that addresses and defines in detail the responsibilities with respect to GTDP and which party is responsible for which quality measures.

13.5 Subcontracting may be permissible under certain conditions, subject to approval by the contract giver, especially for activities such as sampling, analysis, repacking and relabelling.

References

1. ICH harmonised tripartite guideline: Good manufacturing practice guide for active pharmaceutical ingredients – Q7. Geneva: International Conference on Harmonisation of Technical Requirements for Registration of Pharmaceuticals for Human Use; 2000.
2. Good trade and distribution practices for pharmaceutical starting materials. In: WHO Expert Committee on Specifications for Pharmaceutical Preparations: thirty-eighth report. Geneva: World Health Organization; 2004: Annex 2 (WHO Technical Report Series, No. 917).
3. Good manufacturing practice: supplementary guidelines for the manufacture of pharmaceutical excipients. In: WHO Expert Committee on Specifications for Pharmaceutical Preparations: thirty-fifth report. Geneva: World Health Organization; 1999: Annex 5 (WHO Technical Report Series, No. 885).
4. Good manufacturing practices for active pharmaceutical ingredients. In: WHO Expert Committee on Specifications for Pharmaceutical Preparations: forty-fourth report. Geneva: World Health Organization; 2010: Annex 2 (WHO Technical Report Series, No. 957).
5. WHO good distribution practices for pharmaceutical products. In: WHO Expert Committee on Specifications for Pharmaceutical Preparations: forty-fourth report. Geneva: World Health Organization; 2010: Annex 5 (WHO Technical Report Series, No. 957).
6. Guide to good storage practices for pharmaceuticals. In: WHO Expert Committee on Specifications for Pharmaceutical Preparations: thirty-seventh report. Geneva: World Health Organization; 2003: Annex 9 (WHO Technical Report Series, No. 908).

Annex 7

Guidelines on the conduct of surveys of the quality of medicines

1. Introduction

Good quality medicines are essential for efficient disease management. To ensure that good quality medicines are available to patients in their countries, national medicines regulatory authorities (NMRAs) can apply various regulatory instruments. These are:

- authorization/registration for marketing following the assessment of product documentation, inspection to ascertain manufacturers' compliance with the principles of good manufacturing practices (GMP) and approval of product information;
- post-marketing surveillance activities, including maintenance of products' authorization and/or registration through variations or renewals, regular inspections of manufacturers, wholesalers, distributors and retailers, quality control testing and pharmacovigilance;
- implementation of regulatory actions in the event of any quality problem being found.

Quality surveys may serve as a source of information about the quality of medicines available to patients and are an important part of regulatory systems in all countries, whether they are strong or weak. However, it has to be borne in mind that quality surveys that rely only on laboratory testing cannot offer complete assurance that medicines are safe and effective as formulated. Quality surveys can be organized by NMRAs, international organizations, procurement agents, nongovernmental organizations (NGOs) or academic and research groups.

If properly collected, interpreted and used relevant data are vital for the planning of effective interventions to improve the quality of medicines. Surveys give snapshots of the medicine quality situation; however, the accuracy, reliability and interpretation of the data obtained depend on the survey design, organization of sample collection and available resources. Medicine quality surveys are costly and limitations on resources may restrict the number of samples collected, parameters tested, techniques to be used for analysis or number of staff available to conduct the survey and analysis. Therefore it is important to optimize use of resources by focusing on those medicines and parameters that pose a higher risk to patients and apply risk analysis during planning of the survey. Also cooperation with partners, joint organization of surveys in several countries, and sharing testing capacities, experience and information can enhance the effectiveness of quality surveys.

These guidelines outline the steps to consider when preparing and conducting a survey of medicines quality. They provide recommendations and examples of various methodological approaches with a discussion of their advantages and disadvantages, and suggestions on preparation of reports on the results obtained from such surveys.

2. Glossary

The definitions given below apply to the terms used in these guidelines. They may have different meanings in other contexts.

pharmaceutical outlet. Any point (licensed or unlicensed) of sale or provision of medicines for individual patients or other medicine providers.

sample collected in a quality survey. A product in a given presentation (identified by its name, content of active pharmaceutical ingredient(s) (API(s)), dosage form, strength, batch number, production date (if known), expiration date, collection date and name of manufacturer or labelled registration holder) collected at the specific sample collection site. It means that the same product characterized by the same name, content of APIs, dosage form, strength, batch, and from the same manufacturer collected in two different sites represents two samples. Each sample should consist of the number of dosage units (e.g. tablets, capsules, ampoules, vials or bottles) required by the sampling plan.

sampling plan. A plan that contains detailed identification of sites where samples will be collected, medicines to be sampled, minimum number of dosage units to be collected per sample, number of samples to be collected per medicine and total number of samples to be collected in the area for which the sampling plan is prepared. It also contains detailed instructions for sample collectors.

3. Objectives of the survey and initial planning

In general, quality surveys are organized to assess the quality of medicines provided to patients and generate the data that can help to formulate strategies and plans to ensure provision of good quality medicines. They may be organized to confirm that patients are receiving satisfactory medicines and give reassurance that the regulatory system is functional, or when there is a suspicion that patients are not receiving satisfactory medicines. Detailed objectives must be set at the start of planning since all the activities and requirements of the survey should be derived from its objectives. The objectives of a quality survey should reflect the reasons why the survey is being conducted and should be formulated in a way that enables identification of medicines for the survey, sites of sample collection, surveyed areas, regions or countries, and tests to be conducted. Clearly defined objectives are essential for setting the conditions for sampling and testing, which should be described in detail in the survey protocol.

There is a wide range of possible objectives, a few examples of which are given below:

- to evaluate the quality of selected medicines available in the market, in selected areas, regions or countries, at various levels of the distribution/supply chain with the aim of assessing the exposure of patients to poor-quality medicines and proposing appropriate actions;
- to evaluate the quality of specific medicines used in the treatment programme;
- to compare the quality of domestically produced and imported medicines in order to recommend appropriate regulatory actions and adjust pharmaceutical policy in the country concerned;
- to identify possible causes of inferior quality of specific products to which patients are exposed and to propose possible strategies and implementation plans to address the problems identified by the survey;
- to test the quality of selected medicines in order to support the NMRA in identification of manufacturers that are not in compliance with quality standards and regulatory measures;
- to find out if, within a selected category of medicines, any spurious/falsely labelled/falsified/counterfeit (SFFC) products have penetrated the market in selected areas, regions or countries, what the possible health impacts may be for patients, and to propose possible strategies and implementation plans to prevent harm to patients.

To ensure that a survey provides the necessary information it is essential, in addition to a primary objective, to set appropriate and relevant questions to be addressed in the survey. Some examples of such questions include:

- What proportion of sampled medicines fails quality testing?
- What proportions of sampled medicines fail quality testing at different levels of the regulated distribution chain and in the informal market?
- What proportions of medicines sampled from different geographical regions fail quality testing?
- What proportions of sampled domestically produced and imported medicines fail quality testing?
- Which specific quality tests do the selected medicines fail?
- Are any of the deficiencies critical, i.e. could they substantially affect treatment efficiency and/or cause harm to patients?
- Are there treatment failures related to a specific disease, which can be associated with low-quality medicines?

- What is the registration status of the sampled products and what proportions of registered and unregistered products fail quality testing?
- What are the supply chains by which poor-quality medicines are distributed and what are the market segments they serve?
- Are there any indicators of poor storage and distribution conditions that influence quality of sampled medicines?
- Are there poor-quality medicines in the selected area, e.g. at the border checkpoint?
- What is the proportion of poor-quality medicines being sold and/ or the proportion of pharmaceutical outlets selling poor-quality medicines in a particular area?
- Does the proportion of poor-quality medicines or the proportion of pharmaceutical outlets selling poor-quality medicines exceed a predetermined level?
- Has there been a change in the quality of a medicine or medicine category, or in an area (in the case of repeated random surveys with consistent design)?

Setting reasonable objectives and an appropriate design for a survey needs initial planning. Some examples of questions that should be considered in the planning phase are given below.

- *What is already known about the quality and risk of inferior quality of the target medicines?*

  The information may be available from the scientific literature, alerts on medicines quality, or a search of published studies (e.g. in PubMed or Google Scholar). When an NMRA is involved in the survey it is important to gather information from inspectors, assessors, laboratory and pharmacovigilance experts and to design the survey in cooperation with such a multidisciplinary team. Discussions with pharmacists and other health-care professionals may also help to prioritize surveys.

- *What is the distribution/supply system of the target medicines?*

  Distribution/supply chains vary between countries and even within a country they may be different for different categories of medicines. In order to design the survey properly it is important to understand how the target medicines are supplied in the surveyed area and how they reach patients. Knowledge of the distribution/supply chain of the target medicines enables risk-based selection of the sampling sites that best serve the survey objectives. Complex supply chains pose a higher risk of quality deterioration and should be prioritized in market surveillance activities. Information on distribution/supply chains should be available to NMRAs, ministries of health, provincial health departments and health centres or other governmental organizations. In the public domain, some information can be found on the World Health Organization (WHO) Essential Medicines and Health Products Department website (http://www.who.int/medicines/areas/coordination/partnerscoordination/en/). Several international NGOs are mapping pharmaceutical outlets in various areas and publishing the information on their websites, e.g. Population Services International (PSI) (http://www.psi.org/) or, specifically for antimalarials, ACTWatch (http://www.actwatch.info/). If the survey is intended to focus on unlicensed outlets, an initial investigation may be necessary to identify and map the relevant locations.

- *What health-seeking behaviour is associated with the target medicines?*

  For some surveys it may also be important to understand where different categories of patients tend to buy their medicines and what kind of product they buy. In many countries the medicines market is heavily segmented with different markets for people with different spending power and different ethnicity. For example, the wealthier people may go to pharmacies or private clinics, whereas the poorest go to grocery shops or street peddlers, and people in the middle-income category may go to hospitals. There will also be brands of the same product sold at different prices aimed at different market segments. If such information is needed, an initial pre-survey should be performed.

- *What is the overall volume of use of the target medicines?*

  The higher the volumes of a particular medicine used the bigger the impact the inferior-quality medicine will have on patients. Therefore medicines with high consumption volumes should be prioritized in market surveillance activities. It may be difficult to obtain data on consumption volumes in some countries but estimates based on distribution volumes or information from various disease control programmes can be used.

- *What registered medicines are available in the surveyed area?*

  It may be useful for the evaluation of survey results to have available lists of registered medicines in the surveyed countries. These lists can often be obtained from NMRAs or ministries of health and sometimes may be published on their websites. Additionally, most countries make available unregistered medicines under certain conditions, e.g. specific medicines may be used in public health programmes or donated.

- *What brands of the target medicines are available in the surveyed area or in the selected outlets?*

  If the objective of the survey is to obtain an overall impression of the quality of medicines available on the market, samples produced by as many manufacturers as possible should be collected and it may be necessary to visit several sampling sites. Often, it is very difficult to know in advance how many brands of a specific medicine (containing the same API in the same dosage form) are sold in a particular market or what their market share is. A pilot study asking for a product list at the selling points may help in collecting the data needed to better plan the survey.

For correct understanding and proper interpretation of the results and conclusions of the survey, its limitations should always be stated and explained.

4. Survey management and time frame

Ideally, the authorities (ministry of health and/or NMRA) of target countries should be involved and should agree with the survey plan before it is implemented. The responsibilities and tasks of the people who have key roles in the survey organization (e.g. principal survey coordinator and the local coordinators in individual areas or countries) should be identified at the beginning and should include those with the responsibility for monitoring the conduct of the survey, performing analysis, processing results and preparing the final report. Lines and means of communication should be agreed in advance.

The primary aim of a medicines quality survey is to reduce harm to patients and enforce medicines quality standards. Surveys are organized for market surveillance or to generate new scientific knowledge. Normally they do not require ethical approval; however, such approval may be needed for an epidemiological survey. As the requirements for ethical clearance vary between countries, the regulations on ethical approval in the target countries should be verified before planning a specific survey.

It is recommended that before sample collection starts, a meeting with local coordinators is organized to explain and discuss the project and the survey protocol, and to provide detailed instructions to ensure survey consistency.

After data analysis and before publication of the report it is useful to hold a meeting with appropriate stakeholders to discuss the results, conclusions and actions needed.

Timing of sample collection is important since seasonal changes in environmental conditions may have an influence on the quality of the medicine collected. It is possible that falsified antimalarials are more common during the malaria season, or that access to outlets in rural areas may be impeded in the rainy season, for example as a result of floods or landslides.

Issues such as the use of the results and their public availability should be clearly understood by the responsible authorities and all parties involved in the survey from the beginning. Relevant regulatory measures in individual countries lie within the responsibility of the NMRA, when applicable in collaboration with the police or other enforcement bodies (with respect to falsified medicines or criminal negligence). Therefore, if an NMRA does not organize the survey directly, it should be provided with the results before their publication to be able to investigate in line with the regulatory practice and legislation with the relevant manufacturer and, if appropriate, adopt necessary regulatory measures.

A publication plan including authorship of any papers to be submitted for peer-reviewed publication and a distribution list of those to whom the report will be disseminated should be agreed at the beginning of the survey. A policy should be adopted concerning public release of data that might be considered confidential. The default position should be to distribute the data as widely and openly as possible.

The survey protocol should include the plan of survey activities and the personnel responsible for the completion of the different steps within the estimated time frames (Table A7.1). It is important to plan the financial resources expected for the whole survey before it commences.

Table A7.1
Example plan of survey activities

Activity	Time frame	Responsible person
Selection of areas/regions/countries and medicines to be surveyed		
Preparation of survey protocol		
Agreement with authority/authorities in surveyed country/countries		

Table A7.1 *continued*

Activity	Time frame	Responsible person
Seeking ethical clearance for an epidemiological survey		
Selection of testing laboratory/laboratories		
Finalization of testing protocol in agreement with testing laboratory/laboratories		
Meeting held with local coordinators from the target areas to discuss the survey protocol		
Preparation of detailed sampling plans		
Preparation and pilot test of data collection instructions and procedures, if needed		
Training and supervision of personnel collecting samples		
Collection of samples and transport to testing laboratory/laboratories in a manner that assures sample chain of custody and maintaining samples in a state of control, to preclude compromising the samples during shipment or transfer to the laboratory		
Database of information on collected samples (including scanned pictures or photographs of the dosage form, label and package leaflet)		
Testing of samples		
Compilation of results		
Data analysis		
Report drafting		
Meeting with appropriate stakeholders to discuss the results and the actions needed		
Report finalization		
Distribution and publication of the results		

5. Methodology

All surveys should be conducted according to a predefined survey protocol. Inadequate instructions on the protocol or noncompliance with the protocol, e.g. insufficient sample size, incorrect sampling and/or testing, may lead to inaccurate results and policy recommendations. Careful consideration of the methodology and ethical issues should guide the survey preparation and the people involved should comply with the instructions and with appropriate ethical standards.

In principle, in addition to the background and explanation of the survey objectives and limitations, the survey protocol should contain information on the following.

5.1 Selection of areas to be sampled

A number of different geographical areas should be sampled unless the objectives expressly justify targeting only one area. Samples should be collected in various locations, as situations in rural and suburban areas often differ. Depending on the survey objectives, the following variables may be considered when selecting areas to be surveyed:

- population density;
- incidence or prevalence of the disease for which the target medicines are indicated;
- level of risk of poor-quality medicines, e.g. the risk may be higher along trade routes across country borders, in areas where poor-quality medicines have been previously found, areas where formal health services are limited, and in areas where the NMRA has few or no resources to monitor the distribution of medicines;
- degree of urbanization;
- income level of the population in the target area;
- areas with complex distribution systems;
- areas with outlets selling predominantly unregistered and/or illegal medicines.

Sampling several countries according to the same survey protocol gives a broader picture of the quality of medicines in the region and enables comparisons between countries to be made.

Selection of the sampled areas should be explained and justified.

5.2 Selection of medicines to be surveyed

The category of medicines to be surveyed may be characterized in various ways, e.g. according to their content of APIs, therapeutic group classification, formulation, the specific programme under which they are supplied, or the manufacturer or distributor declared on the label. If collection of commonly used products is required, a pre-survey investigation of treatment-seeking behaviour may be necessary. Collaborating with other actors, such as national disease control programmes, may help to identify products commonly used.

Selection of medicines is driven by the survey objectives and public health considerations. The potential public health impact of poor-quality medicines should be a key guide for selection. To optimize use of available resources the survey should focus on medicines posing most risk to patients, e.g. where the therapeutic index is narrow, substandard quality could lead to a significant change in the health outcome, or certain categories may be particularly vulnerable to counterfeiting. To estimate risks posed by individual medicines an analysis should be performed. Aspects to consider may include:

- probability of occurrence of a quality problem, taking into account:
  - complexity of manufacture,
  - stability of the medicine – risk of quality deterioration under local conditions of storage, distribution and use,
  - compliance of manufacturers of the target medicines with GMP principles,
  - complexity of distribution chain for the target medicines and likelihood of non-compliance with good distribution practices (GDP) principles and approved storage conditions during distribution and storage;
- exposure of patients to the medicine and seriousness of potential health impairment, considering:
  - extent of exposed population – number of patients and length of treatment, and volumes used,
  - vulnerability of target population – susceptibility of treated population to the undesired effects of the medicine,
  - complexity of the dosage form in relation to the route of administration,
  - therapeutic properties and risk, such as safety margins and risk of side effects, risk of therapeutic failure, acute versus chronic exposure, and risk of development of resistance.

Instructions should be provided to sample collectors with regard to the dosage forms and strengths of the selected medicines to be collected. Unless the objectives of the survey require a focus on a particular brand or brands, instructions should be given to the collectors on how to select samples if several brands are available at the sample collection site.

The number of medicines that should be selected for the survey depends on available resources (both financial and human) and care should be taken to keep the survey manageable.

5.3 Selection of sample collection sites

5.3.1 Types of sample collection sites

Types of pharmaceutical outlets vary greatly both within and between countries and may be classified according to the countries' medicine legislation. To allow comparison between regions and/or countries, outlets can be classed as:

- public (government);
- formal (licensed), i.e. registered private for profit and private not for profit (nongovernmental organizations (NGOs));
- informal (unlicensed).

Another way to classify sample collection sites is according to their level in the supply chain:

- Level 1 – points of entry to the market, e.g. warehouses of importers or manufacturers, central medical stores, NGO central stores, procurement centres or other facilities supplied directly within various programmes, central wholesalers and/or distributors;
- Level 2 – wholesalers and/or distributors, pharmacies and other regulated retailers, dispensing facilities, hospitals, health centres, sub-health centres, district hospitals, clinics, polyclinics, cabinets, treatment centres, health posts and community health workers;
- Level 3 – informal outlets selling medicines outside the approved distribution system, e.g. kiosks, street vendors, grocery shops, drug stores and itinerant sellers;
- Level 4: virtual outlets, e.g. sales of medicines via the Internet.

Sampling should usually be performed in both the public and private sectors as well as in the "informal market", i.e. both licensed and unlicensed outlets should be included. Types of sites for sample collection should be selected in the way that will best serve the survey objectives and the selection should be explained.

Quality of samples collected in the supply chain close to the point of sale to patients (Levels 2 and 3) may be influenced by distribution and storage conditions. However, these samples will be the closest in terms of quality to the medicines that patients actually take. When a medicine at Level 2 or 3 is found to be substandard, possibly due to degradation, subsequent sampling of that medicine at Level 1 may identify the source of the problem in the supply chain.

Samples collected at points of entry to the market (Level 1) should be less affected by the conditions they may encounter during in-country distribution, but are relatively distant from the actual quality of medicines that patients will have access to and take. Sampling at this point in the supply chain has the advantage of determining the quality of products as supplied by manufacturers and allowing quality issues to be detected before the products reach patients. Corrective actions may be more easily taken if the results are quickly available.

Once the types of sample collection sites have been selected, the areas, regions or countries to be sampled need to be mapped and the sites where samples will actually be collected during the survey should be identified (by address and facility type). Good local knowledge of the distribution and supply chain structure for the target medicines and information on where patients obtain medicines is needed. Cooperation with NMRAs and relevant disease control programmes in this respect is crucial. If the survey objectives require collection of samples offered by itinerant sellers, it may not be possible to map their "territory" and a pre-survey investigation, e.g. in households, may be needed. Another option would be to include a list of the outlets where itinerant vendors buy their medicines.

5.3.2 Sampling designs

Various designs can be used for selection of sample collection sites. The choice depends on the objectives of the survey, the risks and consequences of inherent decision errors and biases, and available resources.

5.3.2.1 Convenience sampling

Convenience sampling is a non-probability sampling technique based on the judgement of the survey organizer. The sites, however, should not be selected just because of their convenient accessibility and proximity. There should be defined rules guiding the selection so as to best reflect the survey objectives. Whenever convenience sampling is used, it is necessary to report how the sites were identified and which types and what proportion of the outlets the selection represents.

Convenience samples are simple and do not necessarily need complete lists of outlets in defined areas, which may be difficult to obtain especially for unlicensed or mobile outlets. However, they are inherently prone to biases that have to be considered when interpreting the survey outcomes. Such surveys are predominantly used for selection of sample collection sites, e.g. by NMRAs for market surveillance. To utilize resources in the most efficient way NMRAs focus on outlets where the risk of poor-quality medicines being found is high. When selecting such sites the risk analysis should take into account, for example, how medicines are distributed to the site, transport conditions, storage conditions and handling of products at the site, and experience of the NMRA with the distribution chain and sites.

The results of convenience sampling cannot be generalized to other areas, even within the same country, or reliably interpreted over time. However, such surveys may provide the evidence necessary to support regulatory actions or to signal a quality problem. If convenience sampling does indicate a medicine quality problem, further investigation or regulatory actions can be initiated. If a wider picture is needed, subsequent surveys using probability sampling can be designed. If convenience surveys do not reveal a problem one should bear in mind that this may be a false-negative result. It is important to explain the limitations of this technique in reports and scientific papers.

Despite its limitations, convenience sampling is most suitable for NMRAs to identify high-risk areas for further regulatory actions.

Examples of convenience sampling include some surveys conducted in Africa (*1*, *2*) and South East Asia (*3*, *4*).

5.3.2.2 Simple random sampling

Random sampling is a probability sampling technique that, if the sample size is sufficient, will give reliable estimates (with confidence intervals) of the prevalence of outlets selling poor-quality medicines. Formulas for calculation of sample size for random sampling can be found in the literature (*5*, *6*). The disadvantages of random sampling are the large sample sizes needed, the necessity for complete lists of the locations of the target outlets and the additional costs in terms of labour and time. In addition, it is important to recognize that a random survey will only produce reliable and useful information if the list of outlets and actual within-outlet sampling is consistent with the primary aims of the survey. For example, a random survey of the quality of a medicine in the private sector, when most patients obtain this medicine in the public sector would not be useful, nor would a random survey using overt shoppers for a medicine which the outlet staff know should not be sold to patients. Comparisons with subsequent estimates using this same sampling design should, however, be valid and will allow the evaluation of interventions.

5.3.2.3 Stratified random sampling

Stratified sampling is a probability sampling technique wherein the researcher divides the entire group of subjects to be investigated (e.g. outlets) into different subgroups (layers or strata), then randomly selects the final subjects proportionally from the different subgroups. Stratified sampling can be used to adjust for potential differences, e.g. sales volume, type of customers, or geographical, trade and socioeconomic variables (such as rural versus urban, private versus public outlets and one geographical area versus another) may be considered. Stratification requires adjustment of the sample size calculation. Sampling that is proportional to the number of outlets will be more efficient than simple random sampling. It is important that the randomization procedure is done using formal random number tables or statistical software. This technique has been used in a stratified random survey in Lao People's Democratic Republic (*7*). Other examples of random surveys come from Nigeria (*8*) and the United Republic of Tanzania (*9*).

5.3.2.4 Lot quality assurance sampling

An alternative approach to formal random sampling that is simpler and less expensive, and needs smaller sample sizes, is lot quality assurance sampling (LQAS). This technique can be used to determine whether the prevalence of outlets selling poor-quality medicines exceeds a certain threshold.

LQAS is designed to find out whether a lot of goods meets the desired specifications without having to inspect the entire lot. Thus, the sample size in LQAS is defined as the number of outlets or medicines ("goods") that are selected for each site or region ("lot") and the only outcome is that the site or region is "acceptable" or "unacceptable". Setting the level of risk taken by not inspecting each and every item enables the researcher to accept or reject an entire lot after inspecting a randomly selected sample of items. Therefore the sample size in LQAS is based on defined threshold values that classify good and bad outcomes and the probability of error that the researchers are willing to tolerate.

Acceptable probabilities of error must be specified, i.e. the risk of accepting a "bad" lot (consumer risk) and the risk of not accepting a "good" lot (provider risk). These risks are commonly referred to as Type I (alpha) and Type II (beta) errors, respectively. The former is often set to 0.05. This means that if the null hypothesis (that the site has fewer outlets selling poor-quality medicines than the specified value) is true, there is a 5% chance that a site with an unacceptable proportion of outlets selling poor-quality medicines will be "accepted" or go undetected. In general, Type I risk is set lower than the Type II risk.

Once the threshold values and probabilities of error have been considered, a sample size and decision value can be obtained. The decision value is the number of outlets selling poor-quality medicines that need to be found before an area is considered unacceptable. LQAS still requires random sampling and preparation of complete lists of the locations of the outlets, and has the disadvantage that it does not estimate an exact prevalence. The advantage is that it requires relatively smaller sample sizes. Sampling can stop once the number of outlets selling poor-quality medicine is exceeded, greatly reducing sampling time and costs.

As LQAS will only provide a binary result, formal random sampling may be required to examine longitudinal changes in the prevalence of poor-quality medicines accurately. It can also be useful as a way to monitor the situation when the exact prevalence of poor-quality medicines is known.

There has been almost no discussion as to what proportion of outlets selling poor-quality medicines should be regarded as unacceptable. Ideally there should be zero-tolerance for outlets selling poor-quality medicines, as even a 1% prevalence of such medicines for potentially fatal diseases, such as malaria, tuberculosis and HIV, is disastrous for individual patients.

Examples of this approach are described in several publications (*10*, *11*). Sampling procedures and tables for lot acceptance by parties who receive goods manufactured by others can be found in the international standards, e.g. ANSI/ASQ Z1.4 and Z1.9 or ISO 2859 and ISO 3951 series.[1]

5.3.2.5 Sentinel site monitoring

Sentinel site monitoring involves following the quality of medicines in a particular locality over time. There are no common rules as to whether these sites should be chosen on the basis of potentially important variables such as rural versus urban and private versus public outlets, or as to sampling design (i.e. convenience or random samples or LQAS). The power of this methodology resides in allowing longitudinal changes to be followed in one place, but data from fixed sentinel site monitoring should be interpreted with caution. Sentinel site monitoring suffers from the disadvantage that shop owners may soon realize that they are being sampled, change their behaviour accordingly and thus cease to be representative. Examples of this approach include the survey in the Mekong region (*12*).

5.4 Sampling plans

Sampling plans should be prepared for each area, region or country involved in the survey and should be in compliance with requirements identified in the survey protocol. They should specify the:

- individual sites where collectors should collect samples (by facility type and address, possibly including global positioning system (GPS) coordinates);
- medicines to be sampled (by APIs, dosage form, strength, and, if needed, also by package size);

[1] http://asq.org/knowledge-center/Z14.Z19/index.html; http://www.iso.org/iso/home/store/catalogue_tc/catalogue_detail.htm?csnumber=39991; http://www.iso.org/iso/home/store/catalogue_tc/catalogue_detail.htm?csnumber=57490.

- minimum number of dosage units to be collected per sample;
- number of samples to be collected per medicine;
- total number of samples to be collected in the relevant area, region or country.

Sampling plans should also contain detailed instructions for collectors. Examples of sampling plans for surveys organized by WHO can be found in the published survey reports.[2]

5.4.1 Number of dosage units to be collected

The number of dosage units that should be collected per sample depends on the survey objectives, surveyed medicines, tests to be conducted, testing methods to be employed and available resources. To protect the integrity of the samples and avoid quality deterioration before testing, dosage units should normally not be taken out of the original primary and secondary packaging, and only intact and unopened packages should be collected. Sampling plans usually define the minimum number of dosage units to be collected per sample. The appropriate number of packages is collected in relation to the available package size.

In surveys aiming to provide evidence to support regulatory actions, which are often organized by NMRAs or with their participation, pharmacopoeial tests performed in compliance with pharmacopoeial procedures are commonly used. In such surveys the principles of good practices for pharmaceutical quality control laboratories (*13*) should be followed and the number of dosage units per sample should allow:

- the planned tests to be conducted;
- investigation and confirmatory testing of samples found to be out-of-specification (OOS);
- sufficient retention samples to be used in case of dispute.

To fulfil these requirements, suitably large numbers of dosage units per sample should be collected (e.g. 100 tablets, 40 injection solution ampoules or powder for injection vials, depending on the medicine and the requested tests), which may be difficult to obtain from some outlets. Requests for such large quantities of products may also suggest to the outlet owner that the buyer is not an ordinary shopper, in cases where the survey objectives require a mystery-shopper approach. The minimum number of dosage units of each selected medicine to be collected should be agreed with the testing laboratory.

---

2 World Health Organization Prequalification of Medicines Programme. Quality Monitoring (http://www.who.int/prequal/).

The advantage of surveys using pharmacopoeial procedures is the possibility to apply quality acceptance criteria as defined in pharmacopoeias. The disadvantage is that the rather time- and resource-intensive laboratory testing leads to fewer samples that can be included in the survey.

Other types of surveys include quality screening surveys using basic, simple tests, non-destructive techniques (such as Raman and infrared (IR) spectroscopy) or unofficial testing methods (i.e. non-pharmacopoeial or not approved by the NMRA during the registration process) to assess the identity of the API and estimate its content. Such surveys cannot be used as a basis for regulatory actions but may prompt further investigations with appropriate protocols. The advantage is that only a few dosage units need to be collected per sample, a higher number of samples can be collected and the mystery-shopper approach can be used, if needed. The disadvantage is that when testing only a few individual dosage units, the usual pharmacopoeial quality acceptance criteria are difficult to apply, e.g. when estimating the content of the API by testing only a few individual tablets, pharmacopoeial criteria for the assay cannot be used.

Testing of individual dosage units to assess the content of API raises the question of how many dosage units, within a specific medicine sample, need to be analysed. The variability of individual units can be very high, especially within a sample of poor-quality medicine. Various statistical approaches to representative medicine sampling, especially for forensic analysis purposes, have been described. These are published, e.g. by the United Nations (UN) Office on Drugs and Crime (*14*), Scientific Working Group for the Analysis of Seized Drugs (*15*), European Network of Forensic Sciences Institutes,[3] and in other publications (*16*).

Sampling procedures to ensure that representative samples are taken by authorities, procurement agencies, manufacturers or customers, for acceptance of consignments, batch release testing, in-process controls, special controls, inspection for customs clearance, deterioration and adulteration, or for obtaining a retention sample are described in the WHO guidelines for sampling of pharmaceutical products and related materials (*17*).

5.5 Sample collection

5.5.1 Overt sampling versus mystery-shopper approach

The decision on who should collect samples will depend on the survey objectives, the regulatory status of the target medicines and what is known about the knowledge and attitude of the sellers (i.e. whether they know that the outlet

[3] Calculator for qualitative sampling of seized drugs (http://www.enfsi.eu/documents/enfsi-dwg-calculator-qualitative-sampling-seized-drugs-2012).

is selling poor-quality medicines and understand the health, legal and ethical implications). If outlet staff are anxious to avoid poor-quality medicines and are informed about the survey objectives, overt sampling with feedback would allow more data to be collected on poor-quality medicines and their risk factors and lead to a direct improvement in the medicine supply. Overt sampling may be the only possible method in some circumstances, such as when collecting samples at locations where people are seen first by clinicians, or in the public sector.

However, many outlets in countries with weak medicines regulation sell expired or unregistered medicines, which may make outlet staff suspicious and anxious about investigations. If the seller knows or is concerned that his or her stock contains illegal or poor-quality medicines and that the buyer is potentially linked to the NMRA, this may influence which medicines are offered. An additional concern is that in many resource-poor countries the medicine market is heavily segmented with different markets for people with different spending power and ethnicity. Even within a single outlet there will often be several different brands of the same medicine at different prices aimed at different market segments. In such cases a covert, mystery-shopper approach may be appropriate (*18*). The identity and purpose of the buyer should not be generally known by the outlet being evaluated. Sampling should usually be performed by nationals of the country concerned although there may be some situations, such as suspicion that migrant workers may take inferior medicines, where this would not be applicable. It may not be safe for people living in the same wider community to act as purchasers. In contrast, in some remote rural locations, it would be difficult for someone who is not local to request medicines as this would cause suspicion. The safety of those acting as mystery shoppers should be considered, a risk assessment performed and instructions appropriate to local conditions need to be developed.

The mystery shopper mimics a "normal shopper" from the community in which the outlet is located and should dress, speak and behave appropriately for that community. Shoppers should use a standard scenario, e.g. pretending to be a visitor from another part of the country who needs some medicines for a specified disease, for a specific reason and for a stereotypical patient. Mystery shoppers should be prepared to explain the real purpose of their visit to protect themselves if their identity is revealed.

After leaving the survey site the mystery shopper should record details of each purchase. Price, name of the provider and/or outlet, and an estimation of temperature at the site should be documented as well as the conditions of the purchase, e.g. how many people were in the outlet, how long the purchase took, the nature of the interaction between the mystery shopper and outlet staff, whether it was easy to convince the provider to sell medicines, and any other information needed to meet the survey objectives. All medicines collected should be properly identified and stored, e.g. in a plastic bag labelled with the name of the outlet.

The mystery shopper should brief the local coordinator for the surveyed area upon his or her return from each outlet. The local coordinator should transcribe the reported interaction together with a translation if appropriate. Translations should use a meaning-based method, rather than a literal or interpretative approach. The original text with translation should be double-checked for accuracy by other members of the team and kept.

Examples of overt sampling include some surveys in Asia (*19*, *20*) and an example using the mystery-shopper approach can be found in the report of a survey conducted in Lao People's Democratic Republic (*7*).

5.5.2 Instructions to sample collectors

The local coordinator for each area, region or country will arrange for training of collectors to familiarize them with the project, survey protocol, sampling plan and instructions for collection of samples. Staff from the NMRA and different national disease control programmes may provide a useful insight into the survey planning. Instructions and procedures for data collection should be well understood by the collectors (translated into the language of the collectors, pilot-tested and revised, if needed). The following principles should be stated in detailed instructions for collectors.

- The minimum number of dosage units per sample and number of batches to be collected from each collection site for each selected medicine as indicated in the sampling plan should be adhered to.
- The target medicines, their dosage forms, strengths and package sizes should be defined. As outlets may have more than one brand of a particular medicine available, instructions should be provided on how to decide which to choose if a selection has to be made. It should be taken into consideration that mystery shoppers requesting a very specific brand or product may alert sellers. However, such an approach may be required if evidence suggests that only one brand of an essential medicine is affected by falsification or substandard production. It may be useful to consider using a specific written prescription for a number of items including the target medicine. This can reduce the suspicion that might be raised by a verbal request. Using the written prescription format may also enable the quality of dispensing, labelling directions and counselling to be studied.
- All units of one sample should have the same batch number.

- The medicine samples should not be taken out of the original primary and secondary packaging (although removal from large secondary packs is appropriate). Containers such as bottles and vials should not be opened. Where medicines are sold without package leaflets, or in unlabelled plastic bags coming from large-sized boxes (locally repacked), or as individual dosage forms, this should be recorded.
- Ideally, samples collected should have at least six months remaining before expiry to allow sufficient time for chemical analysis. However, the frequency of expired medicines is also an important outcome measure and any expired medicine found in the outlet should be recorded.
- The medicine labels and package leaflets should not be removed or damaged.
- Each sample should be recorded separately using the sample collection form (for an example see Appendix 1). Whenever the required information is not available this should be noted in the appropriate space on the sample collection form; any observed abnormalities should also be recorded.
- Each sample should be identified by a unique sample code, defined on the sample collection form and specified on all original packages belonging to the respective sample. It should be written legibly and should not obscure the basic product information. The sample collection form and all packages belonging to one sample should be kept together (e.g. blisters inserted in a dedicated zip-lock plastic bag or an envelope marked with the appropriate sample code and trade name of the product). For large surveys, barcode systems may be helpful to reduce errors.
- When overt sampling is used, manufacturer's batch certificates of analysis should be collected with the samples, if available, and kept with the sample collection form.
- Storage conditions at the site (temperature, humidity, access of light and any other observations) should be described in the sample collection form. When overt sampling is used collectors can measure the temperature if it is not controlled at the site. Mystery shoppers can estimate and record the temperature.
- Samples should be collected and kept under controlled conditions in line with the product label requirements. The cold chain has to be maintained, where required. Samples should be kept protected from light, excessive moisture or dryness. Safety measures against theft should be taken; medicine boxes should be kept in a locked area.

The period within which samples should be collected and the deadline for sending the last sample to the testing laboratory should be clearly indicated and adhered to.

Normally samples of collected medicines should be paid for by collectors. The cost of collected samples needs to be taken into account when determining the numbers of samples to be collected. In some countries, NMRA inspectors have legal power to collect samples from the market without reimbursement.

Collectors should be mindful of the stock of sampled products held in outlets, and of the potential difficulties of replenishing sampled medicines through the supply chain, so as not to jeopardize the availability of these medicines to patients. If there is a risk of product shortage after sampling, replacement of the sampled amount should be arranged immediately after the survey or, less desirably, collection of that particular product from that outlet should be omitted.

For surveys seeking to determine the proportion of poor-quality medicines sold to patients, data on product-specific sales volumes from the outlets may be necessary. These data can be collected after sampling, especially when the mystery-shopper approach is used, and sellers should be informed about the survey. This approach requires the support of the NMRA as data on sales volumes are better collected by inspectors or by officers of the authority.

5.6 Storage and transportation of samples

Storage and transportation of the samples to the testing laboratory should be done according to the requirements set out in paragraph 2.3 of *WHO Guidelines for sampling of pharmaceutical products and related materials* (*17*). Transportation should be as quick and direct as possible so as not to jeopardize the quality of the collected samples.

- The samples should be kept in their original packaging and stored under the conditions specified on the label; freezing should be avoided and, where required, the cold chain should be maintained.
- For transport, all samples should be packaged adequately and transported in such a way as to avoid breakage and contamination. Any residual space in the container should be filled with a suitable material.
- For temperature-sensitive medicines, temperature data loggers may be included within shipments to document maintenance of an appropriate temperature during prolonged transit.
- A covering letter, copies of sample collection forms and, if available, copies of the manufacturer's batch certificate of analysis should accompany the samples.

- Where collectors do not transport samples directly to the testing laboratory, samples, with the accompanying documents, should be sent by a courier service. The documentation with each shipment should clearly indicate that the samples are being sent for laboratory testing purposes only, will not be used on humans or animals, have no commercial value and will not be placed on the market. If the country where the laboratory is located requires permission for importation of samples, the laboratory or NMRA of that country may be able to assist to avoid long clearance procedures. The staff of the testing laboratory should be informed of the shipment and provided with the tracking number assigned by the courier service to enable them to follow the shipment and arrange collection as soon as possible.
- Copies of sample collection forms and, if available, copies of manufacturer's batch certificates of analysis should also be sent to the principal survey coordinator or the person preparing the survey report.

5.7 Testing

5.7.1 Testing laboratory

It is important that only quality control laboratories with demonstrated capability to produce reliable test results are used in quality surveys. Therefore laboratories for testing should be carefully selected and should meet the following criteria:

- the laboratory works in compliance with WHO *Good practices for pharmaceutical quality control laboratories* (*13*), is preferably a WHO prequalified[4] laboratory or is a laboratory where other evidence of equivalent working standards is available;
- the laboratory is capable and competent to perform the tests required by the testing protocol;
- the laboratory should have sufficient capacity and should agree to test the required number of samples within the specified period for the cost specified according to the available budget.

The choice of the testing laboratory or laboratories should be explained in the survey protocol, reports and publications. One or more laboratories may be used for testing the samples collected during the survey. If several laboratories are testing collected samples, samples should be divided in such a way that all

[4] The list of WHO-prequalified laboratories can be found at www.who.int/prequal.

samples containing the same APIs are assigned for testing to the same laboratory. Many countries do not have a fully functioning quality control laboratory and should consider making arrangements with a laboratory abroad. The appropriate arrangements with the laboratory have to be made in advance.

Within the usual selection procedure and the resulting agreement the following should be clearly specified in addition to the usual elements of such agreements (such as deadlines and financial arrangements):

- medicines and numbers of samples to be tested, tests to be conducted and specifications to be used, according to the testing protocol. If more than one testing laboratory is selected, a specific testing protocol should be prepared for each laboratory;
- responsibilities of the laboratory during the survey as specified in section 5.7.4;
- confidentiality declaration made by the laboratory;
- acceptance of a possible audit of the laboratory, access to records and retained samples.

Following conclusion of the agreement(s), the principal survey coordinator should inform the local coordinators in the areas, regions or countries participating in the survey about the following:

- name and address of the laboratory or laboratories;
- the contact person(s) in the laboratory; and
- medicines assigned for testing to the particular laboratory.

The laboratory normally starts testing only when all the samples containing the same API in the same dosage form have been received. Therefore it is important to set and adhere to the deadline for sending samples to the testing laboratory.

5.7.2 Tests to be conducted

Laboratory testing of all collected samples should be performed according to the testing protocol, which is a part of the survey protocol, and should be agreed with the testing laboratory or laboratories. Depending on the survey objectives, target medicines and available resources, the tests to be done on samples collected in the survey may include:

- verifying the identity;
- performing complete pharmacopoeial or analogous testing;
- performing special or specific tests.

If testing is expected to provide a full picture of the quality of target medicines, it should be performed according to a pharmacopoeial or analogous monograph and the following tests are, in principle, included:

- appearance, visual inspection;
- identity;
- assay for APIs declared on the label;
- test for related substances;
- for solid dosage forms – dissolution or disintegration, uniformity of dosage units (by mass or content), fineness of dispersion, for dispersible tablets;
- for liquid dosage forms – pH value and volume in containers or extractable volume;
- for parenteral products – sterility and bacterial endotoxins tests.

Inclusion of tests for uniformity of content for single-dose dosage forms, or for sterility and bacterial endotoxins, which are costly and time consuming, and necessitate the collection of more dosage units, should be considered in relation to the target medicines and available resources. It is impossible to achieve 100% certainty about sterility of the product through testing only and inspections and enforcement of compliance with GMP principles may be more efficient tools for verification in some cases.

The packaging of each collected sample, labelling and package leaflets should be inspected visually for any signs of being an SFFC product. The World Health Professionals Association has published a checklist that may be used for this purpose (*21*). Laboratory analysis is not always successful in identifying falsified or substandard medicines and any suspicious product that is identified should be further examined in cooperation with the NMRA in the country of collection and the manufacturer declared on the label of the suspicious sample (for guidance on conducting such investigations see the WHO guidelines[5]).

Information on labels and in package leaflets can also be checked for quality and completeness of essential information, and compliance with requirements and approved product information in the country of collection can be verified. However, when more than one country is involved in the survey, it should be kept in mind that requirements for information to be provided on medicines labels and package leaflets may differ between countries.

[5] Testing of "suspect" substandard/spurious/falsely-labelled/falsified/counterfeit medicines (QAS/15.634) (draft in preparation).

Screening methods do not provide a full picture of the quality of medicines and may be more likely to underestimate non-compliant findings than laboratory testing methods (*1*). However, they do enable testing of a large number of samples in the field, e.g. to search for SFFC medicines. It is recommended that outcomes of screening are verified by laboratory testing, at least for a random selection of those samples that pass screening and for all those that fail.

5.7.3 Test methods and specifications

Test methods and specifications should be selected in the way that will best serve the survey objectives. In general, when samples from different manufacturers are collected in a quality survey, all samples containing the same APIs in the same dosage form are tested using the same method and specification to enable comparison of samples from different manufacturers. This specification is then used to decide on compliance or non-compliance of tested samples for the purposes of the survey. It should be noted that individual manufacturers may use different specifications and different methods for testing of their products and those specifications and methods may be approved by regulatory authorities in the countries concerned. Non-compliance with the specification selected for the survey does not therefore necessarily imply non-compliance with the specifications approved in the country but it indicates to the respective NMRA the need to look at the product and conditions of regulatory approval more closely and discuss these with the manufacturer or registration holder.

Wherever appropriate, pharmacopoeial methods and specifications should be used. A national pharmacopoeia may be applicable if a survey is organized in one country. If several countries are involved, widely accepted pharmacopoeias (such as the *British Pharmacopoeia*, *European Pharmacopoeia*, *The International Pharmacopoeia* or the *United States Pharmacopeia*) may be appropriate. In spite of efforts to harmonize pharmacopoeias there are still many differences between them. When a monograph for the particular medicine being tested is available in more than one pharmacopoeia the ability of the different methods and specifications to reveal quality problems should be considered and the monograph selected accordingly. Suitability of test methods for the intended use should be appropriately verified.

If no monograph for the target medicine exists in a pharmacopoeia or the existing monographs do not cover the desired tests, a validated method of the laboratory should be used.

When samples from one manufacturer only are tested in a survey, that manufacturer's methods and specifications can be used, if available to the testing laboratory. The performance of such methods under the conditions of the testing laboratory should be verified.

If samples suspected of being an SFFC product are tested, pharmacopoeial methods may not be sufficient and further examination should be conducted (for guidance on such investigations see WHO guidelines[6]).

Once the tests to be performed and the methods and specifications to be used have been selected, the testing protocol should be finalized. For each of the target medicines the protocol should contain the list of tests to be conducted, reference to methods to be used and specifications to be employed. Examples of testing protocols used for surveys organized by WHO can be found in the published survey reports.[7]

5.7.4 Receipt and testing of samples by a testing laboratory

When samples are received, the testing laboratory should:

- inspect each sample to ensure that the labelling is in conformity with the information provided in the sample collection form or test request; an electronic databank (e.g. scanned pictures or photographs of the medicines, e.g. of the tablets, packaging and package leaflet) is recommended;
- store the samples according to the conditions set out on the product labels, including compliance with any cold chain requirements;
- conduct quality testing in line with the testing protocol and in compliance with WHO *Good practices for pharmaceutical quality control laboratories* (*13*), including appropriate verification of test methods, investigation and documentation of each OOS result according to the laboratory standard operating procedure. If the OOS result is confirmed, it should be reported without delay to the principal survey coordinator who should receive both the results and the investigation report;
- prepare complete analytical test reports and certificates of analysis containing the information listed in Appendix 2. The principal survey coordinator should define the format of the outcome (e.g. separately for each sample or as a tabulated report);
- keep document(s) received with the samples, records of testing of each sample including all raw data, and retention samples according to the requirements defined by the principal survey

[6] Testing of "suspect" substandard/spurious/falsely-labelled/falsified/counterfeit medicines (QAS/15.634) (draft in preparation).

[7] For details of the various studies carried out using the protocol referred to, see: http://apps.who.int/prequal/

coordinator (e.g. for at least six months if the sample complied with the specifications, or for at least one year or until the expiry date (whichever is longer) if it did not comply) and archive data according to the agreed conditions.

6. Data management and publication

To allow proper interpretation, the data obtained during collection and testing of samples should be summarized and appropriately organized in a database (using Excel sheets or software for epidemiological studies), linking each sample with all the data gathered and ensuring consistency and security. Suitable precautions should be taken to avoid errors. For analysis of large sets of data, statistical software may be used. If relevant, personal identification of individuals who participated in the survey (e.g. buyers and sellers) should be entered in the database using codes only.

The NMRAs of countries involved in the survey should be informed immediately about confirmed OOS results. NMRAs should carry out their investigations with the involvement of the relevant manufacturer, registration holder or other party (e.g. procurement organizations). It should be kept in mind that if the testing methods and specifications approved during the registration process differ from those used in the survey, it may be necessary to retest the product concerned using the approved manufacturer's method, where available. Appropriate measures should be taken to ensure the accuracy of the results.

Once survey results have been compiled, evaluated and summarized they should be shared with the NMRAs involved as they may provide information on medicine quality problems that will alert NMRAs and manufacturers. Before publication of the results, it is useful to hold a meeting with appropriate stakeholders to discuss the results and the actions needed. The WHO Rapid Alert System should be informed when results are considered to constitute a public health emergency.

A detailed survey report should be prepared that includes all test results on the collected samples together with their interpretation. An example outline for the survey report content is provided in Appendix 3. Recommendations for items to be addressed in the reports of medicines quality surveys can also be found in the published literature (*22*).

The report should be published as widely and openly as possible. The conclusions and wording should be prepared with caution so as not to cause embarrassment or panic. The risk that patients will stop taking genuine medicines and that the public will lose faith in medicines or the health-care system should be reduced by careful wording. Also any potential harm that might be caused to manufacturers, suppliers or outlets should be considered to avoid any legal actions.

References

1. Survey of the quality of selected antimalarial medicines circulating in six countries of sub-Saharan Africa. Geneva: World Health Organization; 2011 (http://www.who.int/prequal/info_applicants/qclabs/monitoring_documents/WHO_QAMSA_report.pdf, accessed 25 November 2015).
2. United States Pharmacopeia Drug Quality and Information Program. Survey of the quality of selected antimalarial medicines circulating in Madagascar, Senegal, and Uganda – November 2009. Rockville (MD): The United States Pharmacopeial Convention; 2010 (http://www.usp.org/worldwide/dqi/resources/technicalReports, accessed 25 November 2015).
3. Newton P, Proux S, Green M, Smithuis F, Rozendaal J, Prakongpan S, et al. Fake artesunate in Southeast Asia. Lancet. 2001;357(9272):1948–50.
4. Dondorp AM, Newton PN, Mayxay M, Van Damme W, Smithuis FM, Yeung S, et al. Fake antimalarials in Southeast Asia are a major impediment to malaria control: multinational cross-sectional survey on the prevalence of fake antimalarials. Trop Med Int Health. 2004; 9(12):1241–6.
5. Cochran WG. Sampling techniques, second edition. New York: John Wiley and Sons; 1963.
6. Yamane T. Statistics: an introductory analysis, second edition. New York: Harper and Row; 1967.
7. Sengaloundeth S, Green MD, Fernández FM, Manolin O, Phommavong K, Insixiengmay V. A stratified random survey of the proportion of poor-quality oral artesunate sold at medicine outlets in the Lao PDR – implications for therapeutic failure and drug resistance. Malar J. 2009;8:172. doi: 10.1186/1475-2875-8-172.
8. Onwujekwe O, Kaur H, Dike N, Shu E, Uzochukwu B, Hanson K, et al. Quality of anti-malarial drugs provided by public and private healthcare providers in south-east Nigeria. Malar J. 2009;8:22. doi: 10.1186/1475-2875-8-22.
9. Kaur H, Goodman C, Thompson E, Thompson KA, Masanja I, Kachur SP, et al. A nationwide survey of the quality of antimalarials in retail outlets in Tanzania. PLoS One. 2008;3(10):e3403.
10. Khojah HMJ, Pallos H, Yoshida N, Akazawa M, Tsuboi H, Kazuko K. The quality of medicines in community pharmacies in Riyadh, Saudi Arabia. A lot quality assurance sampling (LQAS)-based survey. Pharmacol Pharm. 2013;4(7):511–9. doi: 10.4236/pp. 2013.47074.
11. Lemeshow S, Taber S. Lot quality assurance sampling: single- and double-sampling plans. World Health Stat Q. 1991;44(3):115–32.
12. Phanouvong S. Mekong Malaria Initiative. Antimalarial drug quality monitoring and evaluation. Indicators. Rockville (MD): United States Pharmacopeia Drug Quality and Information Program; 2004 (http://pdf.usaid.gov/pdf_docs/pnadh147.pdf, accessed 25 November 2015).
13. Good practices for pharmaceutical quality control laboratories. In: WHO Expert Committee on Specifications for Pharmaceutical Preparations: forty-fourth report. Geneva: World Health Organization; 2010: Annex 1 (WHO Technical Report Series, No. 957 (http://www.who.int/prequal/info_general/documents/TRS957/GPCL_TRS957_Annex1.pdf, accessed 25 November 2015).
14. United Nations Office on Drugs and Crime. Guidelines on representative drug sampling for use by national drug analysis laboratories. New York: United Nations; 2009 (http://www.unodc.org/documents/scientific/Drug_Sampling.pdf, accessed 25 November 2015).
15. Scientific working group for the analysis of seized drugs (SWGDRUG). Recommendations. United States Department of Justice Drug Enforcement Administration; 2011 (http://www.swgdrug.org/Documents/SWGDRUG%20Recommendations%206.pdf, accessed 25 November 2015).
16. Hoffman CG, Frank RS, Hinkley SW. Representative sampling of drug seizures in multiple containers. ASTM International. 1991;36(2).

17. WHO guidelines for sampling of pharmaceutical products and related materials. In: WHO Expert Committee on Specifications for Pharmaceutical Preparations: thirty-ninth report. Geneva: World Health Organization; 2005: Annex 4 (WHO Technical Report Series, No. 929).

18. Madden JM, Quick JD, Ross-Degnan D, Kafle KK. Undercover careseekers: Simulated clients in the study of health provider behavior in developing countries. Soc Sci Med. 1997;45(10):1465–82.

19. ACTwatch. Outlet survey. Kingdom of Cambodia. 2011 Survey Report. Washington (DC): Population Services International; 2011 (http://www.actwatch.info/sites/default/files/content/outlet-reports/ACTwatch%20Cambodia%20OS%20Endline_2011.pdf, accessed 25 November 2015).

20. Survey of the quality of anti-tuberculosis medicines circulating in selected newly independent states of the former Soviet Union. Geneva: World Health Organization; 2011 (http://www.who.int/prequal/info_applicants/qclabs/monitoring_documents/TBQuality-Survey_Nov2011.pdf, accessed 25 November 2015).

21. Be aware. Tool for visual inspection of medicines. Ferney Voltaire: World Health Professions Alliance (http://www.whpa.org/Toolkit_BeAware_Inspection.pdf, accessed 25 November 2015).

22. Newton PN, Lee SJ, Goodman C, Fernández FM, Yeung S, Phanouvong S, et al. Guidelines for field surveys of the quality of medicines: A proposal. PLoS Med. 2009;6(3):0252–0257.

Appendix 1

Example of a sample collection form[1]

SURVEY TITLE

Area/region/country: ______________ **Sample code:** ______________
(Area/region/country code/medicine abbreviation/sequence number/sampling date dd/mm/yy)[2]

Name of location/place where sample was taken: ______________

____

Address (with telephone, fax number and email address, GPS coordinates, if applicable): ______________

____

____

Organization and names of people who collected the sample:

1. ______________
2. ______________

Product name of the sample: ______________

Name of active pharmaceutical ingredient(s) (INN) with strength:

____

Dosage form (tablet, injection, powder for injection, etc.): ______________

Package size, type and packaging material of the container: ______________

____

Batch/lot number: ______________

Date of manufacture: ______________ Expiry date: ______________

Regulatory status in the country, registration number if applicable: ______________

____

Name and address of the manufacturer: ______________

____

____

____

[1] The sample collection form should always be kept with the collected sample.

[2] *Area/region/country code*: e.g. for countries, the two-letter code is used for the Internet country top-level domains; *medicines abbreviations* to be established; sample code system can be extended to be appropriate for a collection system in a particular area, region or country.

Quantity collected (number of tablets/ampoules/vials and number of packages):
____

Initial first page:

Product name: ____________________ **Sample code:** ________________

Date the batch was received at the location: ____________________

Storage and climatic conditions at sampling site:

Conditions controlled? Yes ☐ No ☐

Temperature and humidity in the place where the sample was stored at the time of sample collection: ____________________

____

Comments on suitability of premises where products are stored, abnormalities, remarks or observations that may be considered relevant, if any:

____

____

____

____

____

____

____

____

Date:

Signature of person(s) taking samples	Signature of representative of the facility where sample was taken (*only for overt sampling, optional*)
1. ________________	________________
2. ________________	

Note: Samples collected must remain in their original primary and secondary packaging, intact and unopened.

Appendix 2

Content of the analytical test report/certificate of analysis

- Name and address of the laboratory performing the sample testing
- Name and address of the originator of the request for testing
- Number/code of the analytical test report/certificate of analysis
- Sample reference number assigned by the laboratory and sample code assigned at the time of sampling (specified in the sample collection form and packages belonging to one sample)
- Date on which the sample was received
- Name of the area, region or country where the sample was collected
- Sample product name (trade name as it appears on the label), dosage form, APIs, strength, package size (e.g. number of tablets in one blister and number of blisters in the secondary packaging, volume in one ampoule and number of ampoules in secondary packaging)
- Description of the sample (describing both the product and the primary and secondary packaging, type and packaging material of primary container); if there is any sign of unsatisfactory handling during transportation, this should be mentioned
- Batch number of the sample, expiry date and, if available, date of manufacture
- Number of units received for the sample
- Name and full address of the manufacturer (as specified on the label or in the package leaflet)
- Reference to the specifications used for testing the sample, including the limits
- If a reference substance was used for quantitative determination, this substance should be specified (e.g. *The International Pharmacopoeia*, *British Pharmacopoeia* or *United States Pharmacopeia* reference substance or working standard)
- Results of all the tests performed; for the evaluation and interpretation of results it is useful to request numerical results wherever possible, any observation made during testing, and the following details:
  - for content uniformity, all results for individual units,
  - for dissolution test, results for all tablets tested,

  - for assay, results of each individual sample preparation (usually 3 sample preparations), the average and the relative standard deviation; in the case of an OOS result followed by retesting, also the investigation report and results of retesting

- Conclusion as to whether or not the sample complies with the specifications set for the survey
- Date on which the test was completed
- Signature of the head of the laboratory or authorized person

Appendix 3

Outline of the content of a survey report

Glossary and abbreviations

Executive summary

1. Introduction

1.1 Background
1.2 Objectives of the survey

2. Methodology

2.1 Survey period
2.2 Selection of medicines for sampling and testing
2.3 Selection of areas, regions or countries
2.4 Sampling design and selection of sample collection sites
2.5 Sample collection and transportation
2.6 Testing laboratories
2.7 Quality tests performed and test methods and specifications used
2.8 Definition of compliance of samples with standards

3. Results

3.1 Overview of samples collected
 3.1.1 Medicines
 3.1.2 Manufacturers and batches
 3.1.3 Sites of sample collection
 3.1.4 Storage and transportation conditions
3.2 Registration status of sampled products
3.3 Compliance with specifications
 3.3.1 Overall results
 3.3.2 Results of specific quality tests for individual products

4. Discussion

4.1 Testing methods and data quality
4.2 Limitations of methodology
4.3 Interpretation of the results
4.4 Recommendations

5. Conclusions

6. Other information (conflict of interests, funding)

References

Attachments – Detailed test results tabled for individual samples

Annex 8

Collaborative procedure between the World Health Organization (WHO) Prequalification Team and national regulatory authorities in the assessment and accelerated national registration of WHO-prequalified pharmaceutical products and vaccines

1. Definitions

Collaborative procedure (Procedure)[1]

Procedure for collaboration between the World Health Organization (WHO) Prequalification Team (WHO/PQT) and interested national regulatory authorities (NRAs) in the assessment and accelerated national registration of WHO-prequalified pharmaceutical products and vaccines.

Participating authorities or participating NRAs

NRAs that voluntarily agree to implement this collaborative procedure and accept the task of processing applications for registration of WHO-prequalified pharmaceutical products and vaccines in accordance with the terms of the Procedure. A list of participating authorities is posted on the WHO/PQT website (for pharmaceutical products at http://www.who.int/prequal/, and for vaccines at http://www.who.int/immunization_standards/vaccine_quality/expedited_review/en/).

Pharmaceutical product

Any substance or combination of substances marketed or manufactured to be marketed for treating or preventing disease in human beings, or with a view to making a medical diagnosis in human beings, or to restoring, correcting or modifying physiological functions in human beings.

Vaccine

A vaccine is a biological preparation that improves immunity to a particular disease. A vaccine typically contains an agent that resembles a disease-causing microorganism and is often made from weakened or killed forms of the microbe, its toxins, one of its surface proteins or genetically-engineered material. The agent stimulates the body's immune system to recognize the agent as foreign, destroy it and "remember" it, so that the immune system can more easily recognize and destroy any of these microorganisms that it later encounters.

[1] Collaborative procedure between the World Health Organization (WHO) Prequalification of Medicines Programme and national medicines regulatory authorities in the assessment and accelerated national registration of WHO-prequalified pharmaceutical products appeared as Annex 4 (WHO Technical Report Series, No. 981, 2013).

2. Background information

National assessment of applications for registration of pharmaceutical products and vaccines (marketing authorization) is the key regulatory process that enables NRAs to evaluate and monitor the quality, safety and efficacy of pharmaceutical products and vaccines. For most countries the approach to registration of pharmaceutical products and vaccines is a combination of two components:

- the NRA's own assessment of application documentation combined with verification of compliance with relevant good practices by inspections (mostly focusing on good manufacturing practices (GMP) and inspections of manufacturing sites) and testing of product characteristics when applicable;
- consideration by the NRA of decisions and outcomes of assessments and inspections made by NRAs in other countries, and for vaccines also official batch release by the national control laboratory performing the oversight of the vaccines.

Consideration of the outcomes of assessments and inspections by authorities, whose regulatory decisions are based on acceptable standards, substantially contributes to savings in regulatory resources and improvements in the quality of regulatory decisions, while retaining the prerogative of NRAs to conclude their assessment by sovereign decisions, which reflect their own judgement of the benefit–risk balance as it relates to their specific country situation and the legislation in place. Taking into consideration the regulatory decisions of other NRAs requires setting up a system that will permit:

- identification of reference authorities whose regulatory decisions are based on acceptable standards and identification of documents associated with such regulatory decisions, which are relevant to the regulatory environment in the country wishing to rely on such decisions;
- assurance that the product for which the decision has been taken by the reference NRA is the same (see section 3.2) as the product being assessed or, if it is not the same, that a clear understanding exists of the differences between the products subjected to assessment in the two regulatory environments;
- efficient use of available scientific expertise and human and financial resources to decide, with reasonable certainty, on the benefit–risk profile of an evaluated product when used in a given country;
- the choice by each NRA of the approaches that will make best use of the resources, workload and competence of individual NRAs.

Approaches could range from completely independent data reviews and inspections to adoption of regulatory decisions of reference authorities without any further scientific review. A pragmatic approach is to verify whether the product submitted for registration is the same (see section 3.2) as the product already prequalified and assess only those areas which relate to use of the product in the country concerned and where failure to comply with regulatory standards could pose health risks (e.g. stability data). In the other areas, the outcomes of reference authorities may be adopted.

To enhance timely access to prequalified products in countries, to ensure that the product in countries is the same as the one which is prequalified and to provide a model for regulatory information exchange among countries, this Procedure has been developed based on the above-mentioned considerations. In line with the *Procedure for prequalification of pharmaceutical products* (*1*) and the *Procedure for assessing the acceptability in principle of vaccines for purchase by United Nations agencies* (*2*) it aims to provide a convenient tool for NRAs wishing to enhance their premarketing evaluation and registration system by taking advantage of the scientific assessment work conducted by WHO/PQT. For pharmaceutical products the present procedure is complementary to the WHO/PQT collaborative procedure with NRAs in inspection activities (http://www.who.int/prequal, "Inspections").

The collaborative procedure was first piloted in June 2012 and is currently in use for pharmaceutical products (http://www.who.int/prequal, "Collaborative Registration"). For vaccines another procedure for expedited review of imported prequalified vaccines for use in national immunization programmes was published in 2007 and has been implemented for national registrations since 2010. However, this procedure did not include collaborative arrangements with the NRAs. In 2010 WHO/PQT piloted an expedited registration procedure that involved sharing of the WHO/PQT assessment reports with the NRAs.

Enhanced collaboration and information exchange between NRAs and WHO/PQT benefits all partners. Subject to the agreement of the WHO prequalification (PQ) holders concerned, NRAs have access to assessment outcomes that are not in the public domain and that have been prepared in conformity with the WHO recommended standards on which the *Procedure for prequalification of pharmaceutical products* (*1*) and the *Procedure for assessing the acceptability in principle of vaccines for purchase by United Nations agencies* (*2*) are based. Such reports and relevant WHO documents help NRAs to make their decisions and also assist in training national regulatory staff. At the same time, feedback from NRAs on the information and documentation received from WHO/PQT under the Procedure allows WHO/PQT to improve its work and ensures that the outcomes of its assessments are relevant to NRAs. As a consequence patients and vaccinees benefit from this collaboration by gaining faster access to pharmaceutical products and vaccines that have been found acceptable in principle for procurement by United Nations (UN) agencies. The collaborative registration procedure can be of particular relevance when implemented for pharmaceutical products and vaccines in emergency situations.

Depending on available resources, participating authorities have the opportunity to participate in the assessment process and in inspections organized by WHO/PQT.

This collaborative procedure also benefits manufacturers of prequalified pharmaceutical products and vaccines through faster and better harmonized regulatory approvals in participating countries. This Procedure, when combined with the WHO/PQT collaborative procedure with NRAs in inspection activities, alleviates the burden of additional national inspections on manufacturers.

3. Principles of collaboration

3.1 This collaborative procedure is applicable to:

- pharmaceutical products that have been assessed and inspected by WHO/PQT in line with the procedures and standards available at www.who.int/prequal ("Information for applicants") and have been found to be acceptable in principle for procurement by UN agencies as listed in the *List of WHO prequalified medicines*, available at www.who.int/prequal. The Procedure is not applicable to pharmaceutical products that have been listed as prequalified on the basis of approval by stringent regulatory authorities (SRAs).[2] For such products the principal part of the assessment has been performed by SRAs and WHO/PQT is not in possession of assessment and inspection reports that can be shared;
- vaccines that have been assessed and inspected by WHO/PQT in line with the procedures and standards available at http://www.who.int/immunization_standards/vaccine_quality/pq_system/en/ and have been found to be acceptable in principle for procurement by UN agencies as listed in the *List of WHO prequalified vaccines*, available at http://www.who.int/immunization_standards/vaccine_quality/PQ_vaccine_list_en/en/. This Procedure is applicable to

[2] Products listed as prequalified according to the procedure described in the Guidelines on submission of documentation for prequalification of finished pharmaceutical products approved by stringent regulatory authorities. In: WHO Expert Committee on Specifications for Pharmaceutical Preparations: forty-eighth report. Geneva: World Health Organization; 2014: Annex 5 (WHO Technical Report Series, No. 986).

vaccines that successfully passed either the standard or streamlined prequalification process: http://www.who.int/immunization_standards/vaccine_quality/pq_revision2010/en/).

Although the Procedure mostly serves to accelerate the assessment and registration of prequalified multisource (generic) pharmaceutical products it is applicable to vaccines and any pharmaceutical product for which the safety and efficacy has been documented to WHO/PQT by the submission of preclinical and clinical data.

The Procedure has three major stakeholders: WHO/PQT, interested NRAs and those WHO PQ holders or applicants[3] who agree that this Procedure is used for applications for national registration of their WHO-prequalified product submitted to an NRA.

3.2 WHO/PQT and participating authorities receive applications for the same pharmaceutical product or vaccine. Within the context of this Procedure, the same pharmaceutical product or same vaccine is characterized by:

- the same product dossier;[4]
- the same manufacturing chain, processes, control of materials and finished product, and in the case of vaccines also by the same batch release scheme;
- the same active ingredient and finished product specifications;
- the same essential elements of product information for pharmaceutical products,[5] in the case of vaccines by the same product information, packaging presentation and labelling.

[3] If the applicant for national registration is not the same as the WHO PQ holder, the WHO PQ holder must confirm to the NRA and WHO/PQT by an authorization letter (as per the template annexed to Appendix 3, Part A) that the applicant is acting for, or pursuant to rights derived from, the WHO PQ holder and that the WHO PQ holder agrees with the application of the procedure in the country concerned.

[4] Submission of dossiers in common technical document (CTD) format as required by WHO/PQT is considered a standard. In exceptional situations data can be organized differently in line with specific national or WHO requirements; however, the technical data included in the dossier must be the same. There may be country-specific differences in administrative data, or if required by NRAs under exceptional circumstances, additional technical data can be provided (e.g. bioequivalence with a country-specific comparator).

[5] The essential elements of product information include in particular the indications, contraindications, posology (dosing), special warnings and precautions for use, adverse reactions, storage conditions, primary packaging and shelf life. Differences in brand name, the name of applicant or WHO PQ holder, language, format and degree of detail of the product information, labelling of internal and external packaging, among others, are not considered essential for the purposes of this Procedure. The language of the product information may be different as long as the information content is the same as that approved by WHO/PQT.

3.3 WHO/PQT, with the agreement of the WHO PQ holder, shares the full outcome of prequalification assessments, inspections and, if relevant, also results of laboratory testing, including final assessment and inspection reports, with participating authorities, under appropriate obligations of confidentiality and restrictions on use (see below).

As regards sharing the outcomes of assessments, inspections and results of laboratory testing, only data owned by the WHO PQ holder and WHO are shared. Sharing of any other data (e.g. related to a closed part of the Active pharmaceutical ingredient master file) is subject to additional agreement of the data owners concerned.

3.4 For the purpose of this collaborative procedure, participating authorities accept the product documentation and reports in the format in which they are routinely prepared by WHO in accordance with the *Procedure for prequalification of pharmaceutical products* (*1*) and the *Procedure for assessing the acceptability in principle of vaccines for purchase by United Nations agencies* (*2*). It should be noted, however, that participating authorities may require applicants to comply with specific requirements for local regulatory review. Each participating authority should make such specific requirements public.

3.5 Fees to be paid by the applicants to participating authorities continue to follow standard national procedures. Similarly, the submission by manufacturers of samples for laboratory testing – if required – continues to follow standard procedures as defined in national legislation and/or as defined by NRAs. Participating authorities are advised to refrain from preregistration laboratory testing. Results from the laboratory testing organized in the course of prequalification assessment or inspections will be included in the information package available to each participating authority.

3.6 Consistent with the terms of Appendix 1, Part A and Appendix 3, Part B, each participating authority commits itself:

- to treat any information and documentation provided to it by WHO/PQT pursuant to this Procedure as confidential in accordance with the terms of Appendix 1, Part A, and to allow access to such information and documentation only to persons[6]

6 This includes the focal point(s) and all other persons in the NRA who have access to any information and documentation provided by WHO/PQT.

- who have a need to know for the purpose of the assessment and accelerated registration of the product in question in the country and any post-registration processes that may be required,
- who are bound by confidentiality undertakings in respect of such information and documentation which are no less stringent than those reproduced in Appendix 1, Part A;

- to issue its national regulatory decision on registration of a given prequalified product (whether positive or negative) within 90 calendar days[7] of regulatory time.[8] If the applicant takes a long time to complete missing parts of the documentation without any justification, to provide additional data or to respond to other queries raised by NRAs, or if the applicant fails to provide the NRA with necessary information and cooperation, the NRA is entitled to terminate the Procedure and switch to the normal registration process. Such termination is communicated to the applicant and to WHO/PQT using Appendix 3, Part C.

These commitments are provided by each participating authority to WHO/PQT in writing by entering into the agreement for participation in this Procedure as reproduced in Appendix 1, Part A and are reconfirmed for each pharmaceutical product or vaccine for which collaboration is sought (see Appendix 3, Part B).

Each participating NRA nominates a maximum of three focal points and specifies their areas of responsibility (inspections, assessment of pharmaceutical products, assessment of vaccines). These focal points will access the restricted-access website through which WHO/PQT will communicate all confidential information and documentation. Upon

[7] Participating authorities should issue their national regulatory decisions at the earliest opportunity after being given access to the confidential information and documentation on a given prequalified product. Although a time limit of 90 days of regulatory time is defined in the Procedure, the decision should normally be taken within 60 days. This deadline can be extended to a maximum of 90 days if predefined dates of technical or decision-making meetings do not allow a participating authority to issue its decision within 60 days. If a participating authority does not issue its decision within 90 days of regulatory time and does not communicate valid reasons for the delay to WHO/PQT, WHO/PQT can follow up with the head of the NRA to clarify the situation. The timeline should be reduced as much as possible to facilitate access to products needed in case of emergency situations.

[8] Regulatory time starts after a valid application for the registration according to the Procedure has been received and access to the confidential information has been granted (whichever is the later) and continues until the date of decision on registration. The regulatory time does not include the time granted to the applicant to complete missing parts of the documentation, provide additional data or respond to queries raised by NRAs.

justified request of an NRA to WHO/PQT, the number of focal points can be increased.

Focal points designated by the NRA must sign the undertaking reproduced in Appendix 1, Part B before they will be granted access to the restricted-access website. Any change in designated focal points must be communicated to WHO/PQT in writing without delay and must be accompanied by an undertaking (Appendix 1, Part B) signed by the new focal point(s).

3.7 The decision whether or not to register a given product in a particular country remains the prerogative and responsibility of each participating authority. Accordingly a participating authority may come to a different conclusion from that reached by WHO/PQT or can decide to discontinue the Procedure for a specific product. Within 30 calendar days of having taken its decision, the participating authority reports this decision to WHO/PQT, together with the dates of submission and registration and, if applicable, any deviations from the WHO/PQT's decision on prequalification and the reasons for such deviations[9] and/or any decision to discontinue the Procedure for a specific product. It does so through the restricted-access website by completing the form in Part C of Appendix 3 or providing the same information in another format. The NRA provides a copy of the completed form or the information to the applicant.

3.8 Participation by WHO PQ holders/applicants is voluntary, through the submission to a participating NRA of the expression of interest reproduced in Part A of Appendix 3. For each product such participation will be subject to the WHO PQ holder/applicant accepting the terms of this Procedure, including the confidential exchange of information and documentation between WHO/PQT and the NRA (see Appendix 2).

The WHO PQ holder/applicant can cease participation in this Procedure at any time provided that he or she informs WHO/PQT and the participating NRAs in writing of his or her decision. In such a case the NRA shall cease all use of the information disclosed to it for the respective product(s) as per the terms of the participation agreement (see Appendix 1).

[9] This refers to a decision not to approve the registration of a WHO-prequalified product and to a decision to approve the registration, but with deviations in indications, contraindications, posology (dosing), special warnings and precautions for use, adverse drug reactions, storage conditions and shelf life. For pharmaceutical products differences in brand name, name of applicant or WHO PQ holder, format of product information, level of detail of product information, labelling of internal and external packaging and language of product information are not considered to be deviations from the PQ conclusions.

3.9 The requirements and procedures in case of a variation (as defined in WHO guidelines (*3*)) may differ between NRAs and WHO/PQT. The present collaborative procedure includes a variation procedure (see section 5) which is aimed at promoting consistency between variations accepted by WHO/PQT and variations accepted by participating authorities. There could be situations in which a manufacturer of a WHO-prequalified product submits a variation application to a participating authority and not to WHO/PQT or vice versa. In such a case the conditions of the national registration, which were initially "harmonized" with the WHO PQ decision, may become essentially different through the product life cycle. In such a case a product registered and procured in a participating country would no longer be the same as the WHO-prequalified product because the specifications, manufacturing sites and/or other essential parameters would no longer be the ones accepted by WHO/PQT. The WHO PQ holders/applicants and NRAs are expected to inform WHO/PQT of the differences and the reasons for them, if, due to inconsistencies in variations, the nationally-registered product is no longer the same as the WHO-prequalified product.

As a result, applicants are required to submit to participating authorities without delay, at the latest 30 calendar days after acceptance of the variation by WHO/PQT, those variations which are subject to national regulatory requirements. WHO/PQT will inform the NRAs that have registered individual prequalified products, through the restricted-access website, about variations to the prequalification status of such products if and when regulatory action is deemed to be justified. Participating authorities are encouraged to follow the outcomes of the WHO variation procedures for nationally-approved WHO-prequalified products.

If a national variation procedure results in the nationally-registered product being no longer the same (see section 3.2) as the WHO-prequalified product, or in the event that a variation of a WHO-prequalified product is not followed by the same variation of the nationally registered product (in the case that the particular variation is subject to national regulatory requirements), the participating authority informs WHO/PQT of the situation by submitting the form in Appendix 4, clearly specifying the deviations. The deadline for informing WHO/PQT is 30 days after the NRA has been informed by WHO/PQT about variation outcome. The variation approved by WHO/PQT will be considered by WHO/PQT as accepted by the NRA on a non-objection basis 30 days after information-sharing, unless and until the NRA informs WHO/PQT otherwise. Other participating NRAs, which have registered the WHO-prequalified product in question pursuant to this Procedure, will be made aware of such deviations through the restricted-access website. In addition, if the fact that a WHO-prequalified product has been registered in a particular country pursuant to this Procedure has been made public, any subsequent deviations should also be made public.

3.10 If a prequalified product is withdrawn by the WHO PQ holder, or is suspended or delisted by WHO/PQT, WHO/PQT will inform each participating authority that has approved, or is in the process of reviewing the product pursuant to this Procedure, of the withdrawal, suspension or delisting and the reasons for taking this action, through the restricted-access website and subject to the obligations of confidentiality contained in Appendix 1, Part A. Similarly, when an NRA deregisters or suspends the registration of a prequalified pharmaceutical product or vaccine for any reason, it will inform WHO/PQT of this decision and of its reasons through the restricted-access website. Other participating NRAs which have registered the WHO-prequalified product in question pursuant to this Procedure will be made aware of such national deregistration or suspension through the restricted-access website. In addition, if the fact that a WHO-prequalified product has been registered in a country pursuant to this Procedure has been made public, any subsequent deregistration or suspension should also be made public by posting on the WHO/PQT website.

3.11 Participation in this Procedure does not exempt applicants for national registration and holders of national registration from the respective national regulatory requirements. Participating authorities retain the right to assess submitted data and organize site inspections to the extent they deem appropriate. WHO encourages NRAs not to perform repetitive assessment of thoroughly assessed data, but rather to focus on data verification so that they can be assured that the same product is submitted for registration as is prequalified. It is highly recommended not to reinspect the sites that have already been inspected by WHO/PQT inspection teams or by NRAs recognized by WHO as stringent and as functional with respect to inspections of vaccine manufacturing sites.

3.12 Sharing of information related to the Procedure between WHO/PQT, WHO PQ holders/applicants and NRAs is governed by Appendices 1, 2, 3 and 4. Completed Appendices 1 and 2 must be submitted to WHO/PQT without any change in their content. Provision of Appendices 3 and 4 can be substituted by provision of the same information by other means.

4. Steps in the collaboration for national registration of a pharmaceutical product or a vaccine

4.1 The applicant submits the product dossier for a WHO-prequalified pharmaceutical product or a vaccine to a participating NRA. The technical part of the dossier is updated to reflect the data as approved by WHO/PQT during the initial prequalification procedure, and consecutive variation procedures and requalification (where applicable). The applicant must provide the participating authority with:

- an application dossier complying with established national requirements, including the same technical information as that approved by WHO/PQT. To the extent that national regulatory requirements allow, the technical part of the dossier will be identical to the current version of the WHO/PQT dossier.[10] In specific cases the NRA may prefer a dossier which is abbreviated in line with national requirements;
- an expression of interest reproduced in Part A of Appendix 3;
- data and samples according to country-specific requirements;
- any fees that may be payable to the NRA pursuant to national requirements.

Wherever possible, to minimize the workload of the NRA and facilitate the process, applicants should ensure that they express their interest in using the Procedure (Appendix 3, Part A) to the NRA and to WHO/PQT before submitting a national application for registration. If acceptable to NRAs, not only should the technical content of the dossiers be the same, but also the format in which data are presented should closely follow the format in which dossiers are submitted to WHO/PQT, i.e. the common technical document (CTD) format. In the case of vaccines the product summary file format may be also applicable.

In situations where the applicant wishes to apply the Procedure to an application which is already pending within the NRA, the applicant should first update the dossier to ensure that the technical part of the information is the same as that approved by WHO/PQT.

[10] In the case of vaccines that are prequalified by the "Streamlined procedure for vaccines with marketing authorization/licensing granted by eligible NRAs" (as defined in the *Procedure for assessing the acceptability, in principle, of vaccines, for purchase by United Nations agencies*. In: WHO Expert Committee on Biological Standardization: sixty-first report. Geneva: World Health Organization; 2013: Annex 6 (WHO Technical Report Series, No. 978)) the submitted data should reflect essential data submitted to the NRA that granted the authorization/licence and additional documents as provided to WHO.

4.2 For each application under this Procedure, WHO/PQT is informed by the WHO PQ holder/applicant about the submission to the participating NRA by providing a completed copy of Appendix 3, Part A. The WHO PQ holder provides WHO at this time with its written consent for WHO/PQT to provide the product-related information in compliance with the applicable confidentiality requirements to the NRA of the country concerned (see Appendix 2).

4.3 The participating NRA informs WHO/PQT and the respective applicant of each application which it accepts or declines to include in this Procedure (Appendix 3, Part B). It is for the individual NRAs to decide whether to apply the Procedure for individual submissions. The Procedure applies only to applications that the NRA has accepted as complete.

4.4 Within 30 calendar days of receipt of the WHO PQ holder's consent, WHO/PQT shares the most recent product-related information and assessment, inspection and laboratory-testing outcomes through the restricted-access website with the participating authority. This information is subject to the obligations of confidentiality and restrictions on use and may include assessment report(s), variation assessment report(s) if applicable, inspection report(s) of the most recent inspection(s), the letter of prequalification or requalification and results of laboratory testing, if applicable. At the request of the participating authority, WHO/PQT provides explanations and/or more detailed information. If NRAs have significant concerns or questions which would preclude the registration of the prequalified pharmaceutical product or vaccine in their country, questions may be sent to WHO/PQT, preferably within 60 calendar days from the first day of the regulatory time. WHO/PQT will facilitate the problem resolution in cooperation with relevant parties.

4.5 After receiving the information and documentation from WHO/PQT, the participating authority undertakes an accelerated assessment of the product in question. For each application, the participating authority is required to issue the relevant national decision within 90 calendar days of regulatory time.[11] Within 30 days of having taken its decision the participating authority reports this decision, together with an indication of the dates of submission, registration and, if applicable, the length of the non-regulatory time. The participating authority also reports any deviations from the WHO PQ conclusion and the reasons for such deviations, or, if a decision

[11] See footnote 7.

has been made to discontinue the Procedure for a product, the reasons for such discontinuation, to WHO/PQT through the restricted-access website. This report is provided to WHO/PQT using Part C of Appendix 3 and is copied to the applicant. WHO/PQT lists pharmaceutical products and vaccines registered according to this Procedure by participating NRAs on its public website. The steps in the collaboration for national registration of a pharmaceutical product or vaccine are summarized in Figure A8.1.

Figure A8.1
Flowchart showing the principal steps of the collaborative procedure

The NRA confirms to WHO/PQT its interest in participating in the Procedure and nominates focal point(s) for access to the restricted-access website. The NRA completes signs and submits to WHO/PQT the agreement reproduced in Appendix 1, Part A. The focal point(s) who are nominated to access the restricted-access website complete and submit the undertaking reproduced in Appendix 1, Part B, to WHO/PQT.

Appendix 1, Part A and Appendix 1, Part B

↓

WHO/PQT lists the participating NRAs on its public website.

Registration process

The applicant submits the application for national registration of the WHO-prequalified pharmaceutical product or vaccine to the participating authority and informs the authority of its interest in following the Procedure by completing the expression of interest reproduced in Appendix 3, Part A. If the applicant for national registration is not the same as the WHO PQ holder, the WHO PQ holder confirms to the NRA and WHO/PQT by an authorization letter (as per the form annexed to Appendix 3, Part A) that the applicant is acting for, or pursuant to rights derived from, the WHO PQ holder and that the PQ holder agrees with the application of the Procedure in the country concerned.

Appendix 3, Part A

↓

Figure A8.1 *continued*

The WHO PQ holder/applicant informs WHO/PQT about the submission of its application to the NRA(s) (by providing a copy of completed Appendix 3, Part A) and, for each product and country, provides WHO/PQT with its written consent to share the product-related information and documentation, under confidential cover, with the participating authority. The WHO PQ holder completes and signs the consent form reproduced in Appendix 2 and submits it to WHO/PQT.

Appendix 2

↓

The participating authority informs WHO/PQT and the applicant of its consent to apply the Procedure to the application for registration of the product, on the understanding that the application is accepted as complete, or of its refusal by completing and signing Part B of Appendix 3.

Appendix 3, Part B

↓

Within 30 calendar days of receipt of the WHO PQ holder's consent, WHO/PQT provides the participating authority with product-related information and documentation, and provides additional explanations, if requested, through the restricted-access website, and subject to the obligations of confidentiality and restrictions on use in place between WHO/PQT and the NRA.

↓

The participating authority uses the product-related information and documentation provided by WHO/PQT and by the applicant, at its discretion, to come to its conclusion about national registration and makes its decision on the registration within 90 calendar days of regulatory time.[12]

↓

Within 30 calendar days of having taken its decision, the participating authority informs WHO/PQT and the applicant of this decision, together with an indication of the dates of submission and registration and, if applicable, any deviations from the WHO PQ conclusions and the reasons for such deviations, through the restricted-access website. This report is provided to WHO/PQT by completing Part C of Appendix 3.

Appendix 3, Part C

↓

[12] See footnote7.

Figure A8.1 *continued*

WHO/PQT lists pharmaceutical products registered by participating NRAs according to this Procedure on its public website

Post-registration processes

The WHO PQ holder/applicant submits to participating authorities at the latest 30 calendar days after acceptance of the variation by WHO/PQT those variations which are subject to national regulatory requirements. If regulatory action is deemed to be justified, WHO/PQT promptly provides the participating authorities concerned, through the restricted-access website, and subject to the above-mentioned obligations of confidentiality and restrictions on use, with outcomes of its variation assessment and relevant post-prequalification inspection, and any related information it considers relevant. If a national variation procedure results in the nationally-registered product being no longer the same (see section 3.2) as the WHO-prequalified product, or in the event that a variation of a WHO-prequalified product is not followed by the same variation of the nationally-registered product, the participating authority informs WHO of the situation within 30 calendar days of obtaining access to the information and documentation provided by WHO/PQT, by submitting the form reproduced in Appendix 4, clearly specifying the deviations. Other participating NRAs that have registered the WHO-prequalified product in question pursuant to this Procedure will be made aware of such deviations through the restricted-access website.

Appendix 4

↓

WHO/PQT informs the participating authority, through the restricted-access website, and subject to the above-mentioned obligations of confidentiality and restrictions on use, about withdrawals, suspensions or delistings of prequalified pharmaceutical products or vaccines. The participating authority informs WHO/PQT, through the restricted-access website, of national de-registration or suspension (for any reason) of a prequalified pharmaceutical product or vaccine and the reasons for doing so. Other participating NRAs which have registered the WHO-prequalified product in question pursuant to this Procedure will be made aware of such national de-registration or suspension, through the restricted-access website.

Appendix 4

↓

Figure A8.1 *continued*

WHO/PQT removes a product from the list published in line with this procedure: • if the nationally-registered product is no longer the same (see section 3.2) as the WHO-prequalified product, or • if the NRA deregisters a WHO-prequalified product, or • if WHO/PQT delists a WHO-prequalified product. WHO/PQT will also publish the reasons for the removal from the list.

5. Collaboration mechanisms for post-prequalification and/or post-registration variations

5.1 Those post-prequalification variations submitted to WHO/PQT, which are subject to national regulatory requirements, are expected to be submitted to any relevant participating authorities without delay at the latest 30 calendar days after acceptance of the variation by WHO/PQT. Submission of variations to NRAs should respect national regulatory requirements. Applicants for national variations should inform participating authorities that the same application for a variation is being processed by WHO/PQT.

5.2 WHO/PQT promptly shares the outcomes of variation assessment and of related post-prequalification inspection (if applicable), through the restricted-access website, and subject to the above-mentioned obligations of confidentiality and restrictions on use, with the relevant participating authorities, in all cases in which a variation (including "notification" according to WHO/PQT's variation procedures (*3*)) requires regulatory action (e.g. where product quality, safety, efficacy or patient information materials are concerned).

Within 30 days of obtaining access to the information and documentation from WHO/PQT, each participating authority informs WHO/PQT through the restricted-access website if and to what extent a variation of a WHO-prequalified product is not followed by the same accepted variation of the nationally-registered product and, as a consequence, the nationally-registered product is no longer the same (see section 3.2) as the WHO-prequalified product. The variation approved by WHO/PQT will be considered by WHO/PQT as accepted by the NRA on a non-objection basis 30 days after information-sharing, unless and until the NRA informs WHO/PQT otherwise.

5.3 If a national variation procedure occurs independently of a variation submitted to WHO/PQT and results in the nationally-registered product being no longer the same (see section 3.2) as the WHO-prequalified product, the participating authority informs WHO/PQT within 30 days about the subject and outcome of this national variation procedure.

5.4 Deviations under 5.2 and 5.3 above may include change of source of active ingredients or starting materials, manufacturing sites, manufacturing process, product specifications, testing methods, storage conditions, shelf life, packaging material, indications, contraindications, posology (dosing), special warnings and precautions for use, adverse reactions and other changes specified in WHO/PQT guidelines (*3*). Differences in brand name, name of applicant or WHO PQ holder, format of product information, level of detail of product information, labelling of internal and external packaging and language of product information are not considered to be deviations from the conclusions during the prequalification of pharmaceutical products. For vaccines, such changes must be reported to WHO/PQT, which provides its opinion on the extent to which the difference represents deviation from conclusions during prequalification.

5.5 If a national variation procedure results in the nationally-registered product being no longer the same (see section 3.2) as the WHO-prequalified product, or if a variation of the WHO-prequalified product is not followed by a variation of the nationally-registered product and, as a consequence, the nationally-registered product is no longer the same, the WHO PQ holder will inform WHO/PQT of the differences and their reasons.

5.6 WHO/PQT removes a product from the list published in line with this Procedure if the nationally-registered product is no longer the same (see section 3.2) as the WHO-prequalified product.

6. Withdrawals, suspensions or delistings of prequalified pharmaceutical products or vaccines and national deregistrations

6.1 If a WHO-prequalified product is withdrawn by the WHO PQ holder, or if a product is suspended or delisted by WHO/PQT, WHO/PQT will promptly, through the restricted-access website, and subject to the above-mentioned obligations of confidentiality and restrictions on use, inform relevant participating authorities accordingly, providing the reasons whenever needed.

6.2 In the case that a participating NRA deregisters or suspends the registration of a prequalified pharmaceutical product or vaccine for any reason, the participating authority informs WHO/PQT of the decision (together with an indication of the reasons), through the restricted-access website. The information should be provided promptly whenever there are concerns about product quality, safety or efficacy and in all other cases within 30 days. A participating authority is encouraged to consult WHO/PQT before adopting a decision about deregistration or suspension of registration of a WHO-prequalified product.

6.3 In the case that a WHO-prequalified product is deregistered at the national level, or in the case that WHO/PQT delists a prequalified product, WHO/PQT adjusts the information about this product on its website accordingly.

References

1. Procedure for prequalification of pharmaceutical products. In: WHO Expert Committee on Specifications for Pharmaceutical Preparations: forty-fifth report. Geneva: World Health Organization; 2011: Annex 10 (WHO Technical Report Series, No. 961).
2. Procedure for assessing the acceptability, in principle, of vaccines, for purchase by United Nations agencies. In: WHO Expert Committee on Biological Standardization: sixty-first report. Geneva: World Health Organization; 2013: Annex 6 (WHO Technical Report Series, No. 978).
3. *For pharmaceutical products*: WHO guidelines on variations to a prequalified product. In: WHO Expert Committee on Specifications for Pharmaceutical Preparations: forty-seventh report. Geneva: World Health Organization; 2013: Annex 3 (WHO Technical Report Series, No. 981), (and any updates thereto).
   For vaccines: http://www.who.int/immunization_standards/vaccine_quality/variations_pq_vaccine/en/ (and any updates thereto).

Appendix 1

National regulatory authority participation agreement and undertaking for national regulatory authority focal point(s)

Appendix 1, Part A

Agreement to participate in the collaborative procedure between the World Health Organization (WHO) Prequalification Team (WHO/PQT) and national regulatory authorities (NRAs) in the assessment and accelerated national registration of WHO-prequalified pharmaceutical products and vaccines

Details of NRA

Name of NRA: ____________________ ("the NRA")

Postal address: ____________________

____

Country: ____________________ ("the Country")

Telephone number (please include codes): ____________________

Email (please indicate contact details as appropriate for inclusion in the list of participating NRAs maintained on the WHO website): ____________________

Scope of agreement

Applicants for national registration of a particular WHO-prequalified pharmaceutical product or vaccine (hereafter referred to as "Applicants") may express their interest to the NRA in the assessment and accelerated registration of this product ("the Product") in the Country under the "Collaborative Procedure between WHO/PQT and NRAs in the assessment and accelerated national registration of WHO-prequalified pharmaceutical products or vaccines" (hereafter referred to as "the Procedure").[1]

Subject to the NRA agreeing to conduct such assessment and consider such accelerated registration of the Product under the Procedure (by submitting

[1] If the applicant for national registration is not the same as the WHO prequalification (PQ) holder, the WHO PQ holder must confirm to the NRA and to WHO/PQT by an authorization letter (as per the template annexed to Appendix 3, Part A) that the applicant is acting for, or pursuant to rights derived from, the WHO PQ holder, and that the WHO PQ holder agrees with the application of the Procedure in the country concerned.

the form reproduced in Part B of Appendix 3 attached to the Procedure to WHO/PQT through the restricted-acce ss website), the NRA hereby confirms for each such Product that it will adhere to, and collaborate with the WHO/PQT and the Applicant for registration of the Product in accordance with the terms of the Procedure.

Confidentiality of information

Any information and documentation relating to the Product and provided by WHO/PQT to the NRA under the Procedure may include but shall not necessarily be limited to:

- the full WHO/PQT assessment and inspection outcomes (reports) and if relevant, also results of laboratory testing;
- information and documentation on variations (as defined in WHO guidelines[2]), as well as information and documentation on any actions \taken by WHO/PQT or NRAs post-prequalification of the Product;
- all such data, reports, information and documentation being hereinafter referred to as "the Information".

As regards sharing the outcomes of assessments, inspections and laboratory testing, only data owned by the WHO PQ holder and WHO/PQT are shared. Sharing of any other data is subject to additional agreement of the data owners concerned.

WHO/PQT agrees to make such information available to the NRA through a restricted-access website exclusively for the purpose of the assessment and accelerated registration of the Product in the Country and any post-registration processes that may be required, in accordance with and subject to the terms of the Procedure ("the Purpose"). The NRA agrees to treat any Information provided by WHO/PQT as aforesaid as strictly confidential and proprietary to WHO/PQT, the WHO PQ holder/Applicant and/or parties collaborating with WHO/PQT and/or the WHO PQ holder/Applicant. In this regard, the NRA agrees to use such Information only for the Purpose and to make no other use thereof. Thus, the NRA undertakes to maintain the Information received from WHO/PQT in strict confidence, and to take all reasonable measures to ensure that:

[2] *For pharmaceutical products*: WHO guidelines on variations to a prequalified product. In: WHO Expert Committee on Specifications for Pharmaceutical Preparations: forty-seventh report. Geneva: World Health Organization; 2013: Annex 3 (WHO Technical Report Series, No. 981), (and any updates thereto).
For vaccines: http://www.who.int/immunization_standards/vaccine_quality/variations_pq_vaccine/en/ (and any updates thereto).

- the Information received from WHO/PQT shall not be used for any purpose other than the Purpose;
- the Information shall only be disclosed to persons who have a need to know for the aforesaid Purpose and are bound by confidentiality undertakings in respect of such information and documentation which are no less stringent than those contained herein.

The NRA warrants and represents that it has adequate procedures in place to ensure compliance with its aforesaid obligations.

The obligations of confidentiality and restrictions on use contained herein shall not cease on completion of the Purpose.

The obligations of confidentiality and restrictions on use contained herein shall not apply to any part of the Information which the NRA is clearly able to demonstrate:

- was in the public domain or the subject of public knowledge at the time of disclosure by WHO/PQT to the NRA under the Procedure; or
- becomes part of the public domain or the subject of public knowledge through no fault of the NRA; or
- is required to be disclosed by law, provided that the NRA shall in such event immediately notify WHO/PQT and the Applicant in writing of such obligation and shall provide adequate opportunity to WHO/PQT and/or the Applicant to object to such disclosure or request confidential treatment thereof (provided always, however, that nothing contained herein shall be construed as a waiver of the privileges and immunities enjoyed by WHO/PQT and/or as submitting WHO/PQT to any national court jurisdiction).

Upon completion of the Purpose, the NRA shall cease all use and make no further use of the Information disclosed to it under the Procedure, and shall promptly destroy all of the Information received from WHO/PQT which is in tangible or other form, except that the NRA may retain copies of the Information in accordance with its established archival procedures, subject always, however, to the above-mentioned obligations of confidentiality and restrictions on use. The Purpose for each product shall be deemed completed as soon as:

- the WHO PQ holder/Applicant discontinues participation in the Procedure for the particular product;

- the Product is deregistered by the NRA and/or delisted by WHO/PQT.

The access right of the NRA's focal point(s) to the restricted-access website will cease automatically upon the NRA ceasing to participate in the Procedure. If and as soon as an NRA focal point is replaced by a new focal point or ceases to be an employee of the NRA, such focal point's access to the restricted-access website shall automatically terminate.

The NRA agrees that it has no right in or to the Information and that nothing contained herein shall be construed, by implication or otherwise, as the grant of a licence to the NRA to use the Information other than for the Purpose.

Timelines

In respect of each Product that the NRA agrees to assess and consider for accelerated registration under the Procedure, the NRA undertakes to abide by the terms of the Procedure, including but not limited to the following timelines for processing each application:

- within 90 calendar days of regulatory time[3] after obtaining access (through the restricted access website) to:
  - the data submitted to WHO/PQT for prequalification of the Product and owned by the WHO PQ holder,
  - the full WHO/PQT assessment and inspection outcomes (reports),

  the NRA undertakes to take a decision on the national registration of the Product;

- within 30 working days of the NRA's decision on national registration of the Product, the NRA undertakes to inform WHO/PQT of this decision and of any deviations from WHO conclusions during prequalification (with an indication of the reasons for such deviations) by completing and submitting the form attached as Appendix 3, Part C to the Procedure to WHO/PQT through the restricted-access website;

[3] Regulatory time starts after a valid application for the registration according to the Procedure has been received and access to the confidential information has been granted (whichever is the later) and continues until the date of decision on registration. The regulatory time does not include the time granted to the applicant to complete missing parts of the documentation, provide additional data or respond to queries raised by NRAs.

- if a national variation procedure results in the nationally-registered product being no longer the same[4] as the WHO-prequalified product, or if and to the extent a variation of a WHO-prequalified product is not followed by a variation of the nationally-registered product and as a consequence, the nationally-registered product is no longer the same as the WHO-prequalified product, the NRA undertakes to inform WHO/PQT thereof (together with an indication of the reasons for such deviations) within 30 days of the conclusion of the national variation procedure or within 30 days of having received access to the information and documentation provided by WHO/PQT, as the case may be (i.e. by completing and submitting the form attached to the Procedure as Appendix 4 to WHO/PQT through the restricted-access website);[5]
- the NRA undertakes to inform WHO/PQT in the case that the NRA deregisters or suspends the registration of the Product in the Country, by completing and submitting the form attached to the Procedure as an Appendix 4, to WHO/PQT through the restricted-access website, and to do so promptly if this decision is based on quality, safety or efficacy concerns, and within 30 days if this decision is based on other reasons.

Focal points for access to restricted-access website

The NRA has designated the person(s) listed below to act as focal point(s) for access to WHO/PQT's restricted-access website. The undertaking(s) completed and signed by the focal point(s) is (are) attached hereto as an Appendix to this agreement.

Any change in designated focal points must be communicated to WHO/PQT without delay in writing and will be subject to the new focal point having signed and submitted to WHO/PQT the undertaking reproduced in Appendix 1, Part B to the Procedure. The NRA also undertakes to inform WHO/PQT if and as soon as a designated focal point ceases to be an employee of the NRA.

[4] Within the context of this Procedure, the same pharmaceutical product/same vaccine is characterized by the same product dossier; the same manufacturing chain, processes and control of materials and finished product, in the case of vaccines also by the same batch release scheme; the same active ingredient and finished product specifications; and the same essential elements of product information for pharmaceutical products, in the case of vaccines by the same product information, packaging presentation and labelling.

[5] If the fact that a WHO-prequalified product has been registered in a country pursuant to this Procedure has been made public, any subsequent deviations should also be made public.

Focal point for inspections

If applicable, this should be the same focal point as for the "WHO/PQT Collaborative Procedure with NRAs in inspection activities" (http://who.int/prequal, "Inspections"). The same person should be designated for inspections of pharmaceutical products and vaccines.

1.

Mr/Ms/Dr

First name (and initials): ______________________

Surname/family name: ______________________

Title in NRA: ______________________

Email: ______________________

Telephone: ______________________

☐ A signed Undertaking is attached.

Focal point(s) for dossier assessment

For dossier assessment, different persons can be nominated for pharmaceutical products and vaccines. The same person may be nominated to be the focal point for inspections and dossier assessment. If additional person(s) are nominated for dossier assessment, please complete the details below.

2.

Mr/Ms/Dr as a focal point for dossier assessment of

pharmaceutical products only ☐

pharmaceutical products and vaccines ☐

First name (and initials): ______________________

Surname/family name: ______________________

Title in NRA: ______________________

Email: ______________________

Telephone: ______________________

☐ A signed Undertaking is attached

3.

Mr/Ms/Dr as a focal point for dossier assessment of vaccines

First name (and initials): ______________________

Surname/family name: ______________________

Title in NRA: ______________________

Email: ______________________________

Telephone: ______________________________

☐ A signed Undertaking is attached

Miscellaneous

The NRA agrees that WHO/PQT may list its name on the WHO/PQT website as a participant in the Procedure. Except as provided hereinbefore, neither party shall, without the prior written consent of the other party, refer to the relationship of the parties under this Agreement and/or to the relationship of the other party to the Product, the Information and/or the Purpose, in any statement or material of an advertising or promotional nature.

This Agreement shall not be modified except by mutual agreement of WHO and the NRA in writing. The NRA furthermore undertakes to promptly inform WHO/PQT of any circumstances or change in circumstances that may affect the implementation of this Agreement.

The parties shall use their best efforts to settle amicably any dispute relating to the interpretation or execution of this Agreement. In the event of failure of the latter, the dispute shall be settled by arbitration. The arbitration shall be conducted in accordance with the modalities to be agreed upon by the parties or in the absence of agreement, with the UNCITRAL Arbitration Rules in effect on the date of this Agreement. The parties shall accept the arbitral award as final.

It is agreed furthermore that nothing contained in this Agreement shall be construed as a waiver of any of the privileges and immunities enjoyed by WHO under national and international law, and/or as submitting WHO to any national court jurisdiction.

Agreed and accepted for pharmaceutical products and vaccines.

For the NRA

Signature: ______________________________

Name: ______________________________

Title: ______________________________

Place and date: ______________________________

Attachments:

Signed Undertaking(s) of NRA focal point(s) (Appendix 1, Part B)

Appendix 1, Part B

Undertaking for NRA focal point(s)

The undersigned:

Mr/Ms/Dr

First name (and initials): ________________________________

Surname/family name: ________________________________

Title in NRA: ________________________________

Name of NRA: ________________________________ ("the NRA")

Country: ________________________________ ("the Country")

Email: ________________________________

Telephone: ________________________________

Applicants for national registration of WHO-prequalified pharmaceutical products or vaccines (hereafter referred to as "Applicants") may express their interest to the national regulatory authority (NRA) in the assessment and accelerated national registration of such products under the "Collaborative Procedure between the World Health Organization (WHO) Prequalification Team (WHO/PQT) and national regulatory authorities in the assessment and accelerated national registration of WHO-prequalified pharmaceutical products and vaccines" (hereafter referred to as "the Procedure").[6]

Subject to the NRA agreeing to conduct such assessment and consider such accelerated registration of a WHO-prequalified product under the Procedure, WHO/PQT will communicate confidential Information (as hereinafter defined) relating to each such product to the NRA, and the NRA will communicate outcomes of the national registration procedure and post-registration actions in respect of such products to WHO/PQT, through a restricted-access website, which can be accessed only by the focal points designated by the NRA, including the undersigned. For the purpose of accessing the restricted-access website and downloading Information and uploading reports in accordance with and subject to the terms of the Procedure, WHO/PQT will provide the undersigned with a secret access code. The undersigned undertakes to treat this access code as strictly confidential and not to disclose it to any other person whatsoever. The undersigned furthermore undertakes

[6] If the applicant for national registration is not the same as the WHO PQ holder, the WHO PQ holder must confirm to the NRA and to WHO/PQT by an authorization letter (as per the template annexed to Appendix 3, Part A) that the applicant is acting for, or pursuant to rights derived from, the WHO PQ holder, and that the PQ holder agrees with the application of the Procedure in the country concerned.

to take all precautionary measures that may be needed to prevent any other person whatsoever from obtaining the aforesaid secret access code and from accessing the restricted-access website (i.e. except for the other designated focal points who have signed this Undertaking).

"Information" as aforesaid means any information and documentation relating to a WHO-prequalified product to be provided by WHO/PQT to the NRA under the Procedure, including but not necessarily limited to:

- the full WHO/PQT assessment and inspection outcomes (reports) and if relevant, also results of laboratory testing;
- information and documentation on subsequent variations (as defined in WHO guidelines[7]), as well as information and documentation on any actions taken by WHO/PQT or NRAs post-prequalification of the Product.

As regards sharing the outcomes of assessments, inspections and results of laboratory testing, only data owned by the WHO PQ holder and WHO/PQT are shared. Sharing of any other data is subject to additional agreement of the data owners concerned.

The undersigned confirms that:

1. the NRA has bound him or her to obligations of confidentiality and restrictions on use no less stringent than those contained in Appendix 1, Part A to the Procedure; and that
2. the aforesaid obligations of confidentiality and restrictions on use shall not cease on completion of the assessment and accelerated registration of any product in the Country, nor on completion of any post-registration processes that may be required, nor on the undersigned ceasing to be an employee of (or ceasing to have another relationship with) the NRA.

The undersigned shall automatically cease having the right to access the restricted-access website when the NRA designates a new focal point to replace the undersigned or when the undersigned ceases to be an employee of the NRA.

This Undertaking shall not be modified except by mutual agreement of WHO and the undersigned in writing. The undersigned furthermore undertakes

[7] *For pharmaceutical products*: WHO guidelines on variations to a prequalified product. In: WHO Expert Committee on Specifications for Pharmaceutical Preparations: forty-seventh report. Geneva: World Health Organization; 2013: Annex 3 (WHO Technical Report Series, No. 981), (and any updates thereto). *For vaccines*: http://www.who.int/immunization_standards/vaccine_quality/variations_pq_vaccine/en/ (and any updates thereto).

to promptly inform WHO/PQT of any circumstances or change in circumstances that may affect the implementation of this Undertaking.

The parties shall use their best efforts to settle amicably any dispute relating to the interpretation or execution of this Undertaking. In the event of failure of the latter the dispute shall be settled by arbitration. The arbitration shall be conducted in accordance with the modalities to be agreed upon by the parties or in the absence of agreement, with the UNCITRAL Arbitration Rules in effect on the date of this Undertaking. The parties shall accept the arbitral award as final.

It is agreed furthermore that nothing contained in this Undertaking shall be construed as a waiver of any of the privileges and immunities enjoyed by WHO under national and international law, and/or as submitting WHO to any national court jurisdiction.

Agreed and accepted by the undersigned:

Signature: ______________________________

Name: ______________________________

Title in NRA: ______________________________

Place and date: ______________________________

Appendix 2

Consent of WHO prequalification holder for WHO to share information with the national regulatory authority confidentially under the Procedure

Reference is made to the attached expression of interest in the assessment and accelerated national registration under the Procedure of the following World Health Organization (WHO) prequalified pharmaceutical product or vaccine (hereafter referred to as "the Product") in ____________________ [country].[1]

☐ pharmaceutical product

☐ vaccine

WHO prequalification details:

WHO prequalification (PQ) reference number: ____________________

Date of prequalification (dd/mm/yyyy): ____________________

Date of requalification (if applicable): ____________________

WHO PQ holder:[2] ____________________

Application details:

Name of entity: ____________________ ("the Applicant")

Street: ____________________

City and country: ____________________

Email: ____________________

Telephone: ____________________

The WHO PQ holder hereby consents to the WHO Prequalification Team (WHO/PQT) providing the following information and documentation to the national regulatory authority (NRA) of ____________________ [country]

[1] Please complete a separate copy of this Annex for each country.

[2] If the applicant for national registration is not the same as the WHO PQ holder, the WHO PQ holder must confirm to the NRA and to WHO/PQT by an authorization letter (as per the template annexed to Appendix 3, Part A) that the applicant is acting for, or pursuant to rights derived from, the WHO PQ holder, and that the PQ holder agrees with the application of the Procedure in the country concerned.

("the NRA") for the assessment and accelerated registration of the Product in the country under the Procedure and to freely discuss the same with the aforesaid NRA for this purpose:

- the full WHO/PQT assessment and inspection outcomes (reports), results of laboratory testing and, if relevant, also assessment and inspections reports of other regulatory bodies, provided that these bodies gave their written consent to the use of such reports for the purpose of the Procedure;
- information and documentation on subsequent variations (as defined in WHO guidelines[3]), as well as information and documentation on any actions taken by WHO/PQT post-prequalification of the Product;
- all such data, reports, information and documentation being hereinafter referred to as "the Information".

As regards sharing the outcomes of assessments and inspections, only data owned by the WHO PQ holder and WHO/PQT are shared. Sharing of any other data is subject to additional agreement of the data owners concerned.[4]

Such consent is subject to the NRA having entered into an agreement with WHO/PQT as per Part A of Appendix 1 to the Procedure and having agreed to conduct the assessment and consider the accelerated registration of the Product under the Procedure, by having submitted the form reproduced in Part B of Appendix 3 to the Procedure to WHO/PQT.

The WHO PQ holder/Applicant commits to submit post-prequalification variations to WHO/PQT and any relevant participating authorities respecting national regulatory requirements. Variations should be submitted to participating authorities at the latest 30 calendar days after acceptance of the variation by WHO/PQT. Participating authorities should be informed about the fact that the same application for a variation is being processed by WHO/PQT. If a national variation procedure results in the nationally-registered product being no longer

---

[3] *For pharmaceutical products*: WHO guidelines on variations to a prequalified product. In: WHO Expert Committee on Specifications for Pharmaceutical Preparations: forty-seventh report. Geneva: World Health Organization; 2013: Annex 3 (WHO Technical Report Series, No. 981), (and any updates thereto).
For vaccines: http://www.who.int/immunization_standards/vaccine_quality/variations_pq_vaccine/en/ (and any updates thereto).

[4] In the case that certain data submitted to WHO/PQT by the WHO PQ holder in relation to PQ of the Product are not in his/her ownership, the WHO PQ holder specifies such data in an annex to this declaration of consent.

the same[5] as the WHO-prequalified product, or if a variation of the WHO-prequalified product is not followed by a variation of the nationally-registered product and, as a consequence, the nationally-registered product is no longer the same, the WHO PQ holder/Applicant will inform WHO/PQT of the differences and their reasons.

For the WHO PQ holder

Signature: ______________________________

Name: ______________________________

Title: ______________________________

Place: ______________________________

Date (dd/mm/yyyy): ______________________________

[5] Within the context of this Procedure, the same pharmaceutical product/same vaccine is characterized by the same product dossier; the same manufacturing chain, processes and control of materials and finished product, and in the case of vaccines also by the same batch release scheme; the same active ingredient and finished product specifications; as well as the same essential elements of product information for pharmaceutical products, and, in the case of vaccines, by the same product information, packaging presentation and labelling.

Appendix 3

Expression of interest to national regulatory authority (NRA) in the assessment and accelerated national registration, acceptance by NRA and notification of Procedure outcomes

Appendix 3, Part A

Expression of interest to the national regulatory authorities (NRAs) in the assessment and accelerated national registration of a World Health Organization (WHO)-prequalified pharmaceutical product or vaccine

In line with the Procedure, the undersigned Applicant[1] expresses its interest in the application of the above-mentioned Procedure by the NRA of ______________________________ [country] ("the NRA") in respect of the following submission for national registration:

☐ pharmaceutical product

☐ vaccine

Application details:

Name of entity: ______________________________ ("the Applicant")

Street: ______________________________

City and country: ______________________________

Email: ______________________________

Telephone: ______________________________

Date of application (dd/mm/yyyy): ______________________________

Product name in national system (if known): ______________________________

National reference number (if known): ______________________________

[1] If the applicant for national registration is not the same as the WHO prequalification (PQ) holder, the WHO PQ holder must confirm to the NRA and to WHO/Prequalification Team (PQT) by an authorization letter (as per the template annexed to Appendix 3, Part A) that the applicant is acting for, or pursuant to rights derived from, the WHO PQ holder, and that the PQ holder agrees with the application of the Procedure in the country concerned.

Product details for pharmaceutical products:

Active pharmaceutical ingredient(s) (API(s)) (international nonproprietary name (INN)): ______________________________

____

Dosage form and strength: ______________________________

Packaging: ______________________________

Manufacturing site(s), including block(s)/unit(s), if appropriate: ______________

____

Product details for vaccines:

Name of vaccine: ______________________________

Composition: ______________________________

____

Packaging: ______________________________

Manufacturing site(s), including block(s)/unit(s), if appropriate: ______________

____

WHO prequalification details:

WHO PQ reference number: ______________________________

Date of prequalification (dd/mm/yyyy): ______________________________

WHO PQ holder: ______________________________

The Applicant confirms that the information and documentation provided in support of the above-mentioned submission for national registration is true and correct, that the product submitted for national registration is the same[2] as the WHO-prequalified product and that the technical information in the registration dossier is the same[3] as that approved by WHO/PQT during the initial prequalification procedure, and consecutive variation procedures and

[2] Within the context of this Procedure, the same pharmaceutical product/same vaccine is characterized by the same product dossier; the same manufacturing chain, processes and control of materials and finished product, and in the case of vaccines also by the same batch release scheme; the same active ingredient and finished product specifications; as well as the same essential elements of product information for pharmaceutical products, and, in the case of vaccines, by the same product information, packaging presentation and labelling.

[3] Only the technical data included in the dossier must be the same. There may be country-specific differences in administrative data, or if required by NRAs under exceptional circumstances, additional technical data can be provided (e.g. bioequivalence with a country-specific comparator).

requalification (where applicable). Minor differences[4] from the information submitted to WHO/PQT are the following:

____

____

____

Subject to the NRA agreeing to conduct the assessment and consider the accelerated registration of the Product under the Procedure, the Applicant:

1. undertakes to adhere to, and collaborate with the NRA and WHO/PQT in accordance with the terms of the Procedure; and
2. will authorize WHO/PQT[5] to provide the NRA confidential access to the following information and documentation and to freely discuss the same with the aforesaid NRA for the above-mentioned Purpose:
   - the full WHO/PQT assessment and inspection outcomes (reports), results of laboratory testing and if relevant, also assessment and inspections reports of other regulatory bodies, provided that these bodies gave their written consent to the use of such reports for the purpose of the Procedure,
   - information and documentation on subsequent variations (as defined in WHO guidelines[6]), as well as information and documentation on any actions taken by WHO/PQT post-prequalification of the Product.

As regards sharing the outcomes of assessments and inspections, only data owned by the WHO PQ holder and WHO are shared. Sharing of any other data is subject to additional agreement of the data owners concerned.

---

4 As defined in section 3.2 of the Procedure, in the case of pharmaceutical products, examples of minor differences which are not considered essential may include differences in administrative information, brand name, name of applicant (provided that the applicant is acting for, and has the authority to represent the WHO PQ holder), format of product information, level of detail of product information, labelling of internal and external packaging and language of product information.

5 If the applicant for national registration is not the same as the WHO PQ holder, then the authorization to WHO/PQT must be provided by the WHO PQ holder or their legal representative.

6 *For pharmaceutical products*: WHO guidelines on variations to a prequalified product. In: WHO Expert Committee on Specifications for Pharmaceutical Preparations: forty-seventh report. Geneva: World Health Organization; 2013: Annex 3 (WHO Technical Report Series, No. 981), (and any updates thereto).
For vaccines: http://www.who.int/immunization_standards/vaccine_quality/variations_pq_vaccine/en/ (and any updates thereto).

3. authorizes the NRA to freely share and discuss all registration-related and Product-related information provided by the Applicant to the NRA, with WHO/PQT, subject to the obligations of confidentiality and restrictions on use as contained in the NRA's participation agreement and focal points' undertakings.

☐ The application for national registration was submitted before the Applicant decided to apply the Procedure to the Product and therefore at the time of submission the registration dossier did not respect conditions of the Procedure. Steps taken to update the submission to the NRA to make the dossier "the same" as required by the Procedure are listed and referenced in the attached letter.

☐ The Applicant is not the WHO PQ holder. An authorization letter from the WHO PQ holder is attached.

For the Applicant

Signature: ____________________

Name: ____________________

Title: ____________________

Place: ____________________

Date (dd/mm/yyyy): ____________________

Template for authorization letter

[To be provided if the applicant is not the WHO PQ holder. Please provide a separate letter for each NRA concerned, with a copy to WHO/PQT.]

This is to confirm that ____________ (*name of applicant*) seeking registration for prequalified product number ____________ (*WHO PQ number*) in ____________ (*name of country*) under the WHO collaborative procedure for accelerated registration of WHO-prequalified products, is acting for, or pursuant to rights derived from ____________ (*name of WHO PQ holder*) and that ____________ (*name of WHO PQ holder*) agrees with the application of the Procedure in the country concerned.

For ____________________ (*name of WHO PQ holder*):

Signature: ____________________

Name: ____________________

Title: ____________________

Date: ____________________

Appendix 3, Part B

Decision on acceptance by the NRA to apply the Procedure to a specified WHO-prequalified product and request for access to product-specific information and documentation

Please complete all fields marked *. For other fields, if there have been changes to the details as completed in Part A, please complete the relevant fields below. Where fields below are left blank, the data in Part A are considered to be valid.

Application details:

Name of entity: ______________________________ ("the Applicant")

Street: ______________________________

City and country: ______________________________

Email: ______________________________

Telephone: ______________________________

*Date of receipt of submission (dd/mm/yyyy): ______________________________

Product name in national system (if known): ______________________________

*National reference number: ______________________________

Product details for pharmaceutical products:

Active pharmaceutical ingredient(s) (API(s)) (international nonproprietary name (INN)): ______________________________

____

____

Dosage form and strength: ______________________________

Packaging: ______________________________

Manufacturing site(s), including block(s)/unit(s) if appropriate: ______________________________

____

Product details for vaccines:

Name of vaccine: ______________________________

Composition: ______________________________

____

Packaging: ______________________________

Manufacturing site(s), including block(s)/unit(s), if appropriate: ______________________________

____

WHO prequalification details:

*WHO PQ reference number: ______________________

Date of prequalification (dd/mm/yyyy): ______________________

WHO PQ holder: ______________________

Please complete either section A or section B below:

☐ **Section A**

The NRA agrees to conduct the assessment and the accelerated registration of the above-mentioned product ("the Product") under the Procedure and requests access to product-specific information, in accordance with and subject to the terms of the Procedure and the Agreement between WHO/PQT and the NRA dated ____ /____ /____ (dd/mm/yyyy).

☐ **Section B**

The NRA has decided not to apply the Procedure to the above-mentioned Product for the following reasons: ______________________

____

*For the NRA of ______________________ (indicate country)

Signature: ______________________

Name: ______________________

Title: ______________________

Place: ______________________

*Date (dd/mm/yyyy): ______________________

Appendix 3, Part C

Notification of outcomes of national registration procedure by the NRA

Product and application details as completed in Parts A and B above apply.

Please complete either section A or section B below:

☐ **Section A**

Registration has been granted under the terms of the Procedure, and the above-mentioned product ("the Product") is identified as follows in the national medicines register:

Name of the Product: ____________________

National registration number: ____________________

Date of registration (dd/mm/yyyy): ____________________

Non-regulatory time (days): ____________________

Product details (if different from those specified in Parts A and B):

Product details for pharmaceutical products:

API(s) (INN): ____________________

Dosage form and strength: ____________________

Packaging: ____________________

Manufacturing site(s), including block(s)/unit(s) if appropriate: ____________________

____

Product details for vaccines:

Name of vaccine: ____________________

Composition: ____________________

Packaging: ____________________

Manufacturing site(s), including block(s)/unit(s) if appropriate: ____________________

____

Registration holder (if different from the Applicant as specified in Parts A and B):

Name of entity: ____________________

Street: ____________________

City and country: ____________________

Email: ______________________________

Telephone: ______________________________

Are the national registration conclusions different from prequalification outcomes?[7] __________ (yes/no)

If you answered yes to the above question, please specify:

Deviation	Reason

Please specify whether registration is subject to specific commitments, the registration is provisional or conditional, use of the Product is limited by specific prescribing restrictions, or additional clinical trials or additional data are required:

____

☐ **Section B**

Please complete as appropriate:

☐ The application for registration of the Product was rejected for the following reasons: ______________________________

☐ The collaborative procedure was discontinued for this application for the following reasons: ______________________________

For the NRA

Signature: ______________________________

Name: ______________________________

Title: ______________________________

Place: ______________________________

Date (dd/mm/yyyy): ______________________________

[7] This refers to deviations in indications, contraindications, posology (dosing), special warnings and precautions for use, adverse drug reactions, storage conditions and shelf life. For pharmaceutical products differences in brand name, name of applicant/PQ holder, format of product information, level of detail of product information, labelling of internal and external packaging and language of product information are not considered to be a deviation from the PQ conclusions.

Appendix 4

Report on post-registration actions in respect of a product registered under the Procedure

☐ Variation of the national registration resulting in the national registration conditions being inconsistent with the WHO/PQT prequalification conclusions

☐ Deregistration or suspension of the registration of the product

Product details:

Product name in national system: ______________________ ("the Product")

National registration number: ______________________

Date of registration (dd/mm/yyyy): ______________________

WHO prequalification details:

WHO PQ reference number: ______________________

Date of prequalification (dd/mm/yyyy): ______________________

WHO PQ holder: ______________________

☐ The national variation procedure has resulted in the nationally-registered Product being no longer the same[1] as the WHO-prequalified product.

Deviation	Reason

[1] Within the context of this Procedure, the same pharmaceutical product/same vaccine is characterized by the same product dossier; the same manufacturing chain, processes and control of materials and finished product, and in the case of vaccines also by the same batch release scheme; the same active ingredient and finished product specifications; as well as the same essential elements of product information for pharmaceutical products, and, in the case of vaccines, by the same product information, packaging presentation and labelling.

☐ The variation notified to the NRA by WHO/PQT has not been followed by a variation of the nationally-registered Product and, as a consequence, the nationally-registered product is no longer the same[1] as the WHO-prequalified product.

Deviation	Reason

☐ The Product has been deregistered or the registration of the Product has been suspended.

Deregistration: ______________________________ (yes/no)

suspension of registration: ______________________ (yes/no)

Effective date: ____ /____ /____ (dd/mm/yyyy)

Reasons:

____

____

____

____

For the NRA

Signature: ____________________________________

Name: ____

Title: ____

Place: ____

Date (dd/mm/yyyy): ______________________________

Annex 9

Guidance for organizations performing in vivo bioequivalence studies

Background

During an informal consultation held in 2014, and at the forty-ninth meeting of the World Health Organization (WHO) Expert Committee on Specifications for Pharmaceutical Preparations, discussion took place regarding the possible revision of the guidance for organizations performing in vivo bioequivalence studies (WHO Technical Report Series, No. 937, Annex 9, 2006). The WHO Expert Committee on Specifications for Pharmaceutical Preparations agreed that in light of the new developments a draft for revision would be prepared.

These new guidelines take into consideration the revision of the multisource guidelines, as well as the creation of new guidance on good data management. The revision will also take into account the experience accumulated in the area of assessing and inspecting bioequivalence (BE) studies since 2006. In areas where the same problems are repeatedly identified by inspectors, the new guidelines provide clarifications, and supplementary details have been added on bioanalysis. The guidelines also put increased emphasis on subject safety and data integrity.

Based on the first working document:[1] this second version incorporates the numerous comments and the feedback received from the public consultation, the WHO Prequalification Team (PQT) and from the Consultation on data management, bioequivalence, GMP and medicines' inspection held in 2015.

WHO/PQT was set up in 2001 to assure that medicinal products supplied for procurement meet WHO norms and standards with respect to quality, safety and efficacy (http://www.who.int/prequal/). Specifically, there is a requirement that the submitted product dossier with all its necessary contents is assessed and found acceptable, and that the manufacturing sites for the finished pharmaceutical product (FPP), as well as the active pharmaceutical ingredient (API), are inspected and found to comply with WHO good manufacturing practices (GMP). Since products submitted to WHO/PQT are usually multisource (generic) products, therapeutic equivalence is generally demonstrated by performing a BE study, for example in a contract research organization (also known as a clinical research organization) (CRO). For prequalification of such

[1] http://www.who.int/medicines/areas/quality_safety/quality_assurance/BE-invivo-studies-guidance-QAS15-622_21052015.pdf?ua=1.

a product it is vital that, in addition to the above-mentioned requirements, the CRO used by the sponsor for BE studies complies with WHO good clinical practices (GCP) and considers relevant elements from WHO good laboratory practices (GLP) and good practices for quality control (QC) laboratories to ensure integrity and traceability of data. In addition, if local legal provisions exist, CROs should be licensed by the respective national medicines authority. Where required by national regulations, BE studies should be authorized by the national regulatory authority. Those involved in the conduct and analysis of BE studies on products to be submitted for prequalification therefore need to ensure that they comply with the relevant WHO norms and standards so that they can be prepared for any inspections by WHO.

Introduction

Multisource pharmaceutical products need to conform to the same standards of quality, efficacy and safety as the originator's (comparator) product. Specifically, the multisource product should be therapeutically equivalent and interchangeable with the comparator product. Testing the BE between a product and a suitable comparator (pharmaceutically equivalent or a pharmaceutical alternative) in a pharmacokinetic study with a limited number of subjects is one way of demonstrating therapeutic equivalence without having to perform a clinical trial involving many patients. In such a pharmacokinetic study any statement about the safety and efficacy of the test product will be a prediction based on measurement of systemic concentrations, assuming that essentially similar plasma concentrations of the active pharmaceutical ingredient (API) and/or of its metabolite will result in essentially similar concentrations at the site of action and therefore an essentially similar therapeutic outcome. The BE study thus provides indirect evidence of the efficacy and safety of a multisource pharmaceutical product. Often this will be the only evidence that the product is safe and efficacious. It is therefore crucial that the BE study is performed in an appropriate manner. Several guidance documents stress the importance of on-site inspections to verify compliance with standards of GCP (*1–3*).

1. Scope

The objective of this document is to provide guidance to organizations that are involved in the conduct and analysis of in vivo BE studies. This guidance supersedes the version published in the WHO Technical Report Series, No. 937, 2006 (*4*).

BE studies should be performed in compliance with the general regulatory requirements and good practices recommendations as specified in the WHO BE guidelines (*5*), GCP (*1*) and GLP (*2*) guidelines. It is acknowledged that GLP formally apply only to nonclinical safety studies. However the WHO BE guidelines require that the validation of bioanalytical methods and the analysis of BE study samples be performed following the principles of GLP. This does not imply that the laboratory in charge of the bioanalytical part of the study should be monitored as part of a national GLP compliance programme.

These guidelines provide advice on the conduct of BE studies and the bioanalysis of study samples. Particular consideration is given to premises, equipment, organization and management. Recommended documents, standard operating procedures (SOPs) and records are listed in Appendix 1, but this is not to be considered an exhaustive list – other documents may be necessary depending on each individual CRO's functional and compliance needs.

These guidelines provide information on:

- organization and management;
- study protocols;
- clinical phase of a study;
- bioanalytical phase of a study;
- pharmacokinetic and statistical analysis;
- study report;
- quality management system.

This document does not replace the above-mentioned GCP or GLP guidelines. It is therefore not a stand-alone document.

2. Glossary

The definitions given below apply to the terms used in this guidance. They may have different meanings in other contexts. Unless otherwise stated, the definitions are reproduced from *Guidelines for good clinical practice for trials on pharmaceutical products* (*1*).

adverse event. Any untoward medical occurrence in a clinical trial subject administered a pharmaceutical product; it does not necessarily have a causal relationship with the treatment.

audit of a trial. A systematic examination, carried out independently of those directly involved in the trial, to determine whether the conduct of a trial complies with the agreed protocol and whether the data reported are consistent with the records on site, e.g. whether data reported or recorded in the case-report forms are consonant with those found in hospital files and other original records.

bioequivalence. Two pharmaceutical products are bioequivalent if they are pharmaceutically equivalent or pharmaceutical alternatives, and their bioavailabilities, in terms of rate (C_{max} and t_{max}) and extent of absorption (area under the curve), after administration of the same molar dose under the same conditions, are similar to such a degree that their effects can be expected to be essentially the same.

calibration curve samples (or calibration standards). A matrix to which a known amount of analyte has been added or spiked. Calibration standards are used to construct calibration curves.

case-report form. A document that is used to record data on each trial subject during the course of the trial, as defined by the protocol. The data should be collected by procedures which guarantee preservation, retention and retrieval of information and allow easy access for verification, audit and inspection.

comparator product (or reference product). The comparator product is a pharmaceutical product with which the multisource product is intended to be interchangeable in clinical practice. The comparator product will normally be the innovator product for which efficacy, safety and quality have been established. If the innovator product is no longer marketed in the jurisdiction, the selection principle as described in *Guidance on the selection of comparator pharmaceutical products for equivalence assessment of interchangeable multisource (generic) products* (5) should be used to identify a suitable alternative comparator product.

contract. A document, dated and signed by the investigator, institution and sponsor, that sets out any agreements on financial matters and delegation/distribution of responsibilities. The protocol may also serve as a contract when it contains such information and is signed. Contracts can also be signed with other parties such as vendors supplying services to the contract research organization.

contract research organization (CRO). A scientific organization (commercial, academic or other) to which a sponsor may transfer some of its tasks and obligations. Any such transfer should be defined in writing.

In the context of this guidance document, bioequivalence studies are often contracted by the sponsor to a CRO, which will perform some of the tasks of the sponsor, but which will also perform the trial. The investigator (clinical part of the study) and the study director (bioanalytical part of the study) are then employees of the CRO.

To facilitate reading, the term "CRO" is used throughout this document to designate any organization performing the trial, even though it is acknowledged that part or all of the study may be performed in-house by the sponsor itself or at a hospital.

ethics committee (6). An independent body (a review board or a committee, institutional, regional or national), constituted of medical professionals and non-medical members, whose responsibility is to verify that the safety, integrity and human rights of the subjects participating in a particular trial are protected and to consider the general ethics of the trial, thereby providing public reassurance. Ethics committees should be constituted and operated so that their tasks can be executed free from bias and from any influence of those who are conducting the trial.

final report. A comprehensive description of the trial after its completion including a description of experimental methods (including statistical methods) and materials, a presentation and evaluation of the results, statistical analysis and a critical, ethical, statistical and clinical appraisal.

good clinical practice. A standard for clinical studies which encompasses the design, conduct, monitoring, termination, audit, analysis, reporting and documentation of the studies and which ensures that the studies are scientifically and ethically sound and that the clinical properties of the pharmaceutical product (diagnostic, therapeutic or prophylactic) under investigation are properly documented.

good laboratory practice. A quality system concerned with the organizational process and the conditions under which nonclinical health and environmental safety studies are planned, performed, monitored, recorded, archived and reported.

informed consent. A subject's voluntary confirmation of willingness to participate in a particular trial and the documentation thereof. This consent should be sought only after all appropriate information has been given about the trial, including an explanation of its status as research, its objectives, potential benefits, risks and inconveniences, alternative treatment that may be available, and of the subject's rights and responsibilities in accordance with the current revision of the Declaration of Helsinki.

inspection. An officially conducted examination (i.e. review of the conduct of the trial, including quality assurance, personnel involved, any delegation of authority and audit) by relevant authorities at the site of investigation and/or at the site of the sponsor in order to verify adherence to good clinical practices and good laboratory practices as set out in this document.

internal standard. Test compound(s) (e.g. a structurally similar analogue or stable isotope-labelled compound) added to calibration standards, quality control samples and study samples at a known and constant concentration to correct for experimental variability during sample preparation and analysis.

investigational labelling. Labelling developed specifically for products involved in a clinical trial.

investigational product (or study product). Any pharmaceutical product (see definition) or placebo being tested or used as a reference in a clinical trial.

investigator. A person responsible for the trial and for the rights, health and welfare of the subjects in the trial. The investigator should have qualifications and competence in accordance with local laws and regulations as evidenced by up-to-date curriculum vitae and other credentials. Decisions relating to, and the provision of, medical or dental care must always be the responsibility of a clinically competent person legally allowed to practise medicine or dentistry.

lower limit of quantification. The lower limit of quantification of an individual analytical procedure is the lowest amount of analyte in a sample that can be quantitatively determined with predefined precision and accuracy.

metadata. Metadata are data that describe the attributes of other data, and provide context and meaning. Typically, these are data that describe the structure, data elements, interrelationships and other characteristics of data. They also permit data to be attributable to an individual. Examples of metadata are the audit trails provided by certain types of software.

monitor. A person appointed by, and responsible to, the sponsor or contract research organization for the monitoring and reporting of progress of the trial and for verification of data.

pharmaceutical product. Any substance or combination of substances which has a therapeutic, prophylactic or diagnostic use, or is intended to modify physiological functions, and is presented in a dosage form suitable for administration to humans.

principal investigator. The investigator serving as coordinator for certain kinds of clinical trials, e.g. multicentre trials.

Note: "principle investigator" also has a specific, but different meaning in good laboratory practices, which is seldom used in bioequivalence studies. To avoid any misunderstanding, the term "principal investigator" will only be used in this guidance document with its good clinical practices meaning.

protocol. A document that states the background, rationale and objectives of the trial and describes its design, methodology and organization, including statistical considerations, and the conditions under which it is to be performed and managed. The protocol should be dated and signed by the investigator, the institution involved and the sponsor. It can also function as a contract.

quality assurance relating to clinical trials. Systems and quality control procedures that are established to ensure that the trial is performed and the data are generated in compliance with good clinical practices and good laboratory practices. These include procedures to be followed which apply to ethical and professional conduct, standard operating procedures, reporting, and professional qualifications or skills of personnel.

quality control samples. A spiked sample used to monitor the performance of a bioanalytical method and to assess the integrity and validity of the results of the unknown samples analysed in an individual batch.

raw data. All records or certified copies of original observations, clinical findings or other activities in a clinical trial necessary for the reconstruction and evaluation of the trial. Such material includes laboratory notes, memoranda, calculations and documents, as well as all records of data from automated instruments or exact, verified copies, e.g. in the form of photocopies or microfiches. Raw data can also include photographic negatives, microfilm, magnetic media (e.g. computer diskettes) and optical media (CD-ROMs).

serious adverse event. An event that is associated with death, admission to hospital, prolongation of a hospital stay, persistent or significant disability or incapacity, or is otherwise life-threatening in connection with a clinical trial.

sponsor. An individual, a company, an institution or an organization that takes responsibility for the initiation, management and/or financing of a clinical trial. When an investigator initiates and takes full responsibility for a trial, the investigator then also assumes the role of the sponsor.

standard operating procedures. Standard, detailed, written instructions for the management of clinical trials. They provide a general framework enabling the efficient implementation and performance of all the functions and activities for a particular trial as described in this document.

study director. According to the Organisation for Economic Co-operation and Development principles of good laboratory practice: the individual responsible for the overall conduct of the nonclinical health and environmental safety study. In a bioequivalence study the individual responsible for the conduct of the bioanalytical part of the study.

study product. see *investigational product.*

test product. Any pharmaceutical product (see definition) or placebo being tested against the reference in a clinical trial. In a bioequivalence study, this is the multisource product being tested against the comparator product.

trial subject. An individual who participates in a clinical trial, either as a recipient of the pharmaceutical product under investigation or as a control. The individual may be:

- a healthy person who volunteers to participate in a trial;
- a person with a condition unrelated to the use of the investigational product;
- a person (usually a patient) whose condition is relevant to the use of the investigational product.

upper limit of quantification. The upper limit of quantification of an individual analytical procedure is the highest amount of analyte in a sample which can be quantitatively determined with predefined precision and accuracy.

validation. Action of proving and documenting, in accordance with the principles of good clinical practices and good laboratory practices, that any procedure, process, equipment (including the software or hardware used), material, activity or system actually and consistently leads to the expected results.

verification of data. The procedures carried out to ensure that the data contained in the final report match original observations. These procedures may apply to raw data, data in case-report forms (in hard copy or electronic form), computer printouts and statistical analysis and tables.

A. GENERAL SECTION

3. Organization and management

Note: the acronym "CRO" is used throughout this document to refer not only to a contract research organization, but also to any organization involved in the conduct of in vivo BE studies or in the analysis of samples or of data from such in vivo BE studies

3.1 Where national requirements exist as to the legal status of a CRO these have to be complied with. This also applies to the research unit which is a subsidiary of the manufacturer.

3.2 The CRO should have an organization chart depicting key positions and the names of responsible persons. The organization chart should be dated, authorized and kept up to date.

3.3 There should be job descriptions for all personnel, including a description of their responsibilities. Every job description should be signed and dated by the staff member to whom it applies.

3.4 There should be a list of signatures of the authorized personnel performing tasks during each study.

3.5 For the bioanalytical part of the trial, the principles of GLP clearly establish the responsibilities of the test facility management. For the clinical part of the trial, the CRO management should be aware that as the investigator is an employee of the CRO, some of the responsibilities usually assigned to the investigator would in a similar way reside with the CRO management. At a minimum, the CRO management should:

- ensure that the principles of GCP and GLP, as appropriate, are complied with in the CRO;
- ensure that a sufficient number of qualified personnel, appropriate facilities, equipment and materials are available for the timely and proper conduct of the study;
- ensure the maintenance of a record of the qualifications, training, experience and job description for each professional and technical individual;
- ensure that personnel clearly understand the functions they are to perform and, where necessary, provide training for these functions;
- ensure that appropriate and technically valid SOPs are established and followed, and approve all original and revised SOPs and ensure the maintenance of a historical file of all SOPs;
- ensure that there is a quality assurance (QA) programme with designated personnel and assure that the QA responsibility is being performed in accordance with the principles of GLP and GCP, as appropriate;
- ensure that an individual is identified as responsible for the management of the archive(s), and ensure that the documents

transferred to the archives are kept under adequate conditions for the appropriate duration;
- ensure that supplies meet requirements appropriate to their use in a study;
- establish procedures to ensure that computerized systems are suitable for their intended purpose, and are validated, operated and maintained in accordance with the principles of GCP and GLP, as appropriate.

4. Computer systems

Note: this section highlights only some of the requirements for computer systems that are specific to BE studies. Organizations involved in BE studies should ensure that the relevant principles of the following guidelines are appropriately followed:

- GAMP 5: A risk-based approach to compliant GxP computerized systems (*7*);
- *Good practices for computerised systems in regulated "GXP" environments, PIC/S guidance* (*8*);
- US Food and Drug Administration (FDA) *Guidance for industry: part 11* (9);
- *EU guidelines for good manufacturing practice and medicinal products for human and veterinary use Annex 11, Computerised systems* (*10*);
- *WHO Guidance on good data and record management practices* (*11*).

General

4.1 Computer systems should be qualified and validated (hardware, software, networks, data storage systems and interfaces (*7–10*). Qualification is the planning, carrying out and recording of tests on equipment and systems which form part of the validated process, to demonstrate that the equipment or system will perform as intended.

Hardware

4.2 There should be a sufficient number of computers to enable personnel to perform data entry and data handling, required calculations and compilation of reports.

4.3 Computers should have sufficient capacity and memory for the intended use.

Software

4.4 There should be access control to the trial-related information entered and stored in computers. The method of access control should be specified (e.g. password protection) and a list of people who have access to the database should be maintained. Secure and unique, individual-specific identifiers and passwords should be used.

4.5 The software programs used to perform key steps detailed in these guidelines should be suitable and validated for the intended use. Whether standard, off-the-shelf software is purchased or bespoke software is developed, developer, vendor and/or service provider qualification and/or validation certificates may be provided but it is the user's responsibility to ensure that the software is validated for its intended use and that it was developed in a controlled manner in accordance with a QA system.

4.6 Formal qualification and validation should generally be carried out by the developer. Performance qualification should take account of the specific user's requirements, of regulatory/guideline requirements for BE studies, of the operating environment in which it will be used, and of how it will be used by an organization's staff in the context of a study. Quality risk management should be applied when deciding which components need to be validated. All phases of their life cycle should be considered. For example, when a CRO decommissions the software in use for high-performance liquid chromatography (HPLC) and mass spectrometric (MS) analysis (e.g. HPLC-MS/MS), it should ensure that the data collected by the system using this software remain fully readable. This could be done, for instance, by having the old software installed on a workstation for inspection and/or verification purposes only.

4.7 There should be SOPs in place for usage of each software program that is used to perform activities of a BE study.

4.8 There should be a system in place for the implementation of regular updates to key software programs (e.g. those used for control and data processing of chromatographic and MS systems) whenever required, following an appropriate risk assessment on the potential impact that it could have on current data and on qualification or validation status.

4.9 Software programs used, frequency of virus testing, storage of data and the procedure for backups and long-term archiving of all relevant electronic data should be specified in writing. The frequency of backups and archiving should be specified. If back-up data are periodically rewritten as part of the back-up procedure, the data from the backups should be archived regularly, preferably before rewriting is done.

4.10 The programs used should be able to provide the required quality and management information, reliably and accurately. Programs necessary for data management include word processing, data entry, databases, graphics, pharmacokinetics and statistical programs. Self-designed software programs must be suitable and validated for their intended use.

4.11 Since data for BE studies are often transferred electronically between organizations involved in the studies, verification that the software used by each organization is compatible with the others and that there is no impact on the data so-transferred, should be conducted prior to commencing key study-related tasks.

4.12 These requirements apply to all systems used in clinical BE studies, e.g. subject database, electronic case report forms, electrocardiogram (ECG) recording software, HPLC-MS/MS software, software used for pharmacokinetic analysis, for statistical analysis and any other relevant system.

Networks

4.13 Networks, including the full client/server architecture and interfaces such as laboratory information management systems, when used, should be appropriately designed, qualified, managed and controlled.

4.14 Access to each component of the system by the different users at any given organization involved in the studies, should be appropriately defined, controlled and documented.

4.15 There should be a documented inventory of all computerized systems on the network, with a clear identification of those which are GXP regulated. Any changes to the network, including the temporary addition or removal of systems from the network, should be documented.

Data management

4.16 Data entry includes transfer of the data from case report forms (CRFs), analytical data and any other data relevant to the reliability and integrity of a study, to the computerized system.

4.17 Data entry procedures should be designed to prevent errors. The data entry process should be specified in the SOP.

4.18 Data validation methodology (proofreading, double data entry, electronic logical control) should be specified in writing and performed.

4.19 Changes to data entered in the database should be made by authorized persons only. Changes should be specified and documented.

4.20 Electronic data should be backed up at regular intervals. The reliability and completeness of these backups should be verified – data should not be selected, rather all data should be comprehensively backed up.

4.21 All of the raw electronic data must be kept. This includes:

- all metadata associated with a computerized system and the equipment associated with it (which includes the audit trails for integration, for results, projects and for the entire instrument);
- validation data and metadata in the form of their source electronic files.

PDF copies are not sufficient on their own, unless it can be demonstrated that these are the raw data and that no alteration was possible after they were generated.

4.22 All electronic records obtained from HPLC and MS analysis (e.g. HPLC-MS/MS) are required to be retained, maintained and backed up. It should be ensured that backup data are exact and complete and that they are secure against alteration, inadvertent erasures or loss. The printed paper copy of the chromatogram would not be considered a "true, exact and complete copy" of all the electronic raw data used to create that chromatogram. Printed chromatograms do not generally include, for example, the sample sequence, instrument method, processing method, integration settings or the full audit trail, all of which were used to create the chromatogram or are associated with its validity. Therefore there should be a greater emphasis on conservation of electronic data than paper data, as paper data are usually not considered the true source data, except, for instance, in the case of paper logbooks where the original record was handwritten.

4.23 If data are transformed during processing steps (such as in the example of re-integration of chromatographic data), it should always be possible to compare the original data with the processed data.

5. Quality management

5.1 The CRO should have appropriate QA and QC systems with written SOPs to ensure that trials are conducted and data are generated, documented and reported in compliance with the protocol, GCP, GLP, GMP and the applicable regulatory requirements.

5.2 QA personnel should be independent of the work they are quality assuring, including:

- conducting or monitoring of the trial;
- conducting bioanalysis;
- performing reporting and pharmacokinetic and statistical analyses.

As a consequence, QA personnel should not be directly involved in trial-related activities, and an in-process audit by QA personnel does not replace oversight by another person when required.

5.3 The QA unit should be responsible for:

- verifying all activities undertaken during the study;
- ensuring that the quality management systems, are followed, reviewed and updated;
- determining that the protocol and SOPs are made available to study personnel and are being followed;
- checking all the study data for reliability and traceability;
- planning and performing self-inspections (internal audits) at regular and defined intervals in accordance with an SOP, and following up on any corrective action as required, to determine if all studies are conducted in accordance with GCP and GLP;
- ensuring that contract facilities adhere to GCP and, if applicable, to GLP: this would include auditing of such facilities, and following up on any corrective action required;
- verifying that the trial report accurately and completely reflects the data from the study and the methods and procedures followed;
- promptly reporting audit findings in writing to management, to the investigator and to the study director, as applicable.

5.4 The CRO should allow the sponsor to monitor the studies and to perform audits of the clinical and analytical study and sites and should provide suitable office space for these activities.

5.5 Both in-process and retrospective QA verifications (e.g. in bioanalysis, as the samples and standards are being prepared and tested) should be performed.

5.6 The quality management system should include root cause analysis, tracking for trends, ensuring all aspects of data integrity and the implementation of appropriate corrective and preventive action (CAPA).

6. Archive facilities

6.1 The CRO should have sufficient and appropriately secure storage space, which should be fireproof, relative humidity-controlled and pest-controlled, for archiving of the trial-related documentation. Archives should also be protected from flooding.

6.2 An SOP should be in place for archiving.

6.3 Access to archive storage areas should be controlled and restricted to authorized personnel.

6.4 Records of document access and return should be maintained.

6.5 The length of time for which study documentation, including raw data, is kept in the archive should be defined in the SOP and may vary depending on country requirements. This period should be specified in the contract between the sponsor and the CRO, which should include provisions for financing of the archiving.

6.6 All data, including both paper and electronic versions, should be easy to retrieve and traceable.

7. Premises

7.1 The facilities should be kept clean and should have adequate lighting, ventilation and, if required, environmental control. Floors, walls and working bench surfaces should be easy to clean and to decontaminate.

7.2 Clinical trials must be carried out under conditions that ensure adequate safety for the subjects. The site selected should be appropriate to the potential risk involved.

7.3 The CRO should have sufficient space to accommodate the personnel and activities required to perform the studies. The trial site must have adequate facilities, including laboratories, and equipment. The facilities used for the clinical phase of the study, including areas listed in paragraph 9.6, should be well organized in order to carry out the activities in a logical order.

7.4 Entry to the facility should be restricted and controlled. There should be alarm systems to detect the exit of subjects from clinical facilities, or the doors should be locked (but only if emergency evacuation can still be ensured). Any entry to and exit from the facility should be recorded.

7.5 Sites where clinical activities take place should include a pharmacy where investigational products should be stored under appropriate conditions with entry and exit restricted by access control. Appropriate entry/exit records of each visit to the pharmacy should be maintained.

7.6 Utilities such as water, air, gas and electricity should be adequate, stable and uninterrupted.

7.7 Access to telephone, email and facsimile facilities should be available to ensure proper communication. The CRO should have the necessary office equipment (printer, copy machine) to perform the required activities.

7.8 Laboratory premises should be designed to suit the operations to be carried out in them. Sufficient space should be provided to avoid mix-ups, contamination and cross-contamination. Adequate storage space suitable for samples, standards, solvents, reagents and records should be available.

7.9 Laboratory premises should be designed to provide adequate protection to all employees and authorized external personnel, including inspectors or auditors, by ensuring their safety while handling or working in the presence of chemicals and biological samples. Inappropriate working conditions can have a negative impact on the quality of the work performed and of the data generated.

The general rules for safe working in accordance with national regulations and SOPs normally include the following requirements.

- Safety data sheets should be available to staff before testing is carried out. Staff working in the laboratory should be familiar with and knowledgeable about the material safety data sheets for the chemicals and solvents that they are handling.
- Smoking, eating and drinking in the laboratory should be prohibited.
- Staff should know how to use the firefighting equipment, including fire extinguishers, fire blankets and gas masks.
- Staff should wear laboratory coats or other protective clothing, including eye protection.
- Appropriate care should be taken when handling, for example, highly potent, infectious or volatile substances.
- Highly toxic and/or genotoxic samples should be handled in a specially designed facility to avoid the risk of contamination.
- All containers of chemicals should be fully labelled and include prominent warnings (e.g. "poison", "flammable" or "radioactive") whenever appropriate.

- Adequate insulation and spark-proofing should be provided for electrical wiring and equipment, including refrigerators.
- Rules on safe handling of cylinders of compressed gases should be observed and staff should be familiar with the relevant colour identification codes.
- Staff should be aware of the need to avoid working alone in the laboratory.
- First-aid materials should be provided and staff instructed in first-aid techniques, emergency care and the use of antidotes.
- Containers containing volatile organic solvents, such as mobile phases or liquid/liquid extraction solvents should be closed with an appropriate seal.
- Volatile organic chemicals should be handled under certified fume-hoods or air extractors and safety and eye showers should be available in the laboratory.

7.10 Premises should have suitable systems in place to dispose of waste, to treat fumes and to protect the environment in conformance with local or national regulations.

8. Personnel

8.1 There should be a sufficient number of medical, paramedical, technical and clerical staff with the appropriate qualifications, training and experience to support the trial and to be able to respond effectively to all reasonably foreseeable emergencies. The number of members of staff required depends on the number and complexity of the trials performed by the CRO. At all stages of the trial, including at night, there should be a sufficient number of appropriately qualified and trained personnel to ensure that the rights, safety and well-being of the subjects are safeguarded, and to care for the subjects in emergency situations.

8.2 The delegation of significant trial-related duties should be documented in writing.

8.3 Contract workers may be employed to perform certain activities. All contract workers who have access to the clinical or bioanalytical areas or who are performing trial-related activities should be provided with adequate information, training and job descriptions. Their contracts should be signed before beginning their work.

8.4 Current curricula vitae and training records should be kept for full-time and contract workers.

8.5 The personnel responsible for the planning and conduct of the study should have appropriate qualifications and sufficient knowledge and experience in the relevant field. They should receive the study-specific information and training required for the performance of their work.

8.6 Records of training and assessment of knowledge of GCP, GLP and any other relevant area or technique should be maintained.

8.7 There should be adequate measures in place to protect personnel from accidental infection (e.g. from accidental needle pricks) while obtaining blood samples from subjects or while handling samples that are derived from blood products (e.g. plasma and its extracts) or while handling or disposing of infectious waste.

B. CLINICAL SECTION

9. Clinical phase

Note: As in vivo BE trials are considered as clinical trials, specifically as a Phase I study, the general requirements and recommendations of GCP apply to all BE trials. Clinical trials must be carried out under conditions that ensure adequate safety of the subjects. The clinical phase of the study can be performed on the premises of a CRO or by contracting suitable premises in a hospital.

9.1 A CRO should have rooms meeting the requirements listed in the sections below.

9.2 There should be sufficient space to accommodate the study subjects.

9.3 Where appropriate, beds should be available for the subjects. The necessity for beds and for overnight stays depends on the type of trial and investigational product and should be specified in the trial protocol. Overnight stays are usually required for the night prior to dosing to ensure adequately controlled conditions and that there is no intake of food or medication within the number of hours that is specified in the trial protocol.

9.4 Systems should be in place in the accommodation facilities so that subjects can alert CRO staff in case of need.

9.5 Facilities for changing and storing clothes and for washing and toilet purposes should be clean, well ordered, easily accessible and appropriate for the number of users. Lockable toilets should be alarmed and doors should be designed to ensure that they can be opened from the outside should there be a medical emergency.

9.6 The study site should have rooms or areas, as appropriate, for the following:

- subjects' registration and screening;
- obtaining informed consent of individual subjects without compromising privacy;
- subjects' housing;
- subjects' recreation;
- pharmaceutical operations (restricted access room, e.g. for storage, repacking, dispensing, documentation) (see also section 14);
- administration of the investigational products and sample collection;
- sample processing (e.g. plasma separation) and storage (freezer);
- controlled access storage of study materials, medication and documentation including CRFs;
- preparation of standardized meals and a dining hall;
- proper care of subjects who require emergency or other medical care, with emergency or first-aid equipment and appropriate medication for use in emergencies;
- archiving.

9.7 Provisions should be made for the urgent transportation of subjects to a hospital or clinic equipped for their emergency care, if required.

9.8 Access to key documents, such as the randomization list, should be restricted to specific personnel, such as the pharmacist in charge of the study. Such documents should be password-secured (if electronic) or kept under lock and key (if in the form of a hard copy) and their distribution should be documented.

9.9 Equipment used should be appropriately calibrated at predefined intervals.

9.10 The adequate function and performance of emergency-use equipment (e.g. defibrillators) should be verified at appropriate intervals.

10. Clinical laboratory

10.1 A suitable clinical laboratory should be used for analysing samples. Whenever possible this should be an accredited laboratory.

10.2 Haematological tests, urine analysis and other tests should be performed during the clinical trial as specified in the study protocol.

10.3 Sample labelling, receipt, storage and chain of custody should ensure full traceability and sample integrity (*9*).

10.4 The CRO should receive information about the analytical methods used in the laboratory, a dated list of laboratory normal ranges and, if available, the accreditation certificate of the laboratory. These should be available for inspection by regulatory authorities upon request.

10.5 The laboratory should provide the CRO with current and signed curricula vitae of the responsible individuals.

10.6 Individual reports should be created by the laboratory for each subject and should be included in the CRFs. Source or raw data for all tests performed should be archived by the laboratory in electronic or paper formats, depending on their source and the laboratory's storage capacity. Electronic formats are preferred.

10.7 Data integrity requirements apply to all tests related to the study (*11*). For instance, raw data should be adequately protected from modification or deletion.

11. Ethics

11.1 Independent ethics committee

Trials must be approved by an independent ethics committee (IEC) (or equivalent) before any study is conducted, according to *WHO operational guidelines for ethics committees that review biomedical research* (*6*), and to the legislation in force. This Committee must be independent from the sponsor, the investigator and the CRO. Detailed minutes should be kept of the discussions, recommendations and decisions of the IEC meetings. The IEC should be given sufficient time for reviewing protocols, informed consent forms (ICFs) and related documentation.

11.2 Informed consent

The following points should be borne in mind in relation to informed consent.

- Information for study participants should be given to them in a language and at a level of complexity appropriate to their understanding, both orally and in writing.
- Informed consent must always be given by the subject and documented in writing before the start of any trial-related activities, in accordance with GCP. If informed consent is also recorded by video, this recording should be retained in accordance with local legal requirements.

- The information must make clear that participation is voluntary and that the subject has the right to withdraw from the study on his or her own initiative at any time, without having to give a reason (compensation should be paid pro rata temporis). If subjects who withdraw from the study offer their reasons for doing so, those reasons should be included in the study records.
- The subject must have access to information about insurance and other procedures for compensation or treatment should he or she be injured or disabled by participating in the trial or during screening.
- The volunteers or subjects should be given the opportunity to discuss with a physician their concerns regarding potential side effects or reactions from the use of the investigational products before participating in the trial. They should also be given the opportunity and sufficient time to discuss their concerns about participating in the trial with individuals outside the CRO, such as friends and family members, if they wish.
- If the ICF is available in several languages (e.g. in English and in the local language, or in several vernacular languages) care should be taken to ensure that all versions of the form contain the same information.

12. Monitoring

Note: monitoring is an essential activity to ensure the quality of the clinical trial.

12.1 The monitor should be appropriately qualified (see section 8: Personnel). The main responsibility of the monitor for a BE study is to ensure that the study is conducted in accordance with the protocol, GCP, GLP and applicable ethical and regulatory requirements. This includes verification of the use of correct procedures for completion of CRFs and verification of the accuracy of data obtained.

12.2 The sponsor can delegate the monitoring function to the CRO. In such cases the CRO should be able to arrange for the monitoring of the trial according to regulatory requirements. In this situation, attention should be paid to the independence of the monitoring function to avoid conflicts of interest and pressure on the monitors. The monitoring reports should always be provided to the sponsor.

12.3 A risk-based approach to monitoring can be considered. However, a pre- and post-study visit, as well as a monitoring visit during the conduct of the trial, are usually performed. The monitor should prepare a written report after each site visit and communicate any issues to the CRO and to the sponsor as quickly as possible, even while the study is being conducted, if possible, to enable prompt corrective action. Such communications and corrective actions should be documented.

12.4 When the monitoring is delegated to the CRO, SOPs should be available to describe:

- the designation of monitors, who should be independent from the personnel performing the trial;
- procedures for the monitoring visit;
- the extent of source data verification, including with regard to accountability of the investigational products and adherence to the protocol.

The extent of the monitoring, including the number of visits to be performed, should be agreed with the sponsor.

12.5 Separate SOPs (with checklists for the monitor) for the initiation visit, routine monitoring visits and a closing visit are recommended.

12.6 Appropriate entry/exit records of each monitoring visit should be maintained.

13. Investigators

13.1 The principal investigator (PI) should have the overall responsibility for the clinical conduct of the study, including clinical aspects of study design, administration of the products under investigation, contacts with local authorities and the ethics committee and for signing the protocol and the final study report.

13.2 The investigator(s) should have appropriate qualifications, be suitably trained and have experience in the conduct of BE studies (the legal status of persons authorized to act as investigators differs between countries) and at least one investigator must be legally allowed to practise medicine.

13.3 The medically-qualified investigator should be responsible for the integrity, health and welfare of the subjects during the trial and for the accurate documentation of all trial-related clinical data.

13.4 The CRO is responsible for selecting investigator(s). If the investigators are not permanent employees of the CRO, external investigators should be contracted and adequately trained.

14. Receiving, storage and handling of investigational products

14.1 CROs should record all the information concerning the receipt, storage, handling and accountability of investigational products at every stage of the trial. CROs must keep records of information about the shipment, delivery, receipt, description, storage (including storage conditions), dispensing, administration, reconciliation, return and/or destruction of any remaining pharmaceutical products. Details of the pharmaceutical product used should include dosage form and strength, lot number, expiry date and any other coding that identifies the specific characteristics of the product tested.

14.2 A suitably qualified person within the CRO or a local pharmacy or hospital pharmacy should assume responsibility for storage, delivery, return and keeping records of the investigational products.

14.3 Pharmaceutical products should be stored under appropriate conditions as specified in the official product information provided by the sponsor.

14.4 All study medication should be kept in a securely locked area accessible only to authorized personnel.

14.5 Randomization should be performed in accordance with an SOP and records should be maintained, including the randomization list and seed, if applicable. The randomization list should normally be accessible only to the person who generates it, a dispensing pharmacist and the statistician, and should not be circulated or made available to other staff members via any medium. A system should be in place to allow the PI or delegated staff to access the randomization list in case of emergency.

14.6 Labelling should be performed in accordance with the following requirements.

- The printing step should be done in a manner that reduces potential risks of mislabelling and in accordance with an SOP.
- Each label should include the following information:
  - name of the sponsor,
  - a statement reading “for clinical trial use only”,
  - trial reference number or study number,
  - batch number,
  - subject identification number (to whom the product is destined to be given),

- study period,
- active ingredient and dosage,
- the storage conditions,
- expiry date (month/year) or retest date,
- identification of the product (i.e. test or reference).

- Compliance of all labels with the randomization list should be verified once they have been printed and prior to labelling of the containers.
- Labels should be pasted onto the container, not on the lid, to ensure that the information is not lost once the lid is removed.
- The system used for labelling and documenting the administration of the product should make it possible to verify that each subject did receive the product dispensed for him or her, for instance, by using labels with a tear-off portion. In this case, labels should be designed in such a way that two identical labels are pasted onto the container and the second label can be easily cut or detached and pasted onto the CRF at the time of dosing (e.g. two labels printed side by side, with only one that is actually pasted onto the container and another that remains attached but unpasted. Using two independent labels – one stuck on the container, one kept loose – should be avoided owing to the risk of mix-ups).
- The empty containers should be labelled separately for the test and the reference investigational products and should remain adequately segregated in a secure area under lock and key to avoid the risk of any potential mix-ups, until the dispensing stage.
- Label reconciliation should be performed.
- Appropriate, detailed records should be maintained for each of the above steps.

14.7 Dispensing and packaging should be performed in accordance with the following requirements.

- The surface on which the product will be handled should be thoroughly cleaned before bringing bottles of the product into the area. Any product containers (full or empty), lone dosage formulations, labelling materials, contaminants, dirt and debris should be removed from the area.
- A second person should verify that the surface area (otherwise referred to as the "line") is indeed clear and clean before bringing in and opening containers of the product.

- Test and reference products should be handled using an appropriate instrument, such as a spatula or spoon, as opposed to gloved hands.
- Tablets should be distributed into each container in accordance with the randomization list for the comparator or for the test product as appropriate. The two products should never be handled at the same time. This also applies to the labelled containers.
- Records should be made of this step in a manner similar to that used for manufacturing batch records, as described in WHO GMP guidelines, i.e. each and every step should be recorded sequentially in detail.
- The surface upon which the product is handled and its surroundings should be cleared and cleaned immediately before and after initiating the dispensing of the next product. It is important to note that this also applies to different products used in the same study.
- Investigational product accountability and dispensing records should be maintained at all times. Each activity should be documented at the time it is performed. This includes:
  - records of doses dispensed and returned or destroyed,
  - records of cleaning and clearance of the area before dispensing,
  - record of verification of adequate cleaning and clearance of the area,
  - record of verification by a second person of each step.

Any factors that could affect the integrity of the data relating to investigational medicinal products and comparators should be recorded, monitored and controlled.

For further guidance on labelling and dispensing, please refer to the *WHO good manufacturing practices: supplementary guidelines for the manufacture of investigational pharmaceutical products for clinical trials in humans* (*12*).

14.8 Dosing should meet the following requirements.

- Dosing should be performed in accordance with an SOP.
- Dosing should be performed under the supervision of the investigator or of a qualified staff member to whom this task has been explicitly delegated in writing.
- Whenever possible, just prior to dosing, a check should be performed to ensure that vial contents match the information on the label.

- The exact time of dosing should be documented.
- To ensure that the subject has swallowed the product, a mouth check should be performed by looking under the tongue, under the lips, in the corners of the mouth and between gums and cheeks, using a tongue depressor or a spatula and a penlight, in the case of solid oral dosage forms. For other dosage forms, verification of adequate administration should be performed by other suitable means. This should be documented.
- If more than one dosage unit is administered, this should be clearly documented.
- Dosing can be documented directly in the CRFs. If re-transcribed in the case of report forms from other documents, the original documents should be retained.
- Investigational product reconciliation after dosing should be verified by a second responsible person.

14.9 The investigator should follow the protocol requirements, the randomization scheme and, where required, blinding. The investigator should ensure that the use of the investigational product is documented in such a way as to ensure appropriate dosage.

14.10 Samples of the product in the original container should be retained for possible confirmatory testing in the future for a period of at least one year after the expiry date of the newest product (test or reference) or in compliance with the applicable national requirements or international recommendations, as appropriate. Sample retention should be defined and described in an SOP and be specified in the contract between the sponsor and the CRO. Dispensed products that were not administered should also be retained.

15. Case report forms

15.1 CRFs should be used to record data on each subject during the course of the trial.

15.2 The CRO should have a procedure for designing CRFs if the sponsor requests the CRO to do so. The use of a standardized format or template is recommended. This should be adapted for each study protocol in accordance with the requirements for that particular study. The CRF should be reviewed against other trial documentation, such as the protocol and trial database, to ensure that appropriate information and data are captured and that the CRF is consistent with other trial documentation.

15.3 The data to be collected on each volunteer should be specified in the trial protocol. Any data to be recorded directly on the CRF (i.e. no prior written or electronic record of data), and to be considered to be source data, should be identified in the protocol.

15.4 CRFs should reflect the actual results obtained during the study and allow easy access for verification, audit and inspection of the data.

15.5 Appropriate procedures should be established and followed to document the investigator's certification of the accuracy of CRFs. Any errors or omissions should be clarified with the investigator, corrected, dated and signed and explained on the CRF.

15.6 Copies of the clinical laboratory reports and all ECGs should be included with the CRFs for each subject and should be submitted together with the dossier, if applicable, in accordance with the requirements of the regulatory authority to which the dossier is submitted.

16. Volunteers and recruitment methods

Note: The selection of subjects should be performed sufficiently far in advance to ensure that a sufficient number of subjects will be available for the study. The last-minute selection of additional subjects may result in noncompliance with the inclusion and exclusion criteria, possibly compromising the safety of the subjects and the integrity of the trial data. The use of a generic screening process to select a pool of subjects that can be enrolled in any BE study conducted at the CRO (unless the protocol foresees specific inclusion or exclusion criteria) can help to achieve this goal.

16.1 Procedures for the recruitment of volunteers should be available and should include a description of the potential methods that can be used by the CRO for this purpose. A database should be maintained on volunteers, to avoid cross-participation and to specify a minimum time that should elapse between a volunteer's participation in one study and the next. Access to the database should be password controlled in order to secure confidential information on volunteers or subjects.

16.2 Identification of volunteers and subjects should be ensured by reliable means. If a biometric system is used, this system should be periodically validated, as well as after any change made to the validated system that could affect its function.

16.3 The informed consent of potential subjects should be obtained for any screening procedures required to determine eligibility for the study in addition to informed consent for participation in the research portion of the study.

16.4 Criteria for subject selection (inclusion and exclusion criteria) and screening procedures should be described in the clinical trial protocol.

16.5 The results of subject screening and of trial participation should be recorded in a validated database maintained by the CRO. If a regional or national volunteer database exists, then this should be checked to find out whether any of the subjects have participated in a previous trial and participation data should be uploaded to this central repository to prevent over-volunteering. Access to the database should be password controlled in order to secure confidential subject information.

16.6 Ideally the CRO's database should record and allow the users to query:

- contact details;
- sex;
- status: e.g. eligible, disqualified, not eligible, quarantined, and the reason for this status if applicable;
- date and place of last study participation, if applicable/if known;
- date of last screening;
- a unique code assigned to the subject which will never change;
- outcome of last trial: e.g. completed, randomized but not dosed, withdrawn for personal reasons, withdrawn for medical reasons.

These data should be backed up daily and be available for review at any time.

16.7 Medical records should be generated for each subject and should include information obtained during each screening visit and from each study in which the subject has participated, which could be relevant for the inclusion and follow-up of the subject in subsequent trials. Access to previous medical records for individual subjects should be available and a consistency check conducted where trial-specific medical records are generated. This is important to ensure that safety issues can be assessed before a subject's enrolment in a study.

17. Food and fluids

17.1 As meals can significantly affect absorption of active pharmaceutical ingredients, fasting and meals should be standardized and adequately controlled and scheduled during the study days. The CRO should be able to arrange for standardized meals, snacks and drinks for the study subjects as described in the clinical trial protocol.

17.2 Records should be maintained of the timing, duration and amount of food and fluids consumed. Prior to samples being obtained from ambulatory subjects, they should be asked about their food and drink consumption, if the protocol contains specific requirements.

17.3 Standardized meals should be designed by a dietitian with appropriate qualifications, training and experience. If such services are contracted out, a formal contract with terms of reference should be available.

18. Safety, adverse events and adverse event reporting

18.1 Appropriate study planning includes adequate evaluation of risk to the subjects. The study should be planned, organized, performed and monitored so that the safety profile will be acceptable, including to the volunteers.

18.2 First-aid equipment and appropriate rescue medication should be available and ready for emergency use at the study site where there should be adequate facilities for the proper care of subjects who require emergency or other medical treatment. Any treatment given to a subject should be documented and included in the CRF and in the supporting documentation, as necessary.

18.3 A medical doctor should be responsible for medical decisions in the case of adverse events and for notifying the relevant health authorities, the sponsor and, when applicable, the ethics committee, without delay in the case of serious adverse events. Appropriate timelines should be respected in accordance with national regulations.

18.4 The CRO should have appropriate adverse event registration and reporting forms, which should be provided to the investigator; these forms can be part of the CRF. If required the sponsor's forms may be used.

C. BIOANALYTICAL SECTION

Note: The measurement of analyte concentrations (API or metabolites) may be performed by the same CRO as conducted the clinical study, or this work may be contracted to another laboratory or CRO.

19. Method development

19.1 The bioanalytical laboratory should provide a detailed description of how a bioanalytical method was developed. The laboratory should keep a copy of any publications used in developing the bioanalytical method. The modifications and adaptations to the published method made by the laboratory should be documented.

19.2 Selection of the internal standard should be justifiable by sound scientific principles. In general, the chemical and physical properties of the internal standard should be as close to those of the analyte as possible. Both stable isotope-labelled and non-isotope-labelled internal standards are acceptable, although the use of a stable isotope-labelled internal standard is recommended when MS methods are used. The selection of a stable isotope-labelled internal standard should take into consideration factors such as the isotope labelling positions in order to limit the risk of exchange reactions.

19.3 The procedure for method development should ensure that methods are created in a manner that will minimize any potential human error.

20. Method validation

The most up-to-date guidelines available from stringent regulatory authorities (SRAs) on the topic of bioanalytical method validation should be followed.

20.1 Validation requirements for the analytical method should be described in the protocol. There should be separate SOPs for analytical method validation.

20.2 Data to support the stability of the samples under the stated conditions and period of storage should be available, preferably before the start of the study.

20.3 Method validation should be performed with at least one run that is comparable in length to those that are expected to be used for analysis of samples.

21. Sample collection, storage and handling of biological material

21.1 The specification of the samples (serum, plasma or urine), sampling method, volume and number of samples should be stated in the clinical trial protocol and in the information provided to the volunteers.

21.2 There should be documented procedures for the collection, preparation, transport or shipping and storage of samples.

21.3 Any specific lighting conditions foreseen by the protocol or other documents should be complied with. This should be documented.

21.4 Actual sampling times and deviations from the prespecified sampling times should be recorded. Deviations should be noted in the study report and should be taken into consideration when calculating the pharmacokinetic parameters.

21.5 Labelling of collected samples should be clear to ensure correct identification and traceability of each sample.

21.6 The conditions for the storage of samples depend on the analyte. However, all storage conditions (e.g. freezer temperature) should be specified in the study protocol, controlled, monitored and recorded throughout the storage period and during transportation. Procedures should be in place to ensure maintenance of sample integrity in case of system failures.

21.7 Records of the storage and retrieval of samples should be maintained.

21.8 It is recommended to keep duplicate or back-up samples, and to store and ship them separately.

21.9 The duration of storage of bioanalytical samples should be specified in the contract between the sponsor and the CRO.

21.10 Local requirements for the handling and destruction of any remaining biological materials should be complied with.

22. Analysis of study samples

The most up-to-date guidelines from SRAs on the topic of bioanalytical method validation should be followed. Additionally:

22.1 The results of the method validation should be available before the initiation of study sample analysis, with the possible exception of the evaluation of the long-term stability of the analyte in matrix. However, these results should be available before the study report is issued and should be submitted with the validation report in the application.

22.2 Each analytical run should include calibration curve (CC) standards, QC samples and subject samples processed simultaneously. The exact sequence of processing should be documented. All samples collected from a given subject during all trial periods should be analysed in the same run unless scientifically justified (e.g. where the limited stability of samples necessitates the analysis of period one samples before period two is conducted).

22.3 Equipment with an adequate capacity should be used to enable all samples in a run to be processed simultaneously, rather than splitting the samples into several extraction batches. However, if using several extraction batches within a single analytical run cannot be avoided, each batch should include QC samples. The acceptance criteria for the analytical run should be defined in an SOP first for the full run, then if the run is acceptable, for each individual extraction batch.

22.4 Every effort should be made during method development to avoid carry-over effects. If carry-over cannot be avoided, procedures should be implemented to limit its influence, for instance, by inserting wash samples into runs after samples with a high concentration.

22.5 With regard to the use of blank plasma in the preparation of CCs and QCs:

- the number of freeze–thaw cycles and the duration of storage that a given blank plasma sample can be submitted to should be limited as much as possible to ensure that there is no degradation and/or any change of its properties. Freezing blank plasma in small volumes should be considered to help limit the number of freeze–thaw cycles for any given blank plasma sample;
- the anticoagulant that was used for the blank plasma should be documented. It should match the anticoagulant that was used in study samples, in nature and in proportion.

22.6 With regard to incurred sample reanalysis:

- incurred sample reanalysis should be performed in line with the European Medicines Agency (EMA) *Guidelines on bioanalytical method validation* (*13*);
- large differences between results may indicate analytical issues and should be investigated.

23. Data processing and documentation

23.1 Integration settings should be science-based and fully justifiable. Smoothing should be kept low enough not to mask possible interferences and changes in peak geometry.

23.2 The different iterations used to obtain a CC should be saved – if a given CC fails, it is not acceptable to exclude CCs which meet acceptance criteria or, similarly, to include CC standards that do not meet criteria, just to make the calibration or the QC standards pass. The source data should contain the original, first evaluation of runs (containing all calibration samples). If several calibration samples are excluded sequentially, the CC obtained at each step should be retained to document that the criteria for excluding the next sample were met. If electronic raw data are used it is acceptable to save only the final calibration if it is possible to revert to the initial calibration during an inspection. The process and criteria for acceptance and exclusion of CC standards should be described in an SOP.

23.3 If the first or last calibration sample is rejected, the calibration range should be truncated, i.e. the second calibration sample becomes the lower limit of quantification (LLOQ) in that run (or the penultimate calibration sample becomes the upper limit of quantification (ULOQ). Samples with a concentration below the revised LLOQ (or above the revised ULOQ) should be reanalysed. Alternatively, the whole run may be repeated, but this is not the preferred option.

23.4 Internal standard variation should be trended and used as part of the verifications of result validity. Significant changes in internal standard response could signal an analytical problem that requires an investigation and/or sample reanalysis. Significant differences between the internal standard results of CC standards or QC standards versus samples could also signal problems affecting the reliability of the results.

23.5 Full audit trails should be activated at all times and on all analytical instruments in a given facility, before, during and after the method validation and the study of interest.

23.6 All original analytical raw data (e.g. calculations, chromatograms and their associated audit trails) should be documented in a manner that will ensure traceability with respect to the sample number, equipment used, date and time of analysis and the name(s) of the technician(s). If several audit trail files are generated, all should be retained (e.g. results table audit trail, project audit trail and instrument audit trail).

23.7 Each data point should be traceable to a specific sample, including sample number, time of collection of the sample, time of centrifugation, if applicable, time when the sample was placed in the freezer and time of sample analysis, to be able to determine whether any aberrant results might have been caused by sample mishandling.

24. Good laboratory practices

24.1 Although most GLP guidelines (*2*) apply formally only to nonclinical safety studies, general principles of GLP should also be followed during the bioanalytical part of BE studies.

24.2 Analysis should be performed in a laboratory with established QA systems (*14*).

24.3 Key sample storage systems or other areas requiring environmental controls should be adequately qualified, calibrated and maintained. There should be an alarm system or an adequate monitoring system to control the temperature of the critical stage areas and key sample storage systems, such as freezers. If there is an automatic alarm system it has to be tested regularly to check its functionality. The daily monitoring and all the alarm checks should be documented. There should be a system in place to ensure that timely and appropriate action is taken following an alarm.

24.4 For the purposes of qualification and requalification, the temperature-mapping of the freezers and refrigerators should be run for between 24 and 72 hours, or more if justified. Remapping should be done after any significant modifications to the storage units.

24.5 Appropriate repairs and/or transfer of samples to other equivalent storage units should be considered whenever an analysis of temperature monitoring records shows unexplained variability outside normal operating limits.

24.6 Balances, other measuring devices and equipment and instruments used during the conduct of a trial should be periodically calibrated and verified before use. They should be fit for their intended purpose.

24.7 There should be SOPs for the operation, use, calibration, checks and preventive maintenance of equipment. Records should be maintained. Items of equipment used during the course of the trial should be identified to enable verification that they have been appropriately qualified and calibrated.

24.8 Chemicals, reference substances, reagents, solvents and solutions should be labelled to indicate identity, purity, concentration (if appropriate), expiry date and specific storage instructions. Information concerning source, preparation date and stability should be available.

D. PHARMACOKINETIC, STATISTICAL CALCULATIONS AND REPORTING SECTION

25. Pharmacokinetic and statistical calculations

25.1 The statistical model underlying any primary BE analysis should be stated in the protocol and/or a statistical analysis plan. It should be made clear which factors are fixed and which are random and whether the model is a mixed effects model, a normal linear model, or another type. If the methods of statistical analysis are amended following approval of the protocol then this should be documented in a protocol amendment and should also be reported in the clinical study report together with the reason for change.

25.2 Calculations should be made by suitably qualified personnel (see section 8: Personnel).

25.3 The means of performing pharmacokinetic and statistical calculations (both software and scripts) should be specified in the study protocol and/or a pharmacokinetic analysis plan and a statistical analysis plan. Data analysis should conform to these requirements. This should include the manner in which area under the curve from time zero to infinity (AUC_{inf}) is derived (i.e. how the points used for extrapolation are selected).

25.4 Calculations should be made using validated software and scripts. Software and scripts should be validated or qualified using an SOP, ideally with datasets of varying complexity and with the alpha level(s) actually in use. Self-designed software should be demonstrated as suitable for intended use. For guidance on the use of computerized systems (see section 4: Computer systems) (*8*).

25.5 Data values input should be double-checked by a second qualified person in accordance with an SOP.

25.6 A database of trial records should be maintained and should ideally be locked as soon as possible after completion of the study. Once it is locked the study can be unblinded and statistical analysis performed. The dates of locking and statistical analysis should be documented and mentioned in the study report, and the process should be defined in a suitable procedure.

26. Study report

26.1 The clinical study report should accurately reflect all the study procedures and results.

26.2 The clinical study report should be well written and presented. All deviations from the protocol in the performance of the study should be reported.

26.3 There should be no discrepancies between the results stated in the report and the actual original (raw) data.

26.4 The report should comply with regulatory requirements as applicable and be presented in a standard format.

26.5 The study report should include a report on the bioanalytical part of the trial, including a description of the bioanalytical method used and the report of the validation of this method.

26.6 The clinical study report should be approved by the investigator and sponsor. The bioanalytical report should be approved by the study director.

26.7 The report should be approved (signed and dated) by the responsible personnel.

26.8 All monitoring and audit reports should be available before release of the final study report.

References

1. Guidelines for good clinical practice for trials on pharmaceutical products. In: WHO Expert Committee on Selection and Use of Essential Medicines: sixth report. Geneva: World Health Organization; 1995: Annex 3 (WHO Technical Report Series, No. 850), pp. 97–137.
2. WHO handbook on good laboratory practice: Quality practices for regulated non-clinical research and development. Geneva: World Health Organization; 2009.
3. OECD series on principles of good laboratory practice and compliance monitoring, number 1: OECD principles on good laboratory practice (as revised in 1997). Paris: Organisation for Economic Co-operation and Development; 1998 (ENV/MC/CHEM(98)17. 26).
4. Additional guidance for organizations performing in vivo bioequivalence studies. In: WHO Expert Committee on Selection and Use of Essential Medicines: fortieth report. Geneva: World Health Organization; 2006: Annex 9 (WHO Technical Report Series, No. 937).
5. Guidance on the selection of comparator pharmaceutical products for equivalence assessment of interchangeable multisource (generic) products. In: WHO Expert Committee on Specifications for Pharmaceutical Preparations: forty-ninth report. Geneva: World Health Organization: 2015: Annex 8 (WHO Technical Report Series, No. 992).

6. WHO Operational guidelines for ethics committees that review biomedical research. Geneva: World Health Organization; 2000 (WHO, TDR/PRD/ETHICS/2000.1) (http://www.who.int/tdr/publications/ documents/ethics.pdf?ua=1, accessed 11 January 2016).
7. The good automated manufacturing practice (GAMP) guide – A risk-based approach to compliant GxP computerized systems (GAMP5). Tampa (FL): International Society for Pharmaceutical Engineering (ISPE); 2009.
8. Good practices for computerised systems in regulated "GXP" environments, PIC/S Guidance. Geneva: Pharmaceutical Inspection Convention Pharmaceutical Inspection Co-operation Scheme; 2007 (PI 011–3, 25).
9. Guidance for industry: part 11, electronic records; electronic signatures – scope and application. US Food and Drug Administration; 2003 (http://www.fda.gov/downloads/RegulatoryInformation/Guidances/ucm125125.pdf, accessed 27 February 2016).
10. EU guidelines for good manufacturing practice and medicinal products for human and veterinary use. Annex 11, Computerised systems. Brussels: European Commission (SANCO/C8/AM/sl/ares(2010)1064599).
11. Guidance on good data and record management practices. In: WHO Expert Committee on Specifications for Pharmaceutical Preparations: fiftieth report. Geneva: World Health Organization; 2016: Annex 5 (WHO Technical Report Series, No. 996).
12. WHO good manufacturing practices: supplementary guidelines for the manufacture of investigational pharmaceutical products for clinical trials in humans. In: WHO Expert Committee on Specifications for Pharmaceutical Preparations: thirty-fourth report. Geneva: World Health Organization; 1996: Annex 7 (WHO Technical Report Series, No. 863).
13. Guidelines on bioanalytical method validation. London: Committee for Medicinal Products for Human Use (CHMP); 2012 (EMEA/CHMP/EWP/192217/2009 Rev.1 Corr.*).
14. Reflection paper for laboratories that perform the analysis or evaluation of clinical trial samples. London: European Medicines Agency; 2012 (EMA/INS/GCP/532137/2010).

Appendix 1

Example list of standard operating procedures at a contract research organization

The following is an example list of the standard operating procedures (SOPs) that should be used at contract research organizations (CROs). This list is not exhaustive as additional procedures may be necessary depending on the functional and compliance requirements at the facility concerned.

All of the documents at the CRO related to a bioequivalence (BE) clinical trial should be controlled (e.g. version date, date approved, etc.) documents. This control is easier if the documents are in the SOP format or are appended to SOPs.

SOPs should be in place at least for all the critical and major operations in the BE/clinical trial.

Number and name of SOP

1. Conduct of BE study
2. Archiving and retrieval of documents related to a BE study
3. Quality assurance of a BE study; audits of clinical and bioanalytical part of the study and the study report
4. Study files
5. Preparation and review of the protocol for the study
6. Amendment to the protocol for the study
7. Protocol deviations/violation recording and reporting
8. Sponsor/CRO quality assurance agreement on conducting the BE study
9. Process for approval of study by ethical committee
10. Bioavailability (BA)/BE report
11. Study report
12. Written informed consent
13. Obtaining written informed consent for screening from study volunteers
14. Allocation of identification numbers to volunteers at various stages in BE study
15. Investigator's brochure
16. Case report form (CRF)
17. Preparation of CRF, review and completion

18. Data collection and CRF completion
19. Adverse/serious adverse event monitoring, recording and reporting
20. Organizational chart for the study
21. Training of personnel
22. Responsibilities of the members of the research team
23. Monitoring of the study by the sponsor
24. Conduct of pre-study meeting.
25. Study start-up
26. Subject management
27. SOP on mobilization of individuals for registration in volunteer bank
28. Eligibility criteria for registration and registration of individuals in volunteer bank
29. Handling of subject withdrawal
30. Allocation of identification numbers to volunteers at various stages in the biostudy
31. Screening of volunteers enrolled for the study
32. Collection of urine samples from subjects for detection of drugs of abuse and transportation of samples to pathology laboratory
33. Custodian duties
34. Payments to research subjects for BE studies
35. Procedures for entry into and exit from clinical unit
36. Handling of subject check-in and check-out
37. Housekeeping at clinical unit
38. Planning, preparation, evaluation and service of standardized meals for bio-studies
39. Distribution of meals to study subjects
40. Operation and maintenance of nurse call system
41. Administration of oral solid dosage form of the investigational product to human subjects during BE study
42. Cannulation of study subjects
43. Collection of blood samples from study subjects
44. Identification of biological samples
45. Recording of vital signs of subjects
46. Operation and verification of fire alarm system
47. Administration of oxygen to subject from medical oxygen cylinder

48. Emergency care of subjects during BA/BE study
49. Availability of ambulance during BA/BE study
50. Centrifugation and separation of blood samples
51. Storage of plasma and serum samples
52. Segregation of bio-samples
53. Transfer of plasma and serum samples to bioanalytical laboratory
54. Procedures for washing glassware
55. Recording temperature and relative humidity of rooms
56. Instructions on operation and maintenance procedures for all the equipment in the clinical unit
57. Numbering the equipment and logbooks for use in the clinical unit
58. Control of access to pharmacy
59. Pharmacy area requirements
60. Authorization related to investigational product storage, dispensing and retrieval from storage for BE study
61. Investigational product receipt, return and accountability documentation
62. Investigational product receipt and return procedures
63. Storage of investigational products in the pharmacy
64. Line clearance before and after dispensing
65. Documentation of line clearance and dispensing; packaging records and release of dispensed products
66. Retention of samples of investigational products
67. Disposal of archived investigational products
68. Disposal of biological materials
69. Procedures for bioanalytical laboratory (SOPs for the different items of equipment, analytical methods, reagent preparation)
70. Out-of-specification in the laboratory
71. Acceptance criteria for analytical runs: acceptance of calibration curves, acceptance of the runs based on quality control samples results
72. Chromatographic acceptance criteria and chromatogram integration
73. Sample re-assay
74. Pharmacokinetic data from bioanalytical data
75. Procedure for statistical analysis in a BE study

Annex 10

WHO general guidance on variations to multisource pharmaceutical products

1. Introduction

A marketing authorization (MA) holder or applicant is responsible for the quality, safety and efficacy (QSE) of a finished pharmaceutical product (FPP) that is placed on the market, throughout its life cycle. After the FPP has been authorized for marketing, the manufacturer will often wish to make changes (variations) for a number of reasons, for example, to respond to technical and scientific progress, to improve the quality of the FPP, to apply updates to the retest period for the active pharmaceutical ingredient (API) or shelf life of the FPP, to meet market requirements such as for scale-up or additional manufacturing sites, or to update product information (e.g. the information on adverse reactions). Such changes, regardless of their nature, are referred to as variations and may require the approval of the national medicines regulatory authority (NMRA) prior to implementation.

NMRAs and MA holders should recognize that:

- any change to the manufacture of the API or the FPP may impact the QSE of that FPP;
- any change to the information associated with the FPP (i.e. product labelling information) may have an impact on the safe and effective use of that FPP.

This document is intended to serve as a guide for establishing national requirements for the regulation of post-approval changes. The proposed categories of changes and reporting procedures are provided in these guidelines. It is possible that modification of these principles may be justified in light of risk–benefit and legal considerations specific to each NMRA.

2. Scope

This document provides guidance for NMRAs on the regulation of variations to the original MA dossier or MA for an authorized multisource pharmaceutical product on:

- procedures and criteria for the appropriate categorization and reporting of changes; and
- how NMRAs can establish regulatory procedures for the post-approval variations to an authorized FPP.

These guidelines can be used by NMRAs with respect to changes to the quality sections of product dossiers and should be read in conjunction with the

Guidelines on submission of documentation for a multisource (generic) finished product: quality part (*1*) as well as other related WHO guidelines or applicable national guidelines. These guidelines are intended to provide an overview of the principles that NMRAs should consider when establishing pharmaceutical product variation procedures. Specific guidance on data requirements or risk categorization of a particular change cannot be provided since the approach taken by a specific NMRA is intrinsically linked to the regulatory framework and resources available to that NMRA. Nonetheless, illustrative examples of the data required to enable NMRAs to evaluate the impact of the variation on QSE are provided in detail in the *Guidelines on variations to a prequalified product* (*2*) or other national guidelines.

These guidelines are applicable only to APIs manufactured by chemical synthesis or semisynthetic processes and FPPs containing such APIs. APIs produced by fermentation and APIs of biological, biotechnological or herbal origin fall outside the scope of these guidelines. For vaccines, NMRAs may refer to the *WHO Guidelines for procedures and data requirements for changes to approved vaccines* (*3*).

3. Glossary

The definitions provided below apply to the terms used in this guidance. They may have different meanings in other contexts and documents.

active pharmaceutical ingredient. Any substance or mixture of substances intended to be used in the manufacture of a pharmaceutical dosage form, and that, when so used, becomes an active ingredient of that pharmaceutical dosage form. Such substances are intended to furnish pharmacological activity or other direct effect in the diagnosis, cure, mitigation, treatment or prevention of disease, or to affect the structure and function of the body.

active pharmaceutical ingredient starting material. A raw material, intermediate or an active pharmaceutical ingredient (API) that is used in the production of an API and that is incorporated as a significant structural fragment into the structure of the API. An API starting material can be an article of commerce, a material purchased from one or more suppliers under contract or commercial agreement or produced in-house.

biobatch. The batch used to establish bioequivalence or similarity to the comparator product as determined in bioequivalence or biowaiver studies, respectively.

finished pharmaceutical product. A finished dosage form of a pharmaceutical product which has undergone all stages of manufacture including packaging in its final container and labelling.

in-process control. Check performed during manufacture to monitor or to adjust the process in order to ensure that the final product conforms to its specifications.

manufacturer. A company that carries out operations such as production, packaging, repackaging, labelling and relabelling of pharmaceuticals.

marketing authorization holder. For the purposes of this document, the term marketing authorization holder refers to any person or entity that holds the legal responsibility for the product on the market by submission of the required documentation on a product that has been listed after evaluation as registered or approved.

multisource (generic) pharmaceutical product. Pharmaceutically equivalent or pharmaceutically alternative products that may or may not be therapeutically equivalent. Multisource pharmaceutical products that are therapeutically equivalent are interchangeable.

officially recognized pharmacopoeia (or compendium). Those pharmacopoeias recognized by the national regulatory agencies (e.g. national pharmacopoeia (if applicable), the *British Pharmacopoeia*, the *European Pharmacopoeia*, *The International Pharmacopoeia*, the *Japanese Pharmacopoeia* and the *United States Pharmacopeia*).

pilot-scale batch. A batch of an active pharmaceutical ingredient or finished pharmaceutical product manufactured by a procedure fully representative of and simulating that to be applied to a full production-scale batch. For example, for solid oral dosage forms, a pilot scale is generally, at a minimum, one-tenth that of a full production scale or 100 000 tablets or capsules, whichever is the larger, unless otherwise adequately justified.

production batch. A batch of an active pharmaceutical ingredient or finished pharmaceutical product manufactured at production scale by using production equipment in a production facility as specified in the application.

register. A list of all the pharmaceutical products authorized for marketing in a particular country. The medicines regulatory authority of the country in question maintains the register.

registered medicinal products. Pharmaceutical products that have a marketing authorization.

validation. The demonstration, with documentary evidence, that any procedure, process, equipment, material, activity or system leads to the expected results.

variation. A change to any aspect of a pharmaceutical product, including but not limited to, the change of use of a starting material, a change to formulation, method and site of manufacture, specifications for the finished product and ingredients, container and container labelling and product information.

4. General considerations

For any change, the MA holder must consider the potential impact upon the QSE of the FPP. As part of this consideration the MA holder should decide if the information in the original MA needs to be supplemented and whether this requires an official submission to the responsible NMRA or a change in the application dossier, based on the recommendations in these guidelines. Prior to implementing the variation, the MA holder should assess the effects of the variation and demonstrate through appropriate studies the absence of a significant negative effect of the change on the QSE of the FPP. MA holders should be aware that some variations generate subsequent changes that might require the submission of additional consequential variations. Therefore, for any given variation, the MA holder should consider whether it is better to submit more than one variation. In general no variation should be implemented without the approval of the NMRA unless exempted in the national guidelines.

Even well-resourced agencies find it difficult to evaluate all the pharmaceutical changes that are made to all products. This has resulted in a shift towards increased self-assessment of changes by the MA holder. Therefore it is necessary to define those changes that can be made without the NMRA's prior approval (self-assessable changes) and those that require prior approval based on an understanding of the risk and how best to manage this risk. NMRAs may also establish an intermediate category of changes that do not require prior approval but must be notified ("notifiable" changes) and may or may not be subject to assessment.

MA holders are expected to evaluate the specific change that they are planning to make in the context of their particular circumstances to determine the impact on product QSE. In an application to vary the MA, the MA holder advises the NMRA of an intended change and submits appropriate supportive data. To encourage MA holders to give prior notice regarding such changes, submissions for variations should be processed as quickly as possible. The NMRA should consider publication of the timelines for processing the variations.

Implementation of these guidelines should not affect supply of and access to medicines. Therefore NMRAs are strongly encouraged to establish requirements that are commensurate with public health priorities and their own regulatory capacity and resources. Communication of proposed procedures and requirements to the pharmaceutical industry should also be ensured so that they can adequately plan for the implementation of any new guidance.

Regional NMRA associations or networks could serve as forums for sharing information and exchanging experience on technical issues and regulatory decisions. Use of such networks would expand the capacity of individual NMRAs through work sharing and recognition of the decisions of other NMRAs in the network and convergence of regulatory requirements, thus avoiding unnecessary repetition of evaluations of the same variation by multiple NMRAs.

In these guidelines, descriptions of the reporting categories are discussed in section 5; proposed recommendations on the regulatory procedures for the reporting of changes to the NMRAs are discussed in section 8.

5. Reporting categories for quality changes

In order to enhance predictability, guidelines on the data requirements and conditions for the various categories of variations should be established and regularly updated in light of scientific and technical progress, taking into account the impact of the variation on the product QSE and how to manage this risk.

In addition to considering the impact of the change on a product's QSE, NMRAs may also modify the risk classification of a change through the introduction of prerequisites that must be met by the MA holder. In this way a change nominally identified as high-risk may be categorized across several risk categories depending on the conditions applied. Generally speaking the greater the number and specificity of the prerequisites the greater the possibility that the change can be self-assessed by the MA holder.

An additional consideration for NMRAs when designing their variation procedure is the determination of the default risk-category of changes not described in their variation guidance. For example, if an unspecified change defaults to a major variation, then effort should be focused on describing the conditions and data requirements for circumstances where the change might be considered as a lower risk category. In contrast, if a change defaults to a minor variation, then the conditions and data requirements of major changes and low-risk changes must be clearly defined.

The definitions outlined in the following reporting categories are intended to provide examples of change classification strategies that may be adopted by NMRAs for quality-related changes. Examples of specific variations data and conditions requirements can be found in the *WHO guidelines on variations to a prequalified product* (*2*) or other national regulatory guidelines that NMRAs may consult or reference; attention should be given to the default risk category underpinning the specific guidance.

NMRAs should also issue statements that whenever the MA holder is unclear about the categorization of a particular variation, the respective NMRA should be contacted.

Variations may be categorized into major variation, minor variation and notification. NMRAs may decide to have fewer categories or more categories depending on their national requirements.

5.1 Notifications

Notifications can be made for changes to the product that may have no potential or a minimal potential to have a negative impact on the QSE. The MA holder may implement such variations without prior approval by the NMRA. The NMRA may require the MA holder to submit these variations as immediate notifications (i.e. within a specific time frame after implementation) or as annual notifications.

5.2 Minor variations

Minor variations are changes to the product that may have a potential to have a moderate or negative impact on the QSE. Therefore such changes must be submitted to the NMRA with all required documentation prior to implementation. The MA holder may implement the change if no objection letter has been issued within a time period specified by the NMRA.

5.3 Major variations

Major variations are changes to the product that may have a significant potential to have a negative impact on the QSE. A major variation should be reviewed and approved by the NMRA prior to implementation of the change.

Individual changes normally require the submission of separate variations, but to increase efficiency NMRAs may accept grouping of variations under specific circumstances, for example:

- when variations are consequential to each other, e.g. introduction of a new impurity specification that requires a new analytical procedure;
- when the same change affects multiple FPPs from the same MA holder, e.g. addition of a new API manufacturing site for multiple FPPs;
- when all the changes are annual notifications;
- when variations are related to a common technical topic, for example drug master file updates or changes to the analytical procedures and specifications to comply with pharmacopoeias.

MA holders and NMRAs should exercise caution whenever several changes to the same FPP are envisaged. Although each of the individual changes may be classified in a particular category, classification within a higher-risk category may be warranted as a result of the composite effect of these changes. In all such cases, it is recommended that MA holders are able to contact the NMRA prior to submission of the variation application to obtain guidance on classifying such changes.

If changes to the dossier only concern editorial changes, such changes typically need not be submitted as a separate variation but can be included as a notification together with a subsequent variation concerning that part of the dossier. In such a case a declaration should be provided indicating that the contents of the associated sections of the dossier have not been altered by the editorial changes beyond the substance of the variation submitted.

The "timeline" and "implementation of the variation" are subject to the NMRA's specific provisions and should be made publicly available.

6. New applications

Certain changes are so fundamental that they alter the terms of the accepted dossier and consequently cannot be considered as variations. In these cases submission of a new dossier should be considered, in line with applicable national requirements for applications for MA.

Examples of such changes are:

- change of the API to a different API;
- inclusion of an additional API in a multicomponent product;
- removal of one API from a multicomponent product;
- change in the dose and/or strength of one or more APIs;
- change from an immediate-release product to an extended- or delayed-release dosage form or vice versa;
- change from a liquid to a powder for reconstitution or vice versa;
- changes in the route of administration.

7. Considerations for changes in product information and labelling

For any change to product information[1] (summary of product characteristics (SmPC), patient information leaflet (PIL) and/or labels) the NMRA should be notified and submission of the revised product information and/or labelling is expected as per country-specific requirements.

When a variation leads to a revision of the SmPC, the PIL and/or labelling, the updated information should be submitted as part of the variation. NMRAs may request the MA holder to submit a side-by-side tabular comparison of the current and proposed changes.

[1] Different regions and countries use different terminology for product information. In this document, package insert, the PIL and label are used to refer to product information.

Note that a change in the recommendations for use for a multisource product, such as indications or patient population would result in the product no longer being interchangeable with the comparator product. Therefore the NMRAs may need to take this into consideration prior to approval of such changes.

8. Procedures

8.1 General

NMRAs should establish procedures and criteria for adequate oversight of variations to authorized products. These should include written instructions regarding the submission procedures and timelines with action dates, to be consulted by MA holders when they prepare applications for variations. Depending on the category of the variation, different timelines may be applicable.

Regulation of post-approval variations is part of the whole regulatory framework, which includes among other aspects, MA, good manufacturing practices (GMP) inspection and post-marketing surveillance. Different branches of the NMRA often perform these activities. It is essential that these different branches interact and exchange information effectively and that the roles and responsibilities of each branch are clearly defined, particularly when they operate as separate entities. When multiple branches are involved in the evaluation of a variation a formal decision-making process should be in place to discuss, for instance, whether a change may require a GMP inspection or may be reviewed during the next routine inspection. Procedures should also be established so that the outcomes of inspections are verified or taken into account prior to the approval of variations. Good coordination and communication are pivotal.

8.2 Presubmission meetings

NMRAs should establish procedures to allow MA holders the opportunity to obtain advice prior to submitting variations. MA holders should be encouraged to contact the NMRA regarding plans for future changes and proposed filing dates for changes to authorized products to aid NMRAs in the planning and allocation of review resources.

8.3 Proposed documentation for minor variations

Where applicable the following basic information may be included as part of the description of the variation in the immediate notification, or the annual notification where prior approval is not required:

- a covering letter (including a list of changes, describing each in sufficient detail to allow for a quick assessment as to whether the appropriate reporting category has been used);

- an application form;
- a list of subsections of the current dossier affected by the change(s);
- a list and description of each change, reason for change(s) and the date each change was implemented (each change should be described in sufficient detail to allow for a quick assessment as to whether the appropriate reporting category has been used);
- the relevant summary of data from studies and tests performed to assess the effects of each variation on product quality, including (where applicable) a list of cross- references to the change control and change validation protocols and standard operating procedures (SOPs) that were used to assess or demonstrate the effect of the variation;
- copies of the updated subsections of the original dossier.

The description should also include:

- the name(s) of one or more FPP(s) affected or involved in the change (e.g. different label strengths/product presentations);
- reference to any previously approved variations, if the change affected multiple products.

Executed batch records, SOPs and data from studies and tests performed to assess the effects of each change should be kept on file and made available to the NMRA upon request (e.g. during an inspection).

In the case of annual notifications, which represents the lowest risk category, it may be permissible not to request any summary data if the acceptability of the change can be determined without them.

8.4 Proposed documentation for variations requiring prior approval

Where applicable the following basic information may be included in the application for variations requiring prior approval:

- a covering letter (including a list of changes describing each in sufficient detail to allow for a quick assessment as to whether the appropriate reporting category has been used);
- an application form;
- a list of subsections of the original dossier affected by the change(s);
- a document summarizing the current and proposed condition(s) and the reason(s) for the change(s);

- where relevant, a side-by-side comparison of the currently approved and the proposed information;
- replacement of the relevant subsections of the dossier in accordance with the acceptable dossier format for the NMRAs concerned, with the proposed changes clearly annotated;
- copies of the SmPC, PIL and labels, if relevant;
- the relevant summary of data from studies and tests performed to assess the effects of each variation on product quality, including (where applicable) a list of cross-references to change control and change validation protocols and SOPs that were used to assess or demonstrate the effect of the variation;
- registration status and date of the proposed change(s) in other countries and/or agencies that have already approved the variation(s), especially the country of origin and the reference agencies.

8.5 Review procedures

Taking into account the national situation, the capacity of the NMRA and regional harmonization initiatives, the NMRA should adopt a risk-based review strategy for assessment, concentrating most effort on those changes considered to carry the greatest risk. A key factor in reducing workload is to ensure that the variation documentation requirements permit rapid assessment of changes. Moreover, the NMRA may consider whether it will:

- rely on decisions made by other national authorities;
- rely on assessment reports prepared by other national authorities;
- prepare its own full assessment reports;
- use some combination of these approaches.

If the decision of another NMRA is adopted, it is nevertheless essential for certain minimum information to be available. Where the NMRA has granted MA based on a reference NMRA or WHO prequalification it is recommended that any post-approval variations of such products should have prior approval from the initial reference NMRA or WHO prequalification (*4*, *5*), as appropriate.

References

1. Guidelines on submission of documentation for a multisource (generic) finished pharmaceutical product: quality part. In: WHO Expert Committee on Specifications for Pharmaceutical Preparations: forty-eighth report. Geneva: World Health Organization; 2014: Annex 6 (WHO Technical Report Series, No. 986).

2. Guidelines on variations to a prequalified product. In: WHO Expert Committee on Specifications for Pharmaceutical Preparations: forty-seventh report. Geneva: World Health Organization; 2013: Annex 3 (WHO Technical Report Series, No. 981).
3. Guidelines for procedures and data requirements for changes to approved vaccines. In: WHO Expert Committee on Biological Standardization: sixty-fifth report. Geneva: World Health Organization; 2015: Annex 4 (Technical Report Series, No. 993).
4. Guidelines on submission of documentation for prequalification of finished pharmaceutical products approved by stringent regulatory authorities. In: WHO Expert Committee on Specifications for Pharmaceutical Preparations: forty-eighth report. Geneva: World Health Organization; 2014: Annex 5 (WHO Technical Report Series, No. 986).
5. Collaborative procedure between the World Health Organization Prequalification Team and national regulatory authorities in the assessment and accelerated national registration of WHO-prequalified pharmaceutical products and vaccines. In: WHO Expert Committee on Specifications for Pharmaceutical Preparations: fiftieth report. Geneva: World Health Organization; 2016: Annex 8 (WHO Technical Report Series, No. 996).